Regulating
Menstruation

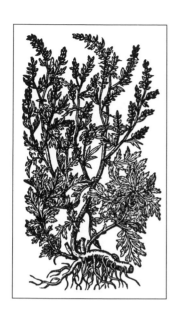

Regulating
Menstruation

Beliefs, Practices, Interpretations

Edited by
ETIENNE VAN DE WALLE
AND ELISHA P. RENNE

The University of Chicago Press
Chicago and London

Etienne van de Walle is professor of demography and a member of the Population Studies Center at the University of Pennsylvania. He coedited *Mortality and Society in Sub-Saharan Africa* (Oxford University Press, 1992).

Elisha P. Renne is assistant professor in the Department of Anthropology and Center for Afroamerican and African Studies at the University of Michigan. She is the author of *Cloth That Does Not Die: The Meaning of Cloth in Bunu Social Life* (University of Washington Press, 1995).

The University of Chicago Press, Chicago 60637
The University of Chicago Press, Ltd., London
© 2001 by The University of Chicago
All rights reserved. Published 2001
Printed in the United States of America

10 09 08 07 06 05 04 03 02 01   1 2 3 4 5
ISBN: 0-226-84743-8 (cloth)
ISBN: 0-226-84744-6 (paper)

Library of Congress Cataloging-in-Publication Data

Regulating menstruation : beliefs, practices, interpretations / edited
by Etienne van de Walle and Elisha P. Renne.
     p. cm.
Includes bibliographical references and index.
   ISBN 0-226-84743-8 (cloth : alk. paper) — ISBN 0-226-84744-6 (pbk. :
alk. paper)
   1. Menstruation—Cross-cultural studies. 2. Menstruation
disorders—Cross-cultural studies. 3. Traditional
medicine—Cross-cultural studies.   I. Van de Walle, Etienne, 1932–   II.
Renne, Elisha P.   III. Title.
   GN484.38.R44 2001
   305.4—dc21
                              00-011205

What extraordinary virtues are ascribed unto plants! *Satyrium et eruca penem erigunt; vitex et nymphea semen exstingunt; sabina fetum educit.* Some herbs provoke lust; some again, as Agnus Castus, waterlily, quite extinguish seed; and that which is much to be admired, that such and such plants should have a particular virtue to such particular parts, . . . for the womb Mugwort, Pennyroyal, Fetherfew, Savine, &c . . .

—Robert Burton,
  The Anatomy of Melancholy
  (1621)

Those diseases that are common both to widows and wives, both to barren women and women that are fruitful, as also to young maids and virgins, proceed from the retention and stoppage of their courses, as the most universal and most usual cause; when they come upon them in a due and regular manner, their bodies are preserved from most terrible diseases; but otherwise they are immediately subject to the falling sickness, the palsy, the consumption, the whites, the mother, the melancholy, burning fevers, the dropsy, inward inflammations of all principal parts, the suppression of the urine, nauseating, vomiting, loathing of meat, yexing, and a continual pain in the head, arising from ill vapors communicated from the matrix to the brain.

—Nicolas Fontanus,
  The Woman's Doctor (1652)

CONTENTS

A chance encounter started the process that culminated in the publication of this volume. The editors, an anthropologist and a demographer, began their collaboration with their accidental discovery of a shared interest in a neglected topic: women's use of substances and practices to stimulate menstruation.

While conducting research on fertility in southwestern Nigeria, Elisha Renne had published a paper in *Social Science and Medicine* (1996) on the extensive use of imported emmenagogues by unmarried women there, chiefly when pregnancy was suspected, to "bring on their menses." Later that year she attended a conference on abortion held in Trivandrum, Kerala, India, under the auspices of the International Union for the Scientific Study of Population. At this conference Elise Levin discussed Guinean women's use of emmenagogues to promote regular menstruation and fertility rather than to induce abortion. Her study suggested a situation more ambiguous than the one originally understood by Renne.

Meanwhile, Etienne van de Walle was writing a paper on the long history of menstrual regularity concerns in the West, eventually published in *Journal of Interdisciplinary History* (1997) under the title "Flowers and Fruits: 2000 Years of Menstrual Regulation." In the course of his research he found a large body of literature addressing the nature and treatment of a disease called menstrual retention. Women, in a wide variety of historical and geographical settings, strove to evacuate bodily humors and manipulate their reproductive system—a practice that may have had demographic implications.

Based on their own findings, Renne and van de Walle believed that the topic of menstrual management was worthy of more attention than it had been receiving from historians, demographers, and anthropologists, although various scholars had begun to study this phenomenon. The pair thought that a conference for these scholars—disparate both in terms of disciplines and of global locales—would perhaps yield additional conclusions. Van de Walle suggested holding the conference on the Internet, as the medium offered attractive new possibilities, particularly for promoting dialogue among scholars working in countries where a wide range of reproductive mores and practices exist. Since the editor-organizers had only elementary computer skills and since they assumed that most of the prospective participants were similarly inexperienced, they wisely decided to keep things very simple. Technological overkill would have easily scared away some prospects, and, as it turned out, a number of the conference participants did not have access to complex technical support.

After consulting with the computer staff at the Population Studies Center of the University of Pennsylvania, Renne and van de Walle supervised the design of a Web page that featured a description of the conference, a list of its participants, access to its abstracts, and a common e-mail address to facilitate communication. A grant to the university by the Andrew W. Mellon Foundation provided funding for a Web page manager, research assistance, the services of a professional editor, and press production.

The conference, "No Menses, No Births: Menstrual Regulation and Its Fertility Implications," took place on 19–22 February 1998. Meetings in real time were avoided to prevent logistical complications arising from different time zones. Instead, the participants committed themselves to on-line "attendance" during the conference period. Papers were posted on the Web, accessible only through the use of a password, and participants exchanged a great deal of information, criticism, and banter via e-mail during and after the event.

Three formal sessions—history, anthropology, and demography— were held. George Alter, Jacob Adetunji, and Philip Morgan accepted the thankless role of discussant. Let their contributions be acknowledged here, as well as those of Henri Leridon, who had initially hoped to coauthor one of the chapters in this volume, but had to limit himself to an advisory role because of his many responsibilities. Pierre Ngom, Denise M. Roth, and John Stanback contributed excellent papers that enhanced the intellectual depth of the conference, but these could not be published here because of space considerations. The logistical success of the conference owed much to Linda Duffy, Web page manager, and to Tim Cheyney, computer advisor at large. Diana Nolan skillfully and gently copyedited the manuscript of the proceedings. The editors would also like to thank Gigi Santow, whose editorial expertise and good humor helped to keep this project on track.

In recent years, two organizations—the Andrew W. Mellon Foundation Program in Anthropology and Demography and the International Union for the Scientific Study of Population Committee on Anthropological Demography—have contributed immensely to fostering cross-disciplinary work among demographers, anthropologists, and historians. This volume provides further testimony to the benefits to be derived from bridging disciplinary divides.

Elisha P. Renne and Etienne van de Walle

Anzi rinnuova come fa la luna . . .
—Boccaccio, *The Decameron,* second day, story 7

When a sexually active woman accustomed to menstruating monthly fails to menstruate and subsequently does something to restore her menses, her actions may be interpreted in several different ways. One obvious explanation is that she thinks she is pregnant and is attempting a very early-term abortion. Another possibility, however, is that she has taken emmenagogues (i.e., substances to promote "proper" menstrual flow) perceived as part of normal reproductive health practice. Another interpretation is that her actions serve as a sort of pregnancy test: if she believes that an established pregnancy would not be affected, resumed menstruation would confirm that she was not pregnant after all (Browner 1985:107).

This ambiguity of women's intentions in such circumstances is rooted in the very nature of menstruation and its absence. Amenorrhea, the absence of menstruation, can be interpreted as either an incapacity to conceive or the result of conception. Some women may welcome the return of their menses because it signals the possibility for future pregnancy, while others welcome it as a sign that they have not conceived. Similarly, women may rejoice (or lament, if they did not want to become pregnant) at the absence of their periods, because it foretells a future birth; or worry because the absence of menses may mean that they cannot achieve biological motherhood. How women interpret and react to menstruation and its absence reflects their individual needs as well as the cultural, social, economic, and political context in which they live. This volume considers what is known of women's options and practices regarding menstrual regulation in different places and times. There is remarkably little knowledge about the prevalence of the problems that these practices attempt to address, but there is probably no society in the world where menstrual irregularity has not been a cause of concern for some women. Both the historical and anthropological record are replete with documents that attest to the importance of these concerns.

A range of practices have been and continue to be used to control the periodicity, consistency, color, and quantity of menses in many historical and contemporary societies all over the world (Newman 1985). In many societies these practices were performed to achieve a sense of balance, as in Greek medical theory, where humors—referring to the bodily fluids: choler, phlegm, bile, and blood—were counterbalanced. In some societies, this need for equilibrium was reflected in a range of bodily states—hot and cold, dry and moist; medicines and foods were also so classified. In other societies, images of bodily balance were conceptualized in terms of worms (Buckley 1985; Kasnitz 1981), the idea being that bodily health is dependent on the presence of these entities but within certain limits. In the nineteenth-century United States and Europe, the idea of balance for bodily health was expressed in terms of balanced "vascular tension"; in other words, blood pressure that was neither too high nor too low. Thus the disorder known as vicarious menstruation, bleeding from orifices other than the uterus among amenorrheic women, was described in gynecological textbooks as "the body's attempt to regain equilibrium" (Skultans 1985:713).

One oft-cited consequence of these imbalances is a blockage of menstrual flow, resulting in a range of health problems. For example, women in one Guinean community attribute changes in the quality of menstrual blood to a blockage in its flow that may lead to infertility (see Levin, this volume). Alternately, free-flowing menses with certain qualities of color, thickness, and frequency are critical if fertility is to be achieved. Considering the pro-natalist tenor of many of these societies, where regular menstruation is promoted by various means and is viewed as a sign of good health, it seems likely that traditional emmenagogues or menstrual stimulators have been used mainly to enhance rather than to limit fertility. Thus while Riddle (1992) has argued that many emmenagogues were used for abortion (or as contraceptives; see also McLaren 1984) during the classical and medieval periods, this conclusion may have overstated the evidence. While it is possible that substances may have been used in such ways and that some might have been effective (McLaren 1984), their use would more likely have been exceptional rather than part of an everyday health regime. That both emmenagogues and abortifacients were used seems to be supported by the fact that some of the substances used as emmenagogues are also cited as abortifacients. For example, the fungus ergot produces an alkaloid that has antifertility effects (*Dispensatory of the United States of America* 1955:512–26).

Significantly, ergot was introduced in U.S. gynecological medicine as a birth facilitator, and was eventually displaced by the forceps in cases of difficult deliveries. An ingredient in many botanical nineteenth- and twentieth-century emmenagogues sold in the United States and Europe, it was also used as an abortifacient there (see Brodie, this volume). Ergot-based emmenagogues continue to be manufactured in India (e.g., EP Forte tablets) and sold in Ghana and Nigeria, where Ergometrine has been documented as being used as an abortifacient (Bleek and Asante-Darko 1986:343; see Renne, this volume).

Popular emmenagogues that were also used as abortifacients in the Western traditional pharmacopeia included savin, pennyroyal, rue, various species of the *Artemisia* genus (including mugwort and wormwood), saffron, and apiol. Some discussion of their pharmacological properties and their effectiveness as emmenagogues or abortifacients is offered by Siedlecky in this volume. However, much skepticism is warranted, as little scientific testing of their effectiveness has been made. Perhaps Potts, Diggory, and Peel (1977:172) say it best, in reference to savin, a substance extracted from a species of juniper and the most popular herbal emmenagogue and abortifacient in the Western tradition:

> The effect of savin in humans, particularly within a few days of the missing period (which appears to have been the common time for administration) has never been scientifically evaluated. Perhaps all that can be said of it is that no other therapeutic agent has been so widely used, for so specific a therapeutic purpose and yet so little studied in animals and never once scientifically investigated in man—or woman.

That some of these substances have dual roles—as both fertility enhancers and fertility inhibitors—is noteworthy, as it relates to an important point raised in several chapters in this volume. While mention of these substances in historical texts presumably gives some indication of their use, the emphasis on one or the other aspect of their dual functions is likely to have changed over time, particularly as women's relationships vis-à-vis production and reproduction have changed. Women whose concern with participating in productive labor overshadowed reproductive labor had reasons to attempt to limit fertility, rather than to enhance it. Indeed, Martin (1987:104–12) suggests that two opposing views of menstruation, expressed in interviews of middle- and working-class American women conducted in the early 1980s, reflect different relationships to life opportunities and different types of work. In one, menstruation is viewed according to a "medical model" of failed conception. In the other, menstruation is seen as part of the process of having children.

These different interpretations of menstruation—as something that is negative, as a "curse," and as failed conception; or as something positive, celebrated as a portent of fertility and part of the reproductive process—suggest not only that different views of menstruation may be held within a single society, but also that such interpretations may change over time. The view of menstrual blood as a harbinger of future fecundity may be aligned with the timing of fertility transition in particular societies; that is, in societies exhibiting a shift toward low-fertility regimens, the use of substances as emmenagogues to promote fertility may be diminished while their use as abortifacients appears to increase. There is evidence in several of the studies in this volume that such a shift has occurred: for example, in the United States during the nineteenth century (see Brodie) and in Bangladesh during the twentieth century (see Johnston). However, such a simple interpretation distorts the evidence, as Martin's interviews show that certain groups within a single society may have quite different views about childbearing and menstruation (e.g., see Buckley 1988; Newman 1985; Skultans 1985).

Furthermore, the objectives of women who use menstrual-regulating substances as fertility enhancers are not always well defined. Indeed, the purpose of their use may have been ambiguously stated, or not stated at all, because the specific mechanisms of fertilization were not known—the result of different views of embryonic development, and different definitions of when life begins (Newman 1985:189). Until pregnancy testing and other means of confirming a pregnancy were developed, women would not have known unequivocally what a missed period meant. A woman might interpret it simply as a delay, and might take a substance to bring on menstruation. Furthermore, the use of such substances might have been left intentionally vague because women wished to avoid confronting the issues of pregnancy and abortion altogether (see Santow, this volume). The ambiguity surrounding the intentions of women using such substances not only provides (as Levin suggests) "a gray area . . . that can provide women with the cultural space . . . to control their fertility," it also provides a means for individual agency and change in the face of prevailing social mores.

THE TERM *MENSTRUAL REGULATION*

The ambiguity regarding the control of menstruation has been invoked more recently by family planning personnel seeking to introduce a new technology (the Karman syringe and cannula) and technique (vacuum aspiration) as a form of post-coital fertility control, ultimately referred to as menstrual regulation. As Dixon-Mueller (1988:131) has observed, the use of such a technique "has blurred the previously accepted boundary, in Western legal terms, between contraception and abortion." Unfortunately, as a result of this terminology, menstrual regulation has recently become a code phrase for early-term abortion and has acquired this meaning almost exclusively in the family planning literature since 1972 (Davis 1972:57).[1]

This situation is not surprising, however. As is often the case with delicate subjects such as reproduction, including menstruation and particularly the controversial subject of abortion, euphemisms may be used in an attempt to divert the attention of political and religious opponents. For example, a recent definition of menstrual regulation states, "Menstrual regulation is a method of establishing non-pregnancy for women whose menstrual period is overdue by a maximum of fourteen days" (IPPF 1997:215).

Ethical concerns emerge in discussing menstrual regulation. On the one hand, open discussions of the evolution of this terminology may endanger programs offering women the possibility of safe early-term abortion. On the other hand, a policy of silence on these matters may misrepresent practices concerning irregular menstruation, about which women need explicit information for making informed decisions. Thus, in the interest of women's reproductive health more generally, we suggest that these issues be considered openly.

The phrase "menstrual regulation," used in connection with a new technology of post-coital fertility control by vacuum aspiration, is of recent origin. While Brodie (in this volume) cites examples of the use of the term *menstrual regulator,* this usage is referring to nineteenth-century emmenagogic preparations. In 1957, the FDA approved the newly synthesized steroids norethindrone and norethynodrel for "menstrual regulation" (i.e., the treatment of menstrual disorders) (Djerassi 1979:250–51). When the agency approved the same compounds for birth control three years later, most Catholic theologians supported their use in regulating the menstrual cycle (Noonan 1986: 474). More recently, however, the term was appropriated (Davis 1972; van der Vlugt and Piotrow 1973) to name the technique of suction curettage using a type of plastic cannula and syringe, developed by Dr.

Harvey Karman in 1970 (Dawn 1975:15).[2] This term was selected for tactical reasons:

> Perhaps one of the greatest contributions that somebody could make to this is a new term that would do for abortion what "family planning" did for "birth control." If we could call this something more acceptable than abortion, we would get the public's attitude changed a little faster. (Davis 1972:57)

The phrase seemed less shocking than "menstrual extraction," which might have been a more appropriate coinage. It has been retained to describe a monthly procedure, self-administered by women with a hand-held suction apparatus.

"Menstrual regulation" gained acceptance in the context of abortion. A classic medical text on abortion published in 1977 includes the following definition:

> Menstrual regulation, menstrual aspiration, very early abortion, *interception,* and pre-emptive abortion are all terms used to describe the surgical evacuation of the uterine contents shortly after the first missed period. Such terms are usually arbitrarily restricted to 14 days after the first missed period. (Potts, Diggory, and Peel 1977:230)

Nonetheless, this usage has reinforced the already considerable ambiguity surrounding absent or irregular menstruation described earlier, namely the boundaries between enhancing and limiting the possibility of a conception. On the one hand, some family planning agencies in the developing world viewed traditional practices of menstrual stimulation as a facade for early abortion procedures that would have been objectionable under a more descriptive terminology. On the other hand, the popular practices that were used in good faith in many societies for regulating the menses and to enhance reproductive health became suspect. Even if the restoration of regular menstruation (and consequently fertility) was the most common reason for the use of emmenagogic medicines, these medicines were also sometimes used in attempts at early-term abortion. Historical and anthropological evidence of the use of such substances is presented in the following sections.

HISTORICAL WRITING ON MENSTRUATION

Much of the literature on menstruation has focused on its association with impurity and pollution in many world cultures (see Buckley and

Gottlieb 1988:3–50 for an overview of these issues). The image of the menstruating woman as a source of pollution dates at least from biblical times (e.g., Lev. 15:19). Many societies exclude menstruating women from public activities and from personal contacts, including sexual intercourse.

But remarkably, there do not seem to have been menstrual taboos in classical Greece, despite the attention Greek physicians devoted to the health implications of regular menses (see van de Walle, this volume). The topic was enormously important in medical discourse, but had little cultural signification. Dean-Jones (1994:226–36) shows that silence about menstruation reigned in nonmedical sources; cultural myths and taboos for menstruation did not exist. She cites texts where both the Hippocratics and Aristotle encouraged a man to have intercourse with his wife while she was menstruating.

In Greek medicine, the idea of menstruation as cleansing dominates the Hippocratic tradition.[3] The terms for menstruation used in antiquity refer to the monthly nature of the menstrual flow. The Greeks and the Romans do not appear to have used metaphors to talk about menses, unless catharsis (which means purification, but is also used in the sense of purgation) would be an example. In his review of terminology, Soranus (1956:16–17) acknowledges that menstruation "is also called *katharsis,* since, as some people say, excreting blood from the body like excessive matter, it effects a purgation of the body." It is important to note that in using the phrase "as some people say," Soranus was not including himself, for he rejected this point of view.

In polite company, the ancients would probably have spoken of "women's things"—*gyneikaia* in Greek and *muliebria* in Latin. The word *flower* (with its positive connotation and the promise of fruit that it implies) was commonly used metaphorically for menstruation in the Middle Ages (van de Walle 1997), although by the midnineteenth century this term had fallen into disuse. Other metaphors have stressed the ideal of regularity: periods, *règles,* or associations with the moon. In the nineteenth century, many menstrual metaphors took on a negative overtone: to be sick, to have a cold, or even to have "the curse." To be sick, in seventeenth-century France, could mean either a pregnancy or menstruation. For example, Madame de Sévigné wrote to her daughter in 1671:

> Today is the sixth of March; I beg you to send word on how you are faring. If you are well, you are sick, but if you are sick, then you are well. I wish, my daughter, that you be sick, so that you will keep your health at least for some time. (Sévigné 1972:1, 177)

The meaning of this cryptic exchange is that "if you have your period, it is good news, it means that you are not pregnant." Jennings, in his frank discussion of menstruation first published in 1808, alluded to the popular name of menses in early nineteenth-century America as a "cold as it is commonly called." But he granted that "[p]erhaps this cannot properly be called a disease, as it is universal to the sex and as there cannot be health without it" (Jennings 1972:38–39).

It appears that the physiological aspects of menstruation dominate its cultural presence in Western historical texts. There is a dissociation between the constant references to menses in medical and pharmaceutical texts concerning women, including lay texts (see Cadden 1993 for the Middle Ages, Crawford 1981 for the seventeenth century, and Lord 1999 for the eighteenth), and their almost total absence in fiction or poetry. Similarly, the herbal products that are cited repeatedly in the technical writings are not featured either as emmenagogues or abortifacients in lay writings.[4]

Menstruation and Health

This paradoxical notion of menstruation as a disease without which the body could not be healthy was probably dominant throughout Western history. Thus amenorrhea without pregnancy was almost unqualifiedly considered an unhealthy condition. Its result was deemed an excess of blood in the body—"plethora"—and the suffocation of the matrix.

The earliest systematic exposition of this position (which is probably even older) came in the Hippocratic treatises. Three of these works, written by the same author and known collectively as *Diseases of Women* since the seventeenth-century edition by Littré (Hippocrates 1962), offer a remarkable and detailed view of female physiology that was to have an influence on the medical literature through the ages. This group of Hippocratic treatises can be interpreted as a cultural construct of a particular society and time. They reveal a gender ideology in which women are assigned the primary task of maintaining their fertility. Thus a coherent paradigm of the causes of disease and health is presented—that correct reproductive functioning was a primary determinant of women's health.

This idea achieved a great authority and a wide diffusion, being cited by subsequent physicians and pharmacologists. It was known and quoted (sometimes critically) by Soranus, Galen, Dioscorides, Pliny, the medieval schools of medicine, and the Arabic physicians. Thus the views of Hippocrates shaped the views contained in the many collections attributed to the school of Salerno and the midwife Trotula (Rowland 1981), and are echoed in the books on midwifery that began to appear from the sixteenth century onward in Western Europe; for example, Eucharius Rösslin's 1513 *Rose Garden for Pregnant Women and Midwives* and Louise Bourgeois's 1609 *Observations* (Rösslin 1994; Bourgeois 1992). It is reasonable to say that any book on official or home medicine for treating women's diseases written in Europe between the fifth century B.C. and the beginning of the twentieth century discusses the retention of menses as a pathology and prescribes the use of herbal substances as its remedy.

This tradition is characterized by an emphasis on the normality of regular menstrual flow, the pathological nature of menstrual retention, and the central position of fertility as an indicator and result of good health. Most of the works in this genre begin (as Hippocrates did) with a description of the menses as a cleaning mechanism and of menstrual retention as a condition that threatens the fertility and the life of a woman. For example, in the English Trotula edited by Beryl Rowland (1981:61), "[t]he first chapter is concerned with the stopping of the blood that women should have in their purgations and be purged of." The text lists a series of procedures and drugs recommended to restore a normal menstrual flow. Later in these volumes, other pathological conditions of women are also addressed. For example, stillbirth or difficult childbirth sometimes requires the use of drugs or mechanical means to extract the fetus, hasten the delivery, or evacuate the afterbirth. The drugs used for these purposes are often the same as those for curing menstrual retention. The English Trotula, under the title "The twelfth chapter is on how to make a woman conceive a child if God wills," states:

> First, if she is full of menstrual blood, have her cleansed with medicines for the retention and suppression of menstruation [a doubtful translation: the original text says 'in retencione menstruorum & in suffocacione menstruorum'], with baths and immersions. Alternatively, take 1 handful each of calamint, catmint, fennel, pellitory, savory, hyssop, artemisia, rue, wormwood, anise, cumin, rosemary, thyme, pennyroyal, and mountain origanum, a gallon of wine, 6 gallons of water, boil them, and have her take this medicine. (146–47)

It is striking that the remedies designed to bring back fertility—artemisia, rue, wormwood, pennyroyal and savin, among others—and the "aperient [openyng]" herbs that are used in the baths and immersions designed to open the veins of the uterus (66–67) are the very emmenagogues that have a dark reputation as abortifacients.

When an allusion is made to contraception or abortion in this early medical literature, it is usually incidental. Whether menstruation was considered as an illness or as bodily purification, menses were generally viewed as a precondition to fertility. Soranus (1956:27), one of the lone voices in antiquity granting that healthy women can be amenorrheic, argued quite clearly that menses are good because they are a precondition for pregnancy. Indeed, when Soranus or Galen provided abortive recipes, they did so with reluctance and only for cases in which the mother's life would be endangered if she continued her pregnancy.

A particular condition of menstrual retention that drew the attention of writers of the modern period was that of young women whose menarche was late, who had "the green sickness," were anemic, or, as the expression went, were "chlorotic" (see in this volume Hull and Hull on anemia in Indonesian women, and Klepp regarding the general absence of chlorosis among well-fed American colonists in the eighteenth century). Curiously, the Greeks had nothing to say on this. Short fragments of a Hippocratic treatise on the sicknesses of young girls survive; in them the author describes a hysteric condition resulting from menstrual retention, a condition normally cured by marriage and childbearing (Hippocrates 1962, vol. 8, pp. 464–71). The ancients were concerned with "plethora" (too much blood), and not with "chlorosis" (too little blood). Bloodletting and the use of emmenagogues were seen as alternative or complementary treatments for young women who were not menstruating and, as a result, had too much blood. By the seventeenth century, however, chlorosis had become the condition of primary concern. Today medical opinion has shifted again and the eating disorder primarily affecting young women, anorexia nervosa, with its attendant absence of menses (see Warriner, this volume), has become a concern. These different perceptions are striking examples of the changing cultural and historical contexts of disease.

Whether the cause of menstrual retention was ascribed to weakness or overabundance of the blood led to very different cures. Louise Bourgeois (1992), for example, distinguished the two conditions, and prescribed different treatments for each. The accepted cure for chlorosis was iron in the form of filings or forge-water, water in which a red-hot iron had been plunged. The accepted cures for suffocation of the matrix were procedures that would facilitate the normal expulsion of blood or substitute for it: pessaries and baths to provoke a mechanical opening of the uterus; purges and emmenagogues to evacuate the blood; and substitute procedures such as bloodletting, leeches, or cupping. In this treatment, Louise Bourgeois came remarkably close to following the Hippocratic tradition. The rationale for these procedures was indicated by the discussion of this issue in the first chapter of her book on midwifery, "Why Some Women Cannot Bear Children." For Bourgeois, menstruation was a prominent factor in reproductive health. She is an unimpeachable witness to the indications for using menstrual stimulants; abortion could not be further from her mind.

This use of menstrual stimulants largely accounts for the paradox reflected in several chapters of this book. Menstrual inducement is commonly used by women in many contemporary pro-natalist societies for the purpose of facilitating subsequent births. It should be added that the ambiguous interpretations of these practices depend, to some extent, on ideas about conception and when life begins. For example, the *Hadith,* an Islamic text, refers to a lump of flesh being animated by the breath of life after 120 days (Musallam 1983:54; see also Hull and Hull for Indonesia and Johnston for Bangladesh, this volume). The assumption, therefore, that menstrual regulation invariably means abortion is misleading, since it may only be that regular menstruation is being restored. This ambiguity also exists because these same societies widely recognize that emmenagogues are potentially dangerous when a woman is pregnant and that they may be used as abortifacients. What is more, the actual intentions of a woman using such substances would not be publicly known. Several authors in this volume explore this fundamental ambiguity, which is especially stressed by Klepp, Brodie, Santow, and Hull and Hull.

Menstrual Regulation in the Nineteenth and Twentieth Centuries: Europe and the United States

The Hippocratic tradition of menstrual stimulation remained vigorous in Europe and the United States from the nineteenth century to 1960. It did not go unchallenged. Although physicians almost universally considered menstrual pathologies as a cause for concern, mainstream gynecologists appeared less enthusiastic about emmenagogues, and even abandoned the use of this term by the early twentieth century (see Siedlecky, this volume). Yet emmenagogues retained an important position in the herbals or self-care manuals, and in the popular medical literature that flourished as a marketing technique for various nostrums (Brodie, and Santow, this volume; Brodie 1994). Despite the militantly moralistic stand taken by this literature, which professed to warn its readers against the perils of abortion, the nineteenth and twentieth centuries also saw an enormous expansion of contraceptive and abortive practices, and a proliferation of products that were quite openly advertised as abortifacients. The good faith of most peddlers in "female pills" was undeniable; but there were those like the infamous Madame Restell who made no secret that they were in the business of helping women to abort (Browder 1988). Madame Restell, like many other advertisers in suspicious-looking publications, dropped hints that left no doubt that abortion was offered. These advertisers were nonetheless careful to protect themselves by warning pregnant women not to use their products. Thus, a typical ad in *The New York Sun* of 1839 read:

> Mrs Restell's celebrated Female Monthly Pills . . . "an infallible regulator or ******. They must not be used when ******." (Browder 1988:11; asterisks in the original)

Such a warning had always been standard in the herbals and the popular health books. In the nineteenth century, it became a double-edged message—a defense against possible legal prosecution and a signal to the initiate.[5]

The sale of emmenagogues that continued in Europe and the United States until the 1960s can thus be interpreted both as a result of the pursuit of cyclical regularity and as the visible part of an underground abortion practice. This ambiguity cannot easily be clarified. A look at the sources of the time suggests that abortion was only part of the story, but the one that has been stressed by critics who gained the moral high ground in the late nineteenth century. Moreover, by the twentieth century, the perceptual gulf between mainstream physicians and their teachings at medical schools, and those using home medicine manuals and materia medica (see Santow, this volume), had increased.

By 1960 the development of hormonal contraceptives and vacuum menstrual regulators made this pharmacopeia obsolete in the West, although an interest in herbal remedies nonetheless persists. Menstrual irregularity became a neglected topic among medical professions, except in the form of "anorexia nervosa"—the new avatar of the chloroses of yesteryear—and in discussions of "premenstrual syndrome" (Martin 1988). Yet the idea of menstruation as bodily cleansing has retained its popularity. The developers of the oral contraceptive pill incorporated this view in allowing a period during its use for the release of blood in what is otherwise an artificial "cycle" (see Potter, this volume).[6] Furthermore, birth control pills are sometimes prescribed to promote regular menstrual periods. Thus, even as these pills are used to reduce fertility, their use is nonetheless related to older beliefs about bodily hygiene that connect cycle regularity with good reproductive health. This idea has a long history not only in Greek medicine and its Western and Middle Eastern descendants but in African and Latin American medicine as well.

ANTHROPOLOGICAL WRITING ON MENSTRUATION

Africa and Latin America

Much of the anthropological literature on menstruation, where it has been discussed at all, has focused on the association of menstruation with pollution and with the related restrictions that exist in many societies (e.g., Balzer 1981; Douglas 1966; Paige and Paige 1981). However, a recent volume on the anthropology of menstruation (Buckley and Gottlieb 1988) has argued that such an emphasis fails to explain cases in which menstruation is positively regarded or menstruating women's restricted movement is viewed as an opportunity. Thus the authors argue that menstrual pollution and taboos must be considered within particular cultural contexts, as their meanings "are ambiguous and often multivalent" (7). Similarly, assumptions relating emmenagogue use with abortion overlook the positive aspects of regular menstruation as a sign of women's fertility and as a prerequisite to good reproductive health. That a woman would rid herself of impurities in the process of menstruating could be, from her own point of view, a form of catharsis or purification rather than of pollution. In some societies, this menstrual purification (and subsequent fertility) is considered beneficial; additionally, as in the case for the Beng of eastern Côte d'Ivoire, menstrual blood is not considered particularly polluting, and few menstrual taboos exist (Gottlieb 1982, 1988:262 n.12; see also Fortes 1949 on the Tallensi).

In other examples from Africa, menstrual blood is interpreted more ambiguously as in the case of the Kaguru of western Tanzania (Beidelman 1997). In this society, any spilled human blood is considered dangerous and polluting, so that considerable effort is made to train young women in the proper means of containing traces of menstrual blood (see also Richards 1956):

> The blood of menstruation (*kutumuka*, "to be involved with," "to be taken up with") is so dangerous that menstruating women may not sleep in their husbands' beds, and, while menstruating, women should avoid entering cultivated fields, attending ritual gatherings, brewing beer, going to court, and many other situations. They should wear dark or unattractive clothing and should not try to appear se-

ductive to men. Nonetheless, the commencement of menstruation by young women is viewed as a positive augur of their fertility.

Yet menstruation is valued by the Kaguru, for it is a sign of fertility. It is thought to mark a plenitude of blood that signifies a readiness to bear children (Beidelman 1997:125).

As with ideas about menstrual pollution and taboos, the ambiguity surrounding menstruation—that it is both vital to fertility and a dangerous sign of social disorder (the loss of human blood)—means that practices and ideas associated with its regulation must be considered within particular sociocultural contexts. The similar but distinctive explanations of menstrual disorders in several African societies illustrate this point.

Menstrual Regulation in Africa

Menstrual disorders—for example, irregular flow (evidenced by either excessive or scanty bleeding), delayed menses, painful menstruation, discolored menses, and amenorrhea—are cause for concern for women in many African societies. Several of the essays in this volume (Levin, Madhavan and Diarra, and Renne) examine some of the ways that women living in Guinea, Mali, and Nigeria address these problems. Their views contrast with medical traditions of the West, since irregular menstruation is often considered a symptom of an underlying condition (such as blockage due to dirt, worms, and witchcraft) rather than its cause. Local herbs, either taken as a remedy at the time a condition is observed or as a prophylaxis to maintain regularity of menses, are often prescribed by traditional healers. Like their emmenagogic counterparts in the West, some of these herbs are also used as abortifacients (see Levin 1996; Renne 1996). In southwestern Nigeria, women use herbal medications to cleanse the womb when menstruation is perceived as discolored or of the wrong consistency. Young, unmarried women also use a range of patent medicines to promote menstruation, primarily when they believe they are pregnant. As elsewhere, African women use various substances to promote both regular menstruation and reproductive health, which may also include the interruption of untimely or unwanted pregnancies. Nonetheless, the continued importance of children in many kin-based African societies puts considerable pressure on its women to give birth, making the need for regular menstruation and reproductive health critical to their social and economic standing.

This pressure may partly explain another aspect of the traditional healer's work regarding menstruation—namely the divination of possible nonphysiological sources of women's menstrual disorders. Indeed, attributions of menstrual disorders to spiritual forces are found in several African societies, although they are not restricted to them (see Cosminsky, Hammer, and Johnston, all in this volume). Western medical explanations for these amenorrhagic complaints—such as the Hausa condition of "sleeping pregnancy" (Kleiner-Bossaller 1993)—attribute them to the social pressure to bear children and to their being a psychological release for women having difficulties conceiving (see also Boddy 1989; Feldman-Savelsberg 1994). Whatever the explanation, when a spiritual being is identified as the source of a menstrual disorder, women take this prognosis seriously and attempt to address the problem.

However, whereas the symptoms of delayed or absent menstruation may be similarly attributed to spiritual forces (and/or to psychosocial pressures), the actual bases of these beliefs and subsequent remedies are quite socioculturally specific. For example, in the matrilineal Ndembu society described by Turner (1967:11), the spiritual forces are perceived as ancestral spirits, mainly identified as members of a woman's matrilineage:

> If a woman suffers from prolonged and painful menstruation she is said to have been "caught by a shade," which has come out in *Nkula* [a form of affliction which results in infertility], and the rite to rid her of the shade is also called Nkula.

The ancestral spirit is said to come out of its grave and then to "sit" on the woman, causing menstrual disorders and infertility; the spirit is propitiated through performance of the ritual Nkula, after which regular menstruation returns and the woman may become pregnant. By performing this ritual, a woman and her husband demonstrate their social commitment to the wife's matrilineage in the hope that they will subsequently be blessed with children.

In the case of Hofriyati women of northern Sudan experiencing menstrual disorder or infertility, they may become possessed by local spirits known as *zaryan*, which make various, often costly, demands of a woman's family for remedying her reproductive problems:

> A woman who is anxious or depressed or whose situation vitiates the ideals and integrity of Hofriyati womanhood is considered a prime target for *zaryan*. . . . Their most common tactics, earlier described are to "seize" or "hold" the womb, and "loosen" or "steal" progeny, bringing about sterility, miscarriage, stillbirth, amenorrhea, menor-

rhagia, or any number of problems affecting women's blood. (Boddy
1989:186–87)

These spirits exist in a world distinct from that of possessed women,
who have a subordinate place in their husband's household and religious worship. Through beliefs and practices associated with *zar* spirit
possession, Hofriyati women acquire an exogenous field of action and
a means of expressing their concerns and demands in a social setting
that largely restricts them.

A final example of spiritual beings' effects on menstruation refers to
beliefs in the powers of witches and wizards (or sorcerers) to expropri-
ate or block menstruation. As discussed in chapters by Renne and Madhavan and Diarra, these supernatural beings (who nonetheless appear
as ordinary ones) may be close relatives, co-wives, or political rivals.
People accused of menstruation-related witchcraft are often in social-
structurally equivocal positions vis-à-vis the accuser, such as a jealous
co-wife (in polygynous societies) or a mother-in-law (in patrilineal
ones). As Rasmussen (1991:759) notes, "Menstruation is a potentially
powerful vehicle of antisocial behavior." Thus Tuareg women in Niger
surreptitiously wash menstrual cloths at night to prevent others from
obtaining this blood. In such cases, a victim's menstrual cloth, perme-
ated with life-giving fluid, may be used by these antisocial beings to
"seize" menstruation, stop its flow, or cause a pregnancy to "go to the
back." It is only with proper propitiations that these menstrual disorders can be remedied.

In considering these examples, it should not be assumed that most
menstrual complaints by African women are attributed to spiritual and
social causes. It is more likely that women would attempt to regularize
delayed or irregular menstruation through herbal means, with spiritual
explanations reserved for more intransigent cases. Menstrual disorders
may thus be interpreted as a reflection of social or spiritual disorders
(MacCormack 1982:17) as well as physiological ones. Furthermore, the
distinctive sociocultural contexts (e.g., the type of social organization
or marriage system) also contribute to the particular forms that spiritual explanations of menstruation have taken in Africa.

Menstrual Regulation in Latin America

Studies conducted in Latin America also mention supernatural causes
for menstrual problems. For example, Browner and Ortiz de Montellano (1986:39) mention witchcraft as a possible explanation for cold
blood and subsequent amenorrhea. What is particularly interesting
about these Latin American studies, however, is the pervasiveness of

the concept of balance of hot and cold. In Cali, Colombia, for example, amenorrhea *(atrazo)* is believed to be caused by cold blood, an indication of imbalance that may be remedied through the use of substances classified as hot (Browner 1985; see Hammer, this volume). Cosminsky, working in rural Guatemala, noted a variation on this theme, in that the condition of delayed menstruation *(detención)* could be caused by too much heat or too much cold (see Cosminsky, this volume). In the former case, cooling medicines would be given, whereas in the latter, hot medicines would be used. Both Cosminsky and Hammer (this volume) note that these systems of medical thought are related to Greek humoral theory, although both suggest that similar physiological concepts existed in the preconquest period. While it is beyond the scope of this volume to investigate these connections, the availability of written records from the early sixteenth century onward offers the possibility of tracing the historical intersections of Spanish-Portuguese medical theories with indigenous ideas about reproductive health.[7]

Another interesting aspect of these studies is the strong pro-natalist tenor shared by many Latin American cultures which, as has been seen, favor the use of emmenagogues to promote fertility and reproductive health. At the same time, herbal abortifacients are well known, suggesting an ambiguity of intentions as noted by Browner (1985:107):

A belief system that equates menstrual delay with poor health allows a certain amount of covert fertility regulation to take place while women are apparently treating minor disturbances in their reproductive systems. Caleñas [women of Cali, Colombia] must practice fertility control discreetly in a society that encourages high fertility and presents the maternal role as the only legitimate one for women. As with any illness, women take the symptom—in this case a missed menstrual period—as the diagnostic clue, and treatments are prescribed to alleviate the symptoms.

This ambiguity surrounding the intentions of those using emmenagogues to regulate their menstruation for reproductive health is also present in family planning programs in several Latin American countries where oral contraceptive pills are widely distributed.

RECENT PRACTICES RELATING
TO MENSTRUAL REGULATION

The stimulation of the menses by synthetic hormonal substances, rather than by herbal products, was a turning point in Western gynecological practice that occurred in the 1960s. Elsewhere in the world, however, the use of progesterone or estrogen to stimulate the menses appears to have gained a foothold in family planning programs alongside traditional medicines. For example, Johnson (this volume) mentions the use of oral contraceptive tablets by women in Bangladesh to bring on menstruation (see also Newman 1985). Hormonal compounds are also reportedly used as a test by women to determine whether their failure to menstruate means that they are pregnant, since such substances will not disturb an established pregnancy. The use of modern drugs to achieve women's traditional goals in this area is illustrated by a story published in the *New York Times* in 1998:

> ABHA, Saudi Arabia, Jan. 19.—A Saudi woman has given birth to septuplets, but she said today that she took a fertility drug to regulate her menstrual cycle and was not trying to have more children. . . . "Whatever comes from God is good," she said today.

Family planning programs have also made use of these hormone-based medicines, such as oral contraceptive tablets, to regulate menstruation. Stanback et al. (1997) describe family planning programs where women are required to demonstrate that they have been menstruating before they are prescribed hormonal contraception, for fear that oral tablets will be misused. And in several countries such as Indonesia (Hull, Sarwono, and Widyantoro 1993), Bangladesh (Amin 1996), and Nigeria (Ladipo et al. 1978; Ojo and Ladipo 1981), menstruation is induced using manual vacuum aspirators. This procedure, referred to as menstrual regulation, is carried out within two weeks of the time when menses were expected. Because a pregnancy has not been definitely established (which in any event depends of prevailing ideas about the time of conception), this method relies on the ambiguous meaning of missing menses. Thus in Bangladesh, a country where abortion is illegal, the practice of menstrual regulation is tolerated by the state, the courts, and women users (Johnston, this volume; Amin et al. 1989; Dixon-Mueller 1988). In Indonesia, where a similar government-sponsored program exists, both the more recent form of menstrual regulation using manual vacuum aspirators and an extensive pharmacopeia of emmenagogues are available to women (Hull and Hull, this volume).

CONCLUSION

The existence of emmenagogues, consisting mainly of herbal substances with the reputation for inducing menses, has been recognized in most societies, both past and present. We are fortunate to have considerable written sources dating from antiquity that testify to their use by women throughout history, even as their importance has waned in the West. More recent studies have shown that in many parts of Africa, Latin America, and Asia, some women continue to use herbal substances to regulate menstruation, equating regular cycles with sound reproductive health. These contemporary studies are not only valuable in their own right, but also suggest possible explanations for such uses in other times and places. One interesting contrast that emerges from these studies relates to the association of menstruation with health. In societies strongly influenced by the Hippocratic model, an absence of menstruation is considered to be a *cause* of disease, whereas in several contemporary non-Western societies (where Soranus's dissenting view of menstruation seems to prevail), its absence is viewed as a *symptom* of ill health.

Furthermore, these contemporary examples provide a welcome corrective to the male point of view that dominates historical European and North American sources. These studies portray the concerns of women whose social situation depends on their reproductive health (and ability to bear children) and proper reproductive timing (such as child-spacing and postmarital pregnancy). Under such circumstances, it is not surprising that young women might anxiously await the onset of menses, and thereafter, want regular menstruation of a certain duration and quality. Older women experiencing amenorrhea without pregnancy might also be concerned about missing menses, since, in several societies, the blockage of menstrual flow is believed to cause disease.

Considering women's perspectives also sheds light on the ambiguity surrounding different interpretations of emmenagogues, their uses in relation to women's fertility and reproductive intentions, and their uncertain efficacy. The chapters in this volume document the wide range of substances and, more recently, mechanical techniques, used for regulating menstruation and subsequent fertility. As has been seen, the broader sociocultural context of women's lives affects how menstruation is perceived—as a sign of fertility, as a respite from an inopportune pregnancy, as a disappointment over a desired one, or as a messy nuisance—and which steps are taken for inducing menstruation when it fails to appear. Some women in societies where high fertility is frowned upon welcome oral contraceptive pills that reduce menstrual flow, whereas women in societies who are concerned with having many children reject such contraceptives on just these grounds (Potter, this volume). In the latter case, women are concerned with regular menstruation. In its absence, they take emmenagogic substances (often of questionable efficacy) with the uncertain hope that these substances will be effective. Since attitudes toward menstruation often reflect local cultural interpretations rather than a biomedical understanding of human physiology, recent biomedical definitions of the concepts relating to menstruation and its regulation are presented in a glossary. These definitions serve as a basis for comparison with the beliefs and practices described in the chapters of this volume.

The historical studies herein suggest a tendency for herbal substances to be used in high-fertility regimes to promote menstruation (and fertility); that tendency shifts to greater use of these substances as abortifacients as fertility declines. It is paradoxical that demographers do not include irregular menstruation as a significant influence on fertility (see Warriner, this volume). The prevalence of pathological amenorrhea has not been accurately measured (using techniques of hormonal assay that are now practical) in large representative populations of women who are not users of oral contraceptives. It is also paradoxical that modern science has not tested the effectiveness of the herbal products that have been used so universally either as emmenagogues or as abortifacients.

Evidence suggests that emmenagogues are sometimes used as abortifacients in high-fertility society just as various methods for inducing menstruation exist in low-fertility ones (Trickey 1998). Several studies in this volume document the coexisting uses of the same substances by women whose intentions might be quite contextually specific but would be voiced as intentionally vague. Moreover, how such substances and their uses are defined may eventually change, reflecting shifting social norms and technological innovations.

OVERVIEW OF THE VOLUME

Part 1 examines beliefs about menstruation, practices for its regulation, and the use of emmenagogues as documented in European and Anglo-American historical and contemporary studies. The first chapter in this section focuses on Greek and Roman medical practices and substances used to induce menstruation. The next three chapters consider menstruation and its regulation through the use of patent medicines and home remedies in the eighteenth- and nineteenth-century United States, as well as the ambiguous usage of various emmenagogues and abortifacients in the West during the late nineteenth and early twentieth centuries. The following two chapters consider contemporary demographic implications of and pharmacological perspectives on menstrual regulation. The section closes with a discussion of the ambiguous role of the birth control pill as a means of regulating both menstruation and fertility.

Part 2 considers seven case studies of contemporary emmenagogue use along with beliefs about menstrual regulation based on ethnographic research. Traditional (primarily herbal) and patent medicines as well as modern contraceptives are used to promote regular menstrual flow in several parts of Africa (with examples from Guinea, Mali, and Nigeria), Latin America (Bolivia and Guatemala), and Southeast Asia (Bangladesh and Indonesia). The chapters about Southeast Asia also refer to menstrual regulation technologies used in government family planning programs that blur the boundaries of normal reproductive health practices associated with regular menstruation and very early-term abortion.

As William James (1975:117) has observed, "Human motives sharpen all our questions, human satisfactions lurk in all our answers, all our formulas have a human twist." The ambiguity surrounding the absence of menstruation and the meanings attributed to its regulation reflect various human motives, satisfactions, and twists. To attribute a single interpretation or meaning to these acts not only overlooks the particularities of specific historical and sociocultural contexts but also discounts the advantage of ambiguity, which has empowered women in different times and different places with a certain reproductive authority.

NOTES

1. There are, nonetheless, some applications for the use of newly developed abortifacients as emmenagogues; recent studies on the use of mifepristone (RU-486) for inducing delayed menstruation have also been conducted (Grimes et al. 1992).

2. The issue of terminology was discussed at the Menstrual Regulation Conference held in Honolulu, Hawaii, 17–19 December 1973, organized to consider the implications of this new technology (van der Vlugt and Piotrow 1974).

3. The release of blood by venesection, a familiar medical procedure during the centuries dominated by the humoral theory of disease, found in the periodic menstruation of women a natural equivalent.

4. For example, savin is more likely to be mentioned in magical spells, and rue as an antidote and a plague medicine. This conclusion comes after a search for the names of the most popular emmenagogues in *Literature Online*, which covers the canon on English literature. For example, in Richard Blackmore's *Prince Arthur* (1695), the magician Merlin uses savin in a spell to destroy the Saxons, and the grave digger who survives the plague of London in Daniel Defoe's *Journal of the Plague Year* (1722) "never used any preservative against the infection other than holding garlic and rue in his mouth, and smoking tobacco."

5. As Hull and Hull (this volume) note in the Indonesian context, such warnings may signal that the substance was a possible abortifacient, "attracting a market seeking this result."

6. Potter also notes that American women sometimes go off the Pill in order to have "a real cleansing bleed" (see also WHO 1981:12).

7. See, for example, Juan de Esteyneffer's *Florilegio Medicinal* ([1719] 1978); also Browner 1985:103 for references.

REFERENCES

Amin, R., G. M. Kamal, S. Firoza Begum, and H. Kamal. 1989. "Menstrual Regulation Training and Service Programs in Bangladesh: Results from a National Survey." *Studies in Family Planning* 20(2):102–106.

Amin, Sajeda. 1996. "Menstrual Regulation in Bangladesh." Paper presented at the International Union for the Scientific Study of Population Seminar on Socio-cultural and Political Aspects of Abortion, Trivandrum, Kerala, India.

Aughterson, Kate, ed. 1995. *Renaissance Women: A Sourcebook*. London: Routledge.

Balzer, Marjorie. 1981. "Rituals of Gender Identity: Markers of Siberian Khanty Ethnicity, Status and Belief." *American Anthropologist* 83:850–67.

Beidelman, T. O. B. 1997. *The Cool Knife: Imagery of Gender, Sexuality, and Moral Education in Kaguru Initiation Ritual*. Washington, D.C.: Smithsonian Institution Press.

Bleek, Wolf, and N. K. Asante-Darko. 1986. "Illegal Abortion in Southern Ghana: Methods, Motives and Consequences." *Human Organization* 45:333–44.

Boddy, Janice. 1989. *Wombs and Alien Spirits*. Madison: University of Wisconsin Press.

Bourgeois, Louise. [1609] 1992. *Observations diverses sur la stérilité, perte de fruits, fécondité, accouchements et maladies des femmes et enfants nouveau-nés*. Paris: Côté-femmes.

Brodie, Janet Farrell. 1994. *Conception and Abortion in Nineteenth-Century America*. Ithaca, N.Y.: Cornell University Press.

Browder, Clifford. 1988. *The Wickedest Woman in New York. Madame Re-stell, the Abortionist.* Hamden, Conn.: Archon Books.

Browner, Carole. 1985. "Traditional Techniques for the Diagnosis, Treatment, and Control of Pregnancy in Cali, Colombia." In *Women's Medicine,* ed. Lucille Newman, 99–123. New Brunswick, N.J.: Rutgers University Press.

Browner, Carole, and Bernard R. Ortiz de Montellano. 1986. "Herbal Emmenagogues Used by Women in Colombia and Mexico." In *Plants in Indigenous Medicine and Diet: Biobehavioral Approaches,* ed. Nina Etkin, 32–47. New York: Gordon and Breach Science.

Buckley, Anthony. 1985. *Yoruba Medicine.* Oxford: Clarendon Press.

Buckley, Thomas. 1982. "Menstruation and the Power of Yurok Women." In *Blood Magic: The Anthropology of Menstruation,* ed. Thomas Buckley and Alma Gottlieb, 187–209. Berkeley: University of California Press.

Buckley, Thomas, and Alma Gottlieb. 1988. *Blood Magic: The Anthropology of Menstruation.* Berkeley: University of California Press.

Cadden, Joan. 1993. *Meaning of Sex Differences in the Middle Ages.* Cambridge: Cambridge University Press.

Crawford, Patricia. 1981. "Attitudes to Menstruation in Seventeenth-Century England." *Past and Present* 91:47–73.

Davis, Geoffrey. 1972. "Menstrual Regulation." *Family Planning Magazine* 21(3):57–59. P. 57 cited in Dawn 1975:4.

Dawn, C. S. 1975. *Menstrual Regulation: A New Procedure for Fertility Control.* Calcutta: Dawn Books.

Dean-Jones, Lesley. 1994. *Women's Bodies in Classical Greek Science.* Oxford: Clarendon Press.

Dispensatory of the United States of America. 1955. 25th ed. Edited by Arthur Osol et al. Philadelphia: Lippincott. Pp. 512–26 cited in Riddle 1992:17.

Dixon-Mueller, Ruth. 1988. "Innovations in Reproductive Health Care: Menstrual Regulation Policies and Programs in Bangladesh." *Studies in Family Planning* 19(3):129–40.

Djerassi, Carl. 1979. *The Politics of Contraception.* New York: W. W. Norton & Co.

Douglas, Mary. 1966. *Purity and Danger.* London: Routledge and Kegan Paul.

Esteyneffer, Juan de. [1719] 1978. *Florilegio medicinal de todas las enfermedades.* Mexico City: Academia Nacional de Medicina.

Feldman-Savelsberg, Pamela. 1994. "Plundered Kitchens and Empty Wombs: Fear of Infertility in the Cameroonian Grassfields." *Social Science & Medicine* 39(4):463–74.

Fortes, Meyer. 1949. *The Web of Kinship among the Tallensi.* London: Oxford University Press.

Gottlieb, Alma. 1982. "Sex, Fertility, and Menstruation among the Beng of the Ivory Coast: A Symbolic Analysis." *Africa* 52(4):34–47.

———. 1988. "Menstrual Cosmology among the Beng of Ivory Coast." In *Blood Magic: The Anthropology of Menstruation,* ed. Thomas Buckley and Alma Gottlieb, 55–74. Berkeley: University of California Press.

Grimes, D. A., D. R. Mishell Jr., and H. P. David. 1992. "A Randomized Clinical Trial of Mifepristone (RU486) for Induction of Delayed Menses: Efficacy and Acceptability." *Contraception* 46(1):1–10.

Hippocrates. 1962. *Oeuvres complètes.* 10 vols, ed. Emile Littré. Amsterdam: Adolf M. Hakkert. [*Nature of Women* is in vol. 7, pp. 312–431; *Diseases of Women,* vol. 8, pp. 10–463.]

Hull, Terence, Sarsanto Sarwono, and Ninuk Widyantoro. 1993. "Induced Abortion in Indonesia." *Studies in Family Planning* 24(4):241–51.

IPPF. 1997. *Family Planning Handbook for Health Professionals: The Sexual and Reproductive Health Approach.* London: International Planned Parenthood Federation.

James, William. 1975. *Pragmatism.* Cambridge: Harvard University Press.

Jennings, Samuel K. [1808] 1972. *The Married Lady's Companion; or, Poor Man's Friend.* New York: Arno Reprints.

Kasnitz, D. 1981. "Work, Gender and Health among Southern Italian Immigrants in Melbourne, Australia." Ph.D. diss., University of Melbourne.

Kleiner-Bossaller, Anke. 1993. "Kwantacce, the 'Sleeping Pregnancy,' a Hausa Concept." In *Focus on Women in Africa,* ed. Gudrun Ludwar-Ene and Mechthild Reh, 17–30. Bayreuth, Germany: African Studies Series, no. 26.

Ladipo, O. A., O. A. Ojo, Sylvia James, and Karen Stewart. 1978. "Menstrual Regulation in Ibadan, Nigeria." *International Journal of Gynaecology and Obstetrics* 15:428–32.

Levin, Elise. 1996. "Menstrual Management and Abortion in Guinea, West Africa." Paper presented at the International Union for the Scientific Study of Population Seminar on Socio-cultural and Political Aspects of Abortion, Trivandrum, Kerala, India.

Lord, Alexandra. 1999. "'The Great *Arcana* of the Deity.' Menstruation and Menstrual Disorders in Eighteenth-Century British Medical Thought." *Bulletin of the History of Medicine* 73, no.1:38–63.

MacCormack, Carol, ed. 1982. *Ethnography of Fertility and Birth.* London: Academic Press.

Martin, Emily. 1987. *The Woman in the Body.* Boston: Beacon Press.

———. 1988. "Premenstrual Syndrome: Discipline, Work, and Anger in Late Industrial Societies." In *Blood Magic: The Anthropology of Menstruation,* ed. Thomas Buckley and Alma Gottlieb, 55–74. Berkeley: University of California Press.

McLaren, Angus. 1984. *Reproductive Rituals: The Perception of Fertility in England from the Sixteenth to the Nineteenth Century.* London and New York: Methuen.

Musallam, B. F. 1983. *Sex and Society in Islam: Birth Control before the Nineteenth Century.* Cambridge: Cambridge University Press.

Newman, Lucile, ed. 1985. *Women's Medicine.* New Brunswick, N.J.: Rutgers University Press.

Noonan, John. 1986. *Contraception: A History of Its Treatment by the Catholic Theologians and Canonists.* Cambridge, Mass.: Belknap Press.

Ojo, O. A., and O. A. Ladipo. 1981. "Menstrual Regulation at University College Hospital, Ibadan, Nigeria." *International Surgery* 66:247–50.

Paige, Karen, and Jeffery Paige. 1981. *The Politics of Reproductive Ritual.* Berkeley: University of California Press.

Potts, Malcolm, Peter Diggory, and John Peel. 1977. *Abortion.* Cambridge: Cambridge University Press.

Rasmussen, Susan. 1991. "Lack of Prayer: Ritual Restrictions, Social Experience, and the Anthropology of Menstruation Among the Tuareg." *American Ethnologist* 18(4):751–69.

Renne, Elisha. 1996. "The Pregnancy That Doesn't Stay: The Practice and Perception of Abortion by Ekiti Yoruba Women." *Social Science & Medicine* 42(4):483–94.

Richards, Audrey. 1956. *Chisungu: A Girl's Initiation Ceremony among the Bemba of Northern Rhodesia.* London: Faber.

Riddle, John M. 1992. *Contraception and Abortion from the Ancient World to the Renaissance.* Cambridge, Mass.: Harvard University Press.

Rösslin, Eucharius. 1994. *When Midwifery Became the Male Physician's Province. The Sixteenth Century Handbook* The Rose Garden for Pregnant Women and Midwives, *Newly Englished.* Trans. Wendy Arons. Jefferson, N.C.: McFarland.

Rowland, Beryl. 1981. *Medieval Woman's Guide to Health. The First English Gynaecological Handbook.* Kent, Ohio: Kent State University Press.

Sévigné, Madame de. 1972. *Correspondance.* 3 vols. Paris: Gallimard.

Soranus. 1956. *Gynecology.* Trans. Owsei Temkin. Baltimore: Johns Hopkins University Press.

Skultans, Vieda. 1985. "Vicarious Menstruation." *Social Science & Medicine* 21(6):713–14.

Stanback, John, Andy Thompson, Karen Hardee, and Barbara Janowitz. 1997. "Menstruation Requirements: A Significant Barrier to Contraceptive Access in Developing Countries." *Studies in Family Planning* 28(3): 245–50.

Trickey, Ruth. 1998. *Women, Hormones and the Menstrual Cycle: Herbal and Medical Solutions from Adolescence to Menopause.* St. Leonard's, New South Wales, Australia: Allen & Unwin.

Turner, Victor. 1967. *The Forest of Symbols.* Ithaca, N.Y.: Cornell University Press.

Vlugt, Theresa van der, and Phyllis Piotrow. 1973. "Menstrual Regulation—What is It?" *Population Reports* (series F) 2:9–23.

———. 1974. "Menstrual Regulation Update." *Population Reports* (series F) 4:49–63.

Walle, Etienne van de. 1997. "Flowers and Fruits: Two Thousand Years of Menstrual Regulation." *Journal of Interdisciplinary History* 28(2):183–203.

WHO [World Health Organization]. 1981. "A Cross-cultural Study of Menstruation: Implications for Contraceptive Development and Use." *Studies in Family Planning* 12(1):3–27.

Stefania Siedlecky

The following definitions underlying the physiology of the menstrual cycle will be used in this volume.

Menstruation (the menses or periods) is the monthly shedding of the lining of the uterus which has been hormonally stimulated during the menstrual cycle to receive a fertilized egg; it normally occurs approximately 14 days after ovulation in the absence of pregnancy. It is the timing of ovulation itself (or of the hormonal surge that provokes it) that leads to variations in the length of the cycle. Menstrual cycles begin at puberty (menarche) and continue until menopause. Anovular cycles, where the ovum fails to complete its development, may occur even in healthy women, mostly in the few years just after menarche or before menopause. These cycles may go unnoticed, or they may result in a missed period or irregular bleeding. A normal cycle lasts 28 days, but variability among women and within an individual is considerable.

An ovum has a life span of less than 24 hours, and **fertilization** can occur only during that time. Fertilization takes place in the fallopian tube; then the fertilized egg, in its first few days of development, passes into the uterine cavity and implants itself into the thickened uterine lining. **Implantation** is completed between the seventh and tenth day after ovulation, or a few days before the due date for the next menstrual bleed, on days 21 to 24 of a normal 28-day cycle. In modern usage, **conception** is a continuous process covering fertilization and implantation. **Contraception** is therefore defined as the deliberate prevention of uterine conception by interfering at any stage in this process, including the prevention of fertilization and of implantation. The World Health Organization defines **pregnancy** thus: "Pregnancy begins when implantation is complete and lasts until expulsion or removal of the conceptus" (IPPF 1994:4).

Amenorrhea is defined as the absence or suppression of menstruation. It occurs naturally before menarche and after menopause, and
during pregnancy and the postpartum period. In this book the term
amenorrhea is used only in reference to women in the childbearing
years from menarche to menopause. While the most frequent cause of
amenorrhea is pregnancy, it can also result from any condition that
disturbs the normal hormonal pattern and, in rare cases, from disease
or damage to the uterine lining. Exactly when a delayed period is identified as amenorrhea, however, is not clear. It is misleading in this regard to talk of *retention of menses,* even though the term appears in
textbooks written before 1900, and the fear of "retained blood" is common in many of the world's populations. True retention occurs in rare
instances in which the monthly bleed banks up behind an obstruction
such as a congenitally imperforate hymen or a blind double uterus, or
as a result of trauma or infection causing adhesions that block the cervix or vagina.

The oral contraceptive, which suppresses ovulation, is designed to
be taken cyclically to imitate the menstrual cycle. The bleeding that
occurs with oral contraceptive use is **withdrawal** or **breakthrough
bleeding,** not true menstruation. Bleeding does not occur after implantation, so breakthrough bleeding indicates that a woman is not pregnant, unless she is threatening to miscarry. Hormone pregnancy tests
relied on this type of bleeding to determine the nonpregnant status;
these tests are now outdated and have been replaced by a more reliable
urine test.

An **emmenagogue** is a drug or herbal product that purports to induce menstruation. The term has sometimes been used when the real
aim of restoring menses was to produce an early abortion. Although
the word is still used in herbal pharmacopeias, it does not appear in
gynecological textbooks, and a whole generation of doctors and medical students has never heard it.

A drug that expels an embryo or fetus after implantation is an **abortifacient.** Abortifacients act by direct toxic effects on the fetus itself; by
generalized toxic effects on the mother and indirectly on the fetus; or
by stimulating uterine activity to expel the fetus. *Ecbolics* were defined
as drugs that hasten the expulsion of the fetus, and *oxytocics* as drugs
assisting in parturition, but the terms are rarely used today. Since these
drugs act by stimulating uterine activity, they may be included in the
definition of abortifacients. To these modes of action we can now add
the interruption of the hormonal balance that maintains the preg-

nancy. In popular usage, the term **abortion** usually refers to induced abortion, while the term **miscarriage** is often reserved for a spontaneous abortion.

The term **menstrual regulation** has been used to cover the regular administration of herbal products or hormones to ensure that bleeding occurs at regular intervals. Nowadays, menstrual regulation usually refers to suction curettage of the uterus at or soon after the expected date of menstruation, before a diagnosis of pregnancy is made.

REFERENCE

IPPF (International Family Planning Federation). 1994. Report from the International Medical Advisory Panel to IPPF Central Council Meeting, 18–20 November.

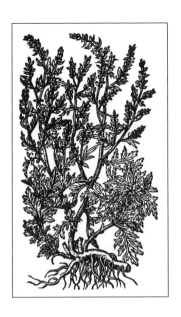

PART 1

HISTORICAL AND
CONTEMPORARY
STUDIES IN THE
WEST

CHAPTER 1

Menstrual Catharsis and the Greek Physician

Etienne van de Walle

Life is short, science is long;
opportunity is elusive,
experiment is dangerous,
judgment is difficult.

—Hippocrates, *Aphorisms*

The corpus of Greek scientific writings, transmitted across more than two millennia, represents a singular intellectual achievement based on the accumulation and interpretation of empirical knowledge. The works of Greek physicians reflect a logical approach to disease and health, and often include the description of cases supporting it. Physicians carefully jotted down the medical history of individual patients, describing symptoms and the day-to-day course of the malady. Botanical and pharmacological lore was collected from folk traditions and organized. These ideas, transmitted through Roman and Arabic writers, exerted an enormous influence on successive generations of physicians even to our days, and still hold sway in much of the world. One topic of this volume, menstrual stimulation, owes much to the humoral theories of Hippocrates and Galen, and to the list of materia medica compiled by Dioscorides.

Because it was largely transmitted through written texts, patiently hand copied and jealously preserved in centers of learning, the core message of the Greek tradition remained remarkably close to the original through the centuries. But inevitably, the content was interpreted and adapted. Translations and commentaries were made available to the practitioners of medicine and pharmacy. And the exact meaning of the originals (for example, the identification of Mediterranean plants for the use of British apothecaries) became the object of speculation. New diseases and new cures were traced back to the urtexts through mental gymnastics. When Renaissance physicians were confronted with the great pox in 1496, they scrutinized Galen and Hippocrates to identify its symptoms in their descriptions: it seemed impossible that this was a new disease, unknown to the Greeks (Arrizabalaga, Henderson, and French 1997:70–84).

Overinterpretations of the Greek texts still exist in present-day discussions of contraception and abortion. Some classicists and historians have seen allusions where probably none existed, as if birth control were a part of the daily life of the Greeks, and commonly alluded to in lay writings. The Greek physicians provided many recipes for gynecological problems ranging from suppressed menses to the retention of a dead fetus or of the placenta, and modern writers have tended to interpret many of those recipes as abortifacients. A historian of pharmacology, John R. Riddle (1992; 1997), has examined in two books the role of plant substances in regulating fertility in antiquity. My own interest owes much to Riddle's studies (van de Walle 1997). Since much of the present chapter is devoted to a work attributed to Hippocrates—*Diseases of Women* (fifth century B.C.)—I will say immediately that I disagree with Riddle's reading on what he interprets as abortive recipes in this work. His interest was pharmacological, and he focused on the recipes rather than on the context in which they were given. He did not ask whether the author had sound reasons, based on his interpretation of the workings of the female body, to recommend these herbal products, nor what effect he intended them to have. He believed that they reflected an old tradition of esoteric female lore, transmitted by male writers without true understanding (Riddle 1992:81).

Diseases of Women is the longest and most systematic exposition of gynecological issues to appear before the academic textbooks of the late nineteenth century. It is difficult to accept that it represents the work of bumbling amateurs who did not understand what they were copying down, and were unknowingly recording widely applied folk recipes. In this chapter I will examine the context in which Greek physicians recommended menstrual stimulants. I start by considering a particular claim that pennyroyal, a mint commonly found throughout Europe, was widely known as an abortifacient, and openly alluded to by classical Greek writers.

THE CASE OF PENNYROYAL

There is mention of pennyroyal in *Peace,* a play by Aristophanes produced in Athens in 421 B.C., at the time of the Peloponnesian War. In the play, Trygaeus has flown on a huge dung beetle to the home of the gods. There he convinces Hermes to release Peace, who has two attendants, Oporas (bizarrely translated in the Loeb edition as Harvesthome), the goddess of fruits and agricultural abundance, and Theorias (translated as Mayfair), the goddess of festivities. To clinch the deal, Hermes gives Oporas in marriage to Trygaeus. The Loeb translation renders the next exchange as follows:

TRYGAEUS: But, Hermes, won't it hurt me if I make
Too free with fruits of Harvesthome at first?
HERMES: Not if you add a dose of pennyroyal.
(Rogers 1972, 2:65)

The verb translated here as "make free with fruits of" (*katelauno*, literally, "to drive down") could be an obscene reference to the sex act.[1] In fact this is the meaning adopted in another translation of *Peace* (The Athenian Society 1931, 1:195):

TRYGAEUS: Tell me, Hermes, my master, do you think it would hurt me to . . . her a little, after so long an abstinence?

Riddle believes that pennyroyal constitutes an allusion to contraception and abortion. Similarly, Scarborough (1991:145) maintains that Aristophanes is emphasizing "the well-known fact that pennyroyal quaffed in solution prevented pregnancies." Is Trygaeus perhaps afraid of having too many children in his marriage? On the contrary, it would be rather strange, and counter to the spirit of the play, that Trygaeus would want to restrain the fertility of his bride after the great loss of life caused by the Peloponnesian War. When the wedding is celebrated at the end of the play, the Chorus celebrates the return of abundance:

And that every field may its harvest yield,
And our garners shine with the corn and wine,
While our figs in plenty and peace we eat,
And our wives are blest with an increase sweet . . .
(Rogers 1972:121)

The Loeb translation greatly embellishes the original, which consists of short and simple verses. The last verse quoted here simply says: "and our wives to bear [children]" [*tas te gunaikas tiktein emin*]. In any case, a contraceptive allusion would make little sense. Trygaeus is the person who is advised to take pennyroyal, after the act. It would make sense in the context if the advice were to take pennyroyal as a restorative after debilitating sex.

By what authority is pennyroyal considered a widely used contraceptive? According to Scarborough (1991:45), the mention of pennyroyal in the Homeric *Hymn to Demeter* confers it "quasi-mythical associations with the functions of birthing and nursing the newborn"; and "pennyroyal's reputation as a female contraceptive and abortifacient is verified in the Hippocratic writers, Dioscorides, and Galen." Pennyroyal entered into the composition of the *kykeon,* or drink given to new initiates, in the mysteries of the cult of Demeter at Eleusis. The modern editor of the *Hymn to Demeter* discounts, however, "ulterior motives for its use at Eleusis" (e.g., as an aphrodisiac) and notes that "it was in fact believed to cure a wide range of ailments, in ancient times (burning thirst, fainting, headaches, coughs, indigestion, fevers, nervous troubles, etc.)" (Richardson 1974:344). Kerényi (1967:179–80) discusses at length the role of pennyroyal in the *kykeon,* citing one opinion about possible hallucinatory properties; he does not mention any connection with fertility. Dioscorides says, as he does for some 80 other plants, that "being drank [pennyroyal] expelleth ye menstrua, & ye seconds [i.e., the placenta], & ye Embrya";[2] there is no suggestion of contraception, and "ye Embrya" may refer to spontaneous fetal deaths. Scarborough (1991:168) gives one reference to a Hippocratic treatise, *Nature of Woman,* paragraph 32, "among many refs." The paragraph is a long enumeration of recipes, mostly of potions and pessaries to restore the menstrual flow or evacuate the placenta (Hippocrates 1962, 8:347).[3] More than 100 plants and substances are mentioned in the section, and pennyroyal is cited once in a recipe toward the end, without special emphasis, as one component among many.

Other recipes in *Nature of Woman,* and in the other Hippocratic treatise that covers the same ground, *Diseases of Women,* give no special importance to pennyroyal. It enters in the composition of a small number of potions and pessaries, but never in a contraceptive context. Its first mention in *Nature of Woman* (p. 17) is in a pessary for women who suffer a hysteric fit. The author comments that the best remedy would be to become pregnant, or, for a young girl, to take a husband. As elsewhere, pennyroyal seems more of a fertility enhancer than a limiter. On page 93 of *Diseases of Women,* it is recommended for women in case of postpartum problems, just before sleeping with their husband, to promote conception. On page 157, it enters into the preparation of an emmenagogic pessary. On page 165, for a woman who has had children and cannot conceive again, the treatise advises: "apply dry pennyroyal in a linen; the woman will drink pennyroyal at the time of going to sleep." A pennyroyal soup cooked with flour and a light decoction of pennyroyal in wine are part of another 7-day treatment to conceive (167). Dried pennyroyal, mixed with honey and applied in wool, enters in the composition of a *peireterion* ("fecundity test," described later) on page 179. However, pennyroyal is also part of an injection to expel a dead embryo on pages 191 and 195. The quotes from Galen are equally unconvincing. One appears in a treatise on venesection, where a number of plant substances are offered as an alternative to bloodletting in cases of a plethora of blood.

Why then was pennyroyal well known to the Athenian public attending the plays of Aristophanes? It is a striking plant, with a distinctive smell, and a reputation as something of a cure-all. It was used as an insect repellent, as the Latin (*pulegium,* from *pulex,* "flee") and French (*pouliot* evokes *pou,* "louse") names suggest; Pliny (1969, 6:91) says that the flowers of pennyroyal were burned to kill fleas. The author of the first treatise on botany, Theophrastus (fifth century B.C.), who does not attribute any particular property to the plant, mentions it in the description of other plants: for example, he notes that dittany looks like pennyroyal. Pennyroyal was a condiment, as attested by its popular English name of pudding grass. St. Jerome wrote that among Indians, it was more valuable than pepper. Hildegarde of Bingen had only good things to say about it, particularly as a medicine for the eyes.[4] For the great English botanists of the seventeenth century, Gerard and Culpeper, it had pro-fertility properties. In the nineteenth century, it appears to have had a reputation as a mild emmenagogue. A concentrated extract, pennyroyal oil has caused deaths among women who used it as an abortifacient, and this may account for its bad name, applied retrospectively by modern-day exegetes to the time of Aristophanes.

The example of pennyroyal suggests that it is risky to see birth control everywhere in the texts of antiquity. It also reveals, however, the existence of a vast medical and botanical literature referring to potions and pessaries for gynecological uses. I now turn to these uses.

DISEASES OF WOMEN

The Treatise

The Hippocratic treatises date mostly to the fourth or fifth centuries B.C. Although Hippocrates is a historical figure, the works attributed to him were probably written by several physicians over an extended period. Dean-Jones (1994) collectively designates the authors of the treatises as "the Hippocratics." The corpus includes more than 50 treatises, and several deal with reproduction, gynecology, and obstetrics. Foremost among these are two treatises, *Nature of Woman* and *Diseases of Women.* On linguistic grounds, they appear to be among the oldest works in the corpus, and to date to the fifth century B.C. (Dean-Jones 1994:10). I will refer to the translation of these texts by Emile Littré, the French lexicographer who edited the Hippocratic corpus in the nineteenth century (Hippocrates 1962).

The treatises illustrate the sophistication of physicians of the time, and the use of feminine verbal forms suggests that they reflect at least in part the practices of midwives. In one of Plato's dialogues, *Theaetetus,* Socrates, whose mother was a midwife, asks, "Is it not true that the midwives give *pharmakia* and incantations to stimulate the labor pains, to facilitate a difficult delivery, or to abort the fetus if it seems necessary to abort it? *[ambliskein]*" (Nardi 1971:56–57). Nevertheless, incantations and *pharmakia,* a word that has given us *pharmacy* but suggests *magic* in many contexts, are completely absent from the Hippocratic treatises (Thivel 1975).[5] Dean-Jones (1994:7) comments that "the Hippocratics were among the first Greek scientists to try to make close observation rather than abstract reasoning the foundation of their theories." The procedures described do not invoke the divinity or mysterious forces, but are entirely rational, supported by the detailed description of cases, and based on the logic of the humoral theory. Indeed, the knowledge is clearly that of learned physicians, not a collection of folk wisdom based on experiences passed from mothers to daughters. In a telling passage from *Diseases of Women,* the author denies his reliance on a female culture that would have presided over gynecology:

> Among women who do not know the source of their pain, the disease often becomes incurable before the physician has been informed by the patient on the origin of her ailment. Indeed, out of modesty, they do not talk even when they know; inexperience and ignorance make them consider it shameful for them. (Hippocrates 1962, 8:127)

The organizing principle of *Nature of Woman* is hard to fathom. It presents a series of diagnoses and remedies for a variety of feminine conditions. As the same ground is covered in *Diseases of Women* in a more detailed and logical fashion, I will focus on that work, and particularly on book 1, the part devoted to the birthing process.

The traditional Greek title of the work, *Gynaikeioon,* means literally "Of Women's Things," but the author specifies in the very first sentence that he will discuss the diseases of women.[6] The tone of the work is unabashedly pro-natalist; the author repeatedly indicates which conditions will result in temporary or permanent sterility, or what should be done in order to conceive. He also points out that childless women are especially vulnerable to certain diseases (for example, p. 126), and that marriage or pregnancy are the natural cures for many ailments: "there are more accidents suppressing the menstrual flow among women who have never been pregnant" (13). There is no recognition that repeated pregnancies present a health hazard, and many preparations to enhance the chances of conception are described. One isolated recipe (involving *misy,* probably a copper oxide, p. 170) is given for a contraceptive *(atokion),* but arguably none for abortifacients, although Littré sometimes translates *ekbolion,* literally "expulsive," as *abortifacient.*[7]

The treatise on *Diseases of Women* includes three separate books—perhaps different treatises by a common author—collected under a common title by Littré. Book 1 is a long (the Greek text occupies 111 pages in the Littré edition) and systematic discourse on the nature and treatment of potential complications in the childbearing process. The second book (86 pages) discusses various pathologies that are not directly connected with childbearing, such as bloody spotting or displacements of the matrix; and the third book (62 pages) is entirely devoted to the nature and causes of sterility in women.

The first part of book 1 consists of a description of pathologies, while the second is a pharmacological appendix of corresponding recipes for treatment (see table 1.1). For instance, paragraphs 1 through 9 in the text, which address various menstrual problems, correlate with paragraph 74 in the appendix, which describes emmenagogic pessaries. There are occasional deviations from this general layout, as one would expect from a work that has been copied many times; for example, an occasional recipe is interpolated in the section on pathology, as is the case for paragraphs 23 and 31, which seem out of place. In addition, the organization of the work is obvious in the beginning, but by the end, both the main text and the appendix consist of short paragraphs

Table 1.1 Topics Covered by Book 1 of *Diseases of Women* (by Paragraphs)

	Main Text Pathology	Appendix Recipes
Menstrual problems	1–9	74
Impediments to conception	10–22, 24	75
Diseases of pregnancy	25–30, 32	31 [76?]
Problems of delivery	33–34	77
Discharges after delivery	35–41	45, 78
Other postpartum problems (e.g., retention of the placenta)	42–54	Passim, 78–92
Varia (e.g., dead fetus)	55–73	78–92

in apparently random sequence. After paragraph 92, the text is altogether unrelated to diseases of women.

The main text and the recipes of book 1 clearly attempt to decompose the birthing process in a stepwise fashion (before conception, during pregnancy, at delivery, in the aftermath of the delivery), although some disorderly accretions or interpolations seem to have occurred before the work reached us. The place where one would expect recipes for treating the diseases of pregnant women is occupied by paragraph 76 with its isolated mention of *misy* as a contraceptive. In *Aphorisms,* the collection of Hippocratic sayings that has served to train physicians well into the modern period (Lloyd 1978), aphorism 4.1 advises against medicating pregnant women, which may explain the absence of recipes for treating pregnant women in *Diseases of Women*. Some of the diseases of pregnancy listed in paragraphs 25–32 stem from tiredness and poor health, and it is possible that the author recognized implicitly that there are occasions when a year's rest brought about by contraception would benefit the woman's future fertility. It is also possible that paragraph 76, which also appears verbatim in *Nature of Woman*, is simply out of place.

Humoral Gynecology

There is little theory explicitly presented in the work, but the underlying ideas are consistent with humoral principles. (For a discussion of the physiology and pathology underlying Hippocrates' work, see Hanson 1990 and Dean-Jones 1994.) The consequence of humoral imbalance—for example, of excessive bile or phlegm in the uterus—is considered at length. In the first paragraph, the author compares the physiology of women and men:

> [B]eing softer by nature, the woman extracts from the belly, on behalf of the body, more fluid in a faster way than the man; and with this softness, when the body is full of blood, if there is no outlet in the state of plethora and warmth of the flesh, this provokes pain. The woman has warmer blood, and hence is warmer than the man. But if the fullness that formed is evacuated, then blood causes neither pain nor heat. Man, who has firmer flesh, is not subject to the abundance of blood that would cause him pain if he did not get rid of a certain amount of blood every month. . . . That the man exerts himself much more than the woman contributes greatly to this situation; tiredness dissipates part of the fluid. (Hippocrates 1962, 8:13–15)

It is in this context that menstrual retention is treated as a major cause of bad health and sterility. Women who have never borne a child are more likely to suffer from menstrual retention:

> When menses are suppressed and cannot find an outlet in a woman who has never been pregnant, a disease occurs. This happens when the uterine opening closed or was displaced or if some part of the sexual organs underwent a contraction. In such a case, the menses will not find an outlet as long as the matrix is not reinstated in its natural condition. (8:15)

It is noteworthy that the author has a mechanistic view of the reproductive organs and the process of menstrual retention. In one well-known representation of the uterus in a Latin version of Muscion in the ninth or tenth century, the matrix appears as a jug or wineskin, whose opening fits into the woman's vagina.[8] Although Hippocrates does not use the analogy of a jug, such an image is useful to understand his views of female anatomy. According to Hippocrates, menstrual retention is the result of closing the neck of the jug; this happens because an accumulation of impurities clogs the outlet. In more frequent cases, however, the problem is that the matrix has shifted within the woman's body, and the opening of the uterus/jug no longer aligns with the vagina. Menstrual blood then will be evacuated by other parts of the body; through the lungs, for example. Similarly, the common cause of infertility (extensively discussed in book 3) is a shift or stoppage of the matrix's neck. The matrix itself is said to wander throughout the body with various ill effects. This phenomenon goes beyond the case of a prolapsed uterus, which also gets a full description (pars. 142–45, 247–48).

The text (notably pars. 123–28) explores at length, and repeatedly, the effects of womb travel to such parts of the body as the head, the heart, the liver, the bladder, the ribs, or the hipbone. Various treatments are proposed, from pessaries to unclog the "jug," to an array of wooden sticks to move the uterus back in position and a leaden rod to keep it aligned with the vagina (pars. 133, 217, and 230). Remarkably, the oral ingestion of an herbal product is not mentioned as a treatment for menstrual retention. In this treatise, Hippocrates does not resort to the systemic explanations that we intuitively adopt, where some potion would restore or alter a function such as menstruation. Potions with poorly understood effects would be magical in nature, *pharmakia*. It is striking that all the medications noted take the form of pessaries, and no potions are prescribed for stimulating the menses, at least in paragraph 74.[9]

A series of "fecundity tests," *peireteria,* are mentioned as ways to ascertain that the womb is open, along the lines of aphorism 5.59:

> If a woman has not conceived and you wish to determine whether conception is possible, wrap her up in a cloak underneath which incense should be burned. If the odor seems to pass through the body to the nose and mouth, then she is not sterile. (Lloyd 1978:226)

In *Diseases of Women,* fecundity is diagnosed if a pessary of garlic gives bad breath to the woman the next day. Pennyroyal appears in the same context, perhaps because of its strong odor.

The author describes at length the consequences of a mechanical obstruction of the uterus. If blood cannot be evacuated through menstruation, it will escape through other parts of the body, such as the lungs, and death will occur after six months. If menstruation resumes after several months, the woman may have been rendered sterile. Insufficient or excessive menstruation also leads to various ailments, and to sterility.

We should note that Hippocrates selects, of the two possible directions of causality, that which goes from menstrual retention to disease. It is easy to see how this association, rather than the opposite one— that disease may cause amenorrhea—corresponds to his general interpretation of female physiology. For the Hippocratic writers, woman is a flawed organism whose humid and soft constitution demands the monthly purgation. Its absence will be deadly, whereas its presence is almost a guarantee of survival. Dean-Jones (1994:144–46) has inventoried the instances of female case studies in the seven books of another treatise, *Epidemics.* Among 91 sick women who could menstruate (i.e., were not pregnant, aborting, giving birth, or nursing), "22 are recorded as having done so, and survived; of the remaining 69, 32 died." Menstruation was associated 100 percent with a successful cure, a rate that is certainly the result of the selection of cases, but reflects also the conviction of the reporting physicians.

Menstrual Catharsis and Abortion

Since Hippocrates has a mechanistic, not a systemic, view of what prevents menstruation, his remedies do not aim at "stimulating" the menses, but rather at removing impediments to their flow. Hence his insistence on pessaries. When he is dealing with the placenta or a dead fetus, however, he considers drugs that may have a systemic effect. This logic suggests that to Hippocrates, menstrual stimulation belongs to a different realm than abortion.

In paragraph 74, where he gives remedies to restore the menses, Hippocrates does not employ the terms used by Dioscorides more than 500 years later: *ago* ("to lead," meaning "to stimulate")[10] and *ekballo*, ("to expel," meaning "to extract"), but rather the verb that one would use for describing the action of a spigot, *kataspan* ("to draw down"). There is no question of emmenagogues, but there is mention of *malthaka*, softening substances to decongest.[11] *Prostheton kathartikon malthakon* can be translated as "pessary to purify by softening." The author opposes it to *drimu* (which Littré translates as *"pessaire acre"*—"sharp pessary"—but might be rendered better as "piercing pessary"), meant to reestablish the flow by "biting through" rather than by softening. The aim is "to evacuate the blood" (*aima ekkenoun*, p. 158). Hippocrates uses a different verb for the actions of expelling the lochia (the discharge that follows a delivery) and the placenta: *ekballo*, "to expel or throw out." Clearly, the action on the menses is not meant to parallel that on the fetus or on the lochia.

In English, the word *abortion* can take the meanings both of spontaneous abortion, or miscarriage, and of induced abortion. A similar ambiguity existed in classical Greek. In at least one passage of the third book of *Diseases of Women* (Hippocrates 1962, 8:456), the author specifies, "if a woman aborts against her will, without intending to get rid of her fruit . . ." According to Nardi (1971:360–62), the verb used by Hippocrates in the passive sense of "to undergo an abortion," *ektitrosko*, in his time meant "to miscarry," although some later authors, including Dioscorides, also used it to refer to an induced abortion. There was another verb referring to an induced abortion, *ambloo* (or the variant *amblisko* used by Plato), but it appears only once in all the Hippocratic works edited by Littré, according to the systematic inventory of words in the Hippocratic vocabulary by Maloney and Frohn (1984). In that passage (Hippocrates 1962, 8:68, par. 25, line 33), the context clearly implies an accidental miscarriage.

Miscarriage is probably the word that the author intended in most instances, but there are two passages where *induced* rather than *spontaneous abortion* would make sense. In both, he describes the physician's reaction to earlier interventions by amateurs. In the first passage, on pages 140–41, he may be discussing a physician's intervention to treat the consequences of a botched abortion. His disapproval is tangible:

When the woman is affected with a great wound as a result of a miscarriage, or when the matrix has been ulcerated by piercing pessaries, which happens in view of the many practices and treatments that women make on their own, or when, the fetus having been corrupted

[using the verb *phtheiro*] and the woman having had no lochial purgation, the matrix is strongly inflamed, closes and cannot provide
an exit to the purgation except for what has initially gotten out with
the child, the patient if treated promptly will heal but will remain
sterile.

On pages 150–53, the author discusses the problems linked with the
lochia and then says the following:

The dangers with the lochia are greater for the woman whose embryo
has been corrupted, since abortions are more painful than live births.
It is indeed not possible that there would be no violence in the expulsion of the embryo, either through a purge, through a drink or food,
or by pessaries, or by any other means. Indeed, violence is bad, it
brings about a risk of ulceration or inflammation of the matrix, and
this is very dangerous.[12]

However, it is possible that these cases all refer to spontaneous abortion.

The active verbs referring to aborting the fetus have a similar ambiguity. *Ekballo,* "to expel," could refer to a dead fetus in a miscarriage,
whereas *phtheiro,* "to corrupt" or "to destroy," refers to the deadly action of external agents on the fetus, which may also result from an
accident. In a widely cited passage, Soranus, a gynecologist of the second century A.D., refers to two types of abortive procedures, using
nouns derived from the same two verbs: *ekbolion* ("expulsive") and
phthorion ("destructive"). *Diseases of Women* never uses *ekballo* or *ekbolion* in the sense of aborting a live fetus, as far as can be ascertained
from text and context; nor are they ever used in reference to the menses. Instead, they are restricted to the realm of the chorion (i.e., the
membrane enveloping the fetus), and, in a few instances, of a dead or
unviable fetus ("a child become livid" or "a child stricken by apoplexy").[13] Furthermore, Hippocrates does not employ the noun *phthorion* in any context in this work or in others (Maloney and Frohn 1984).
The verb *phtheiro* or some composite such as *diaphteiro* appears in a
number of passages, and several times in combination with *ekballo,* as
for example: "to destroy and expel the fetus that is not moving." In
most instances, the verb refers to an accidental corruption of the fetus,
but it is used several times, as noted, in the passages quoted earlier
(pars. 67 and 72).

To summarize our discussion of *Diseases of Women,* Hippocrates
seems to concentrate on the pathologies of the female reproductive
system, and describes induced abortion, if at all, as a cause of disease.

He cites various health consequences of retained, irregular, or defective menses, but the general organization of the work, and the repeated mentions of the risks of sterility resulting from menstrual problems, suggest that his main preoccupation is reproductive success.

POST-HIPPOCRATIC WRITINGS

When reviewing the works of the other great physicians of antiquity, it is difficult to glean from this literature that many centuries had elapsed since Hippocrates' era. Galen, who wrote 6 centuries later, appears to treat Hippocrates as a respected colleague. Five centuries after Galen, Stephanus of Athens comments on the *Aphorisms* as if they had been recently published. Science (meaning the physician's understanding) was long, and life short. Scientific time was flowing very slowly, if at all. And yet, there existed an active intellectual life, as well as conflicting medical theories, teachers and students, medical schools and academies.

It is to the teaching activities of Theophrastus, Aristotle's successor at the head of the Peripatetic school in Athens, that we owe the first treatise on botany, which was almost contemporary with the Hippocratic treatises. Book 9 of his *Enquiry into Plants* is devoted to their medicinal properties, so it is logical to examine what Theophrastus had to say about emmenagogues. The book contains several brief references to emmenagogues and even to abortifacients, but unfortunately the standard Loeb text and translation are quite inadequate (Theophrastus 1916). The text has been expurgated by the prudish editor, who deleted two references to abortion, among other passages. Furthermore, the allusions to menstruation were mistranslated, with *gyneikeia* ("women's things") being rendered as "diseases of women" rather than as "menses." About *khalbane* and *kakhry* Theophrastus writes that they were used "for the menses" (277), and Dioscorides specifically quotes Theophrastus on the subject of the latter plant. In contrast with Hippocrates, who only referred to emmenagogic pessaries, Theophrastus, who must have relied on traditional recipes, appears to reintroduce systemic effects approaching magic. For example, he reports on an abortifacient wine from Achaia (Nardi 1971:135). Dioscorides describes how a similar wine was produced:

> There is also made a wine destructive of Embrya, for amongst ye vines planted, there is planted Veratrum, or wild Cucumber, or Scammonie,

of which ye grape doth take the faculty, & the wine made of them
becomes destructive. (Gunther 1959:621)

Thus it is tempting to hypothesize that the mechanistic views of Hippocrates concerning the release of the menses competed with other
practices relying on a tradition of folk medicine. The notion that the
same plant substances could alternatively be used to stimulate the
menses and to provoke an abortion was alien to the Hippocratic physicians. Later schools of physicians questioned some of these views. Galen, who relied on other physicians' accounts of dissections of the human body, and had dissected animals himself, would deny that the
uterus wandered about in the body (see the reference in Soranus 1956:
9). Soranus simply says, "the uterus is not an animal (as it appeared to
some people)." More important, Soranus reversed the path of causation
between sickness and menstrual retention. He reveals much skepticism
as to whether menstruation effected a purgation of the body with the
phrase "as some people say" (17). He notes that some healthy women
do not menstruate at all; for example, women engaged in singing con-
tests (the equivalent of the amenorrheic ballet dancers and athletes of
our time). The *Gynecology* includes a section entitled "Whether Catharsis of the Menses Fulfills a Helpful Purpose" (23), where he challenges
the use of emmenagogues. Disease would bring about the constriction
of the neck of the uterus and retention of the menses; curing the disease should be sufficient to reestablish the regular flow. Soranus concludes that menstruation probably contributes nothing to health in
itself, and "is useful for childbearing only: for conception does not take
place without menstruation" (27).
    Galen opposed the Methodist school of medicine to which Soranus
belonged (see Temkin's introduction to Soranus 1956). One of the
points of contention was the use of venesection to relieve the symptoms of menstrual retention. In his first treatise on the subject, Galen
argues much like Hippocrates before him:

Does [nature] not evacuate all women every month, by pouring forth
the superfluity of the blood? It is necessary, in my opinion, that the
female sex, who stay indoors, neither engaging in strenuous labor nor
exposing themselves to direct sunlight—both factors conducive to
the development of plethos—should have a natural remedy by which
it is evacuated. This is one of the ways in which nature operates in
these conditions; another is the cleansing that follows childbirth, although the conceptus itself is also an evacuation, since it is nourished
from the blood of the uterus; and the development of milk in the

breasts after delivery is itself also an important factor in eliminating the plethos. (Brain 1986:25–26)

Galen rhetorically addresses Erasistratus, dead two centuries before, who did not follow Hippocrates and did not believe in bloodletting:

If you had the intelligence to understand further what great benefits accrue to the female sex as a result of this evacuation, and what harm they suffer if they are not cleansed, I don't know how you would be able to go on wasting time and not eliminate superfluous blood by every means at your disposal. (26)

The conflict came to a head when Galen was consulted during a visit to Rome, and advised bloodletting "in the case of a certain young woman about 21 years of age who, from suppressed menstruation, had a flushed face, a slight cough, and already some difficulty breathing" (38). Galen diagnosed a case of plethora of blood. The Roman physicians, who were disciples of Erasistratus, recommended ligature of the limbs and fasting. Galen suggested emmenagogic drugs as an alternative to venesection. We note that there was no mention of trying to restore fertility, and that the problem was purely one of plethora following menstrual retention. Even so, a midwife had routinely treated the young woman with herbal drugs "of proven value," and they had failed to be effective. In a third treatise on venesection, Galen lists a series of emmenagogues that could be used to complement bloodletting: mint, pennyroyal, savin, dittany, aloes, and cinnamon (93).

Galen would exert a major influence on Arabic and Western medicine.[14] Meanwhile, the major influence on pharmacology was provided by the work of Dioscorides in the first century A.D.. Dioscorides had traveled extensively in the Mediterranean world with the Roman legions and had collected plant lore from popular traditions and written work. His *Materia Medica* is a monumental compilation of all the properties attributed to some 950 substances, most of them vegetal; claims on the virtues of plants are listed without critical assessment. Among many other properties, 141 substances are listed as emmenagogues, but some of those were also known to expel the fetus or the placenta; a number of them are said to destroy the fetus or kill it. The products are prescribed either as potions or as pessaries. In most instances, the verb used to refer to the action on the menses is *ago* ("to lead"). Goodyear, the seventeenth-century translator of the *Materia Medica,* renders *ago* as "to expel" or "to draw out," but the word is compatible with a more neutral "to release" (Gunther 1959). Many of the products Hippocrates recommended for confecting pessaries to release the menses are mentioned by Dioscorides too, but sometimes for oral or other uses. Although Dioscorides mentions Hippocrates occasionally, and may have known of his gynecological treatises, they do not appear to be a major direct source.

It is fair to conclude, then, that the pathology of menstrual retention, as understood in the West until the twentieth century, was largely transmitted from Hippocratic sources. (For the diffusion of Hippocratic ideas, see Cadden 1993.) But the oral therapy for menstrual retention owes more to Galen and Dioscorides. Part of the attractiveness of this protocol lay in the mysterious, quasi-magical action of plants on the human body, which lent itself to mystical and symbolic interpretations that had little to do with the strong empirical bent of the Hippocratic writers. At least in their gynecological writings, these writers focused on the plight of women who were trying to conceive and bear children. Galen, in the works that helped to impose the practice of bloodletting as a major therapy in medieval and modern times, pays little attention to fertility. He mentions, however, some of the herbal substances used for treating infertility as substitutes for venesection and, in various other treatises, as abortifacients (Nardi 1971:367–86). Because of their organizing principle, the *Materia Medica* of Dioscorides lumped together indiscriminately all the reported properties of plants. The confusion between the emmenagogic and the abortive virtues of plants was the product of an evolution in knowledge, and owed little to the Hippocratic writers.

The various strands of the Greek traditions were widely adopted in Arabic and European medicine. The systemic views dominated, although the Hippocratic influence remained very powerful until the nineteenth century. Among the ideas that can be traced to it are the dominance of menstrual retention as the principal pathology of women; the suffocation of the matrix; the itinerant uterus, bringing about such conditions as "rising of the mother"; vicarious menstruation, when the obstructed blood flows through other organs; and the mole, or false pregnancy.

Arabic physicians reintroduced the Greek influence in Europe. The emphasis in the works of Rhazes and Avicenna (translated in Latin in the thirteenth century) was on menstruation as a necessary purification of the body. There was a certain ambiguity, because the remedies meant to bring about menstruation could sometimes be read as prescriptions for abortion (Jacquart and Thomasset 1988:92). The various works attributed to members of the school of Salerno such as Platearius or the midwife Trotula advocate herbal means to regulate the menses, extract the afterbirth, and assist in difficult deliveries. Here too abortion could be inferred, but the mainstream Western tradition was strongly opposed to the practice. If it was mentioned at all by medical writers, it was with obvious distaste.

NOTES

I acknowledge the help of Wesley Smith, from the Classics Department of the University of Pennsylvania, who made a critical reading of this text. Errors, of course, are mine alone.

1. The *Oxford Greek Lexicon* cites the passage from *Peace* as an example of obscene meaning *(sens. obsc.)* and provides the Latin equivalent *subagitare.*

2. As quoted from the seventeenth-century translation by the botanist John Goodyear, which remains the standard English version of the *Materia Medica* (Gunther 1959).

3. This title was added by Emile Littré in the authoritative nineteenth-century edition and French translation.

4. I obtained the reference to Jerome and Hildegarde by running a search for the word *pulegium* in the *Patrologia Latina* Database on the Internet. This includes the Latin works of fathers and doctors of the church through thirteen centuries. Twenty-two references were found, none of them scandalous.

5. The word *pharmakon* is used occasionally in a context that leaves no doubt that a drug rather than magic is used. For example, Hippocrates (1962, 8:70, 74, 80): "the best *pharmaka* are Ethiopian cumin . . . etc."

6. "Women's things," in other contexts, may refer broadly to the reproductive system, or more specifically to menstruation. In *Diseases of Women,* Hippocrates (1962) occasionally uses *gyneikaia* in the sense of "menses"; see, for example, 8:156.

7. Riddle (1997:62) interprets a recipe in a paragraph devoted to expelling the chorion and the lochia (i.e., postpartum discharges) as that for a "potent uterine abortifacient" (quotation marks in the text).

8. The picture is reproduced in Soranus (1956:9) and in Soranos d'Ephèse (1988). There are multiple representations of the uterus as a vessel in Middle Ages manuscripts or early printed texts, and some are reviewed in Rowland 1981. (See also Cadden 1993:92, 178–79.) It is still represented as such, with a mature child standing up in it, in a 1651 English treatise on midwifery (*The Compleat Midwifes Practice* 1656). The analogy of a jug is used by Hanson (1990); Dean-Jones (1994:65) thinks the wineskin more suitable because of its ability to contract, a property linked with the notion of "the wandering womb."

9. Potions for the lochia following delivery, however, are indicated. Hippocrates calls them *cathatheria*. The absence of oral emmenagogues in *Diseases of Women* is remarkable. In one of the recipes in paragraph 74, the author specifies, "Pessaries to be used if draughts do not bring forth the [menstrual] catharsis" (8:158). See also page 23, where the author mentions a draught that purifies the blood (Littré translates as "that acts on the blood"). *Nature of Woman* provides examples of potions to restore the menses.

10. The expression *agonta aima*, "leading the blood," is used once in the paragraph, but could be used in the sense of "letting flow" rather than "stimulating." The use of the term by Dioscorides may well imply the same unclogging action as described in Hippocrates, whom he quotes repeatedly.

11. In the *Aphorisms*, there are examples of emmenagogues; for example, in 5.28, *gynaikeioon agogon* (Hippocrates 1962, 1:542).

12. I am translating from the French in Littré's classical work. This passage uses the Greek verb *phtheiro*, which implies destruction or corruption rather than expulsion of a fetus.

13. Most of the references appear in paragraph 78, to which Littré gave the general title "Formulas of Preparations Suited to Eliminate the Lochia."

14. Soranus was copied and imitated by Roman and medieval physicians and influenced midwifery and gynecology in the West, but he had less influence on Arabic medicine. When the school of Salerno utilized Arabic texts to address the problems in female reproductive health, the domination of Hippocrates and Galen was reinforced.

REFERENCES

Arrizabalaga, Jon, John Henderson, and Roger French. 1997. *The Great Pox: The French Disease in Renaissance Europe.* New Haven, Conn.: Yale University Press.

The Athenian Society. 1931. *Aristophanes Comedies.* 2 vols. New York: Rarity Press.

Brain, Peter. 1986. *Galen on Bloodletting.* Cambridge: Cambridge University Press.

Cadden, Joan. 1993. *Meaning of Sex Differences in the Middle Ages: Medicine, Science, and Culture.* Cambridge: Cambridge University Press.

The Compleat Midwifes Practice. 1656. In *Early English Books, 1641–1700,* 220:7. Ann Arbor, Mich.: University Microfilms International.

Dean-Jones, Lesley Ann. 1994. *Women's Bodies in Classical Greek Science.* Oxford: University Press.

Gunther, Robert T., ed. 1959. *The Greek Herbal of Dioscorides . . . Englished by John Goodyear.* New York: Hafner Publishing Co.

Hanson, Ann Ellis. 1990. "The Medical Writers' Woman." In *Before Sexuality: The Construction of Erotic Experience in the Ancient Greek World,* ed. David M. Halperin, John J. Winkler, and Froma I. Zeitlin, 309–37. Princeton, N.J.: Princeton University Press.

Hippocrates. 1962. *Oeuvres complètes.* 10 vols, ed. Emile Littré. Amsterdam: Adolf M. Hakkert. [*Nature of Woman* is in vol. 7, pp. 312–431; *Diseases of Women,* vol. 8, pp. 10–463.]

Jacquart, Danielle, and Claude Thomasset. 1988. *Sexuality and Medicine in the Middle Ages.* Princeton, N.J.: Princeton University Press.

Kerényi, Carl. 1967. *Eleusis: Archetypal Image of Mother and Daughter.* Bollingen Series 65-4. Princeton, N.J.: Princeton University Press.

Lloyd, G. E. R., ed. 1978. *Hippocratic Writings.* London: Penguin Books.

Maloney, Gilles, and Winnie Frohn, eds. 1984. *Concordance des oeuvres hippocratiques.* Quebec: Editions du Sphinx.

Nardi, Enzo. 1971. *Procurato Aborto nel Mondo Greco Romano.* Milan: Dott. A. Giuffrè.

Pliny. 1969. *Natural History.* 10 vols. Cambridge, Mass.: Harvard University Press.

Richardson, N. J., ed. 1974. *The Homeric Hymn to Demeter.* Oxford: Clarendon Press.

Riddle, John M. 1992. *Contraception and Abortion from the Ancient World to the Renaissance.* Cambridge, Mass.: Harvard University Press.

———. 1997. *Eve's Herbs: A History of Contraception and Abortion in the West.* Cambridge, Mass.: Harvard University Press.

Rogers, Benjamin B. 1972. *Aristophanes.* 3 vols. Cambridge, Mass.: Harvard University Press.

Rowland, Beryl. 1981. *Medieval Woman's Guide to Health: The First English Gynecological Handbook.* Kent, Ohio: Kent State University Press.

Scarborough, John. 1991. "The Pharmacology of Sacred Plants, Herbs, and Roots." In *Magika Hiera: Ancient Greek Magic and Religion,* ed. Christopher A. Faraone and Dirk Obbink, 138–74. Oxford: Oxford University Press.

Soranos d'Ephèse. 1988. *Maladies des femmes.* Ed. and trans. Paul Burguière, Danielle Gourevitch, and Yves Malinas. Paris: Les belles lettres.

Soranus. 1956. *Gynecology.* Trans. Owsei Temkin. Baltimore: Johns Hopkins University Press.

Theophrastus. 1916. *Enquiry into Plants.* Trans. Arthur Hort. New York: G. P. Putnam's Sons.

Thivel, Antoine. 1975. "Le 'divin' dans la collection hippocratique." In *La collection hippocratique et son rôle dans l'histoire de la médecine,* 59–76. Leiden: E. J. Brill.

Walle, Etienne van de. 1997. "Flowers and Fruits: Two Thousand Years of Menstrual Regulation." *Journal of Interdisciplinary History* 28, no. 2: 182–203.

CHAPTER 2

Colds, Worms, and Hysteria: Menstrual Regulation in Eighteenth-Century America

Susan E. Klepp

An obstruction of the *menses* is often the
effect of other maladies.

—William Buchan, *Domestic Medicine,* 1795

Savin is "hot and dry, opening and attenuating,
and a powerful provoker of the catamenia,
causing abortion and expelling the birth; it is
very good to destroy worms" and in "jaundice,
dropsy, scurvy, rheumatism, &c."

—Culpeper's *Complete Herbal,* [1625] 1826

Respectable married women in eighteenth-century America used emmenagogues in order to restore health. That other purposes may have been involved in married women's use of these sometimes potent drugs was rarely recognized, yet when identical substances and practices were employed by single, separated, or widowed women or were insisted upon by men who were not their husbands, then contraceptive or abortive intentions were assumed. Medical, moral, and social judgments affected emmenagogic usage.

Our knowledge of the historical use of emmenagogues and abortifacients in the thirteen North American British colonies and the early United States is limited. Diaries and letters rarely mention such topics, and there are few medical case histories. Court records preserve a few cases that were uncovered during the prosecution of various crimes. Herbals, pharmacists' advertisements, and home medical guides present a wide array of information on the known techniques of restoring menstruation, but do not usually indicate which methods were commonly practiced, nor under what circumstances. Complicating the

process of rediscovery are the arcane definitions of disease and reproduction used in the past.

Women apparently utilized emmenagogues to restore general mental and physical health, not to enhance their fertility.[1] While contemporaries certainly recognized that the onset of menstruation signaled
the beginning of childbearing capacity and menopause the end, amenorrhea in a healthy adult woman was classified either as a disease symptom or as pregnancy. The best-selling home medical guide, Dr. William
Buchan's *Domestic Medicine* (first edition 1769), did state that barren-
ness might "proceed from various causes, as high living, grief, relax-
ation, &c. but it is chiefly owing to an obstruction or irregularity of
the menstrual flux" (Buchan 1795:545; Rosenberg 1982). Yet diet and
exercise were the recommended cures for infertility, not emmenagogues, because the emphasis was entirely on pernicious effects of
"high living" rather than on the amenorrhea. Other sources also fail
to link emmenagogues to infertility.

Eighteenth-century American women considered amenorrhea as a
disease in its own right, symptomatic of a disease of the internal organs, or indicative of pregnancy. According to medical texts, if disease
accompanied by amenorrhea was diagnosed in a respectable single or
married woman, then treatments focused on "bringing down the
terms" as part of the cure. If pregnancy was diagnosed in a healthy
woman, emmenagogues were not to be employed, especially in unmarried women who had been beguiled by presumably licentious men or
who were of dubious characters themselves. Under these circumstances, emmenagogues could be redefined as abortifacients. They then
might be criminally suspect and their use introduced at trial, if they
were designed to remove evidence of fornication, rape, adultery, or infanticide. Yet for all the attempts by contemporaries to clearly demar-
cate the boundaries between the restoration of health through emmenagogues and interference with pregnancy through abortifacients,
women's intentions in using the substances were truly ambiguous.

Disease categories in the eighteenth century were a matter of considerable dispute among doctors. Apart from a few epidemic diseases
such as smallpox, measles, and influenza, most physicians preferred to
stress systemic or localized imbalances, tensions, or irritability as the
cause of illness. Contemporary "therapy was directed against general
body conditions, whether or not these were associated with particular
names" (Shryock 1960:49–50). Ill health was as much determined by
the mental or emotional state of the patient as by her external physical
symptoms. Symptoms might have multiple meanings and would indicate various therapeutic regimens. Nonprofessionals and botanists

were somewhat more likely to associate specific complaints with a particular organ and treatment. It would be foolish, however, to try to draw substantial distinctions among the beliefs of doctors, pharmacists, botanists, midwives, ladies bountiful (local women called upon in medical crises for their herb lore, supplies of linens, and medical recipe books), and laywomen. Medical practice was quite eclectic; this was as true in the evaluation of amenorrhea as in any other complaint.

If disease definition was uncertain, so too was pregnancy difficult to ascertain. As one early nineteenth-century doctor noted, "An entire suppression of the menses attends almost every case of pregnancy. But as suppressions may be brought on by other causes this cannot be an infallible mark" (Jennings 1972:75). There was no necessary connection between amenorrhea and pregnancy until quickening (when fetal movement can be felt) in the third to fifth month of gestation. Quickening was an entirely subjective test, dependent on the woman's testimony that she felt the fetus move. The other common test of pregnancy involved drawing the breasts of the woman to see if liquid appeared.[2] This was the pregnancy test most often used in court, but it would give a false negative until about 19 weeks' gestation, that is, until the last weeks in which quickening might be expected to occur. Certainly, women either looking forward to or especially fearful of pregnancy seemed capable of an immediate suspicion about their condition, but in other circumstances there was no need to confine evaluations to a single eventuality. One doctor suspected deliberate misrepresentation when he wrote that "[s]ome woman are so Ignorant, They do not know whin she are Conceived with Child, and others so easy, They will nott Confess when they do know it"; yet in this doctor's list of medical indications the symptoms of early pregnancy could be easily read as symptoms of disease (DeBenneville [1760–79?]:124).

If a woman decided her amenorrhea was symptomatic of disease, she had a number of possible diagnoses, one of which was hysteria. In a married woman, hysteria was assumed to be caused by a "sudden suppression of the *menses*," and was accompanied by fatigue, low spirits, and feelings of "oppression and anxiety." The physical symptoms of hysteria included a sensation like that of "a ball at the lower part of the belly, which gradually rises towards the stomach, where it occasions inflation, sickness, and sometimes vomiting" (Buchan 1795:455–56). Another interpretation was that hysteria felt "as if some little animal were [in the bowels] in actual motion with wandering pains" (Jennings [1808] 1972:54). Intestinal cramping during sleep was also hysteric in origin and called for "a pretty strong compression upon the *abdomen*" (Buchan 1795:458–59). In the twentieth century, these emotional associations after a cessation of menstruation might be seen as fear of an unwelcome pregnancy, not as an illness, while the physical symptoms—nausea, cramping, and a swelling belly—are most strongly associated with pregnancy, not with disease.

Amenorrhea could also be traced to catching a cold, and because colds might develop into pleurisy or rheumatism, these too could be identified as the underlying illness. "More of the sex [women] date their disorders [amenorrhea] from colds, caught while they are out of order [expecting menstruation], than from all other causes" (Buchan 1795:529). Colds, pleurisy, and rheumatism were indicated by the congestion of bodily fluids, including menstrual fluids. These diagnoses rest on the ancient theory of the humors: blood, black bile, yellow bile, and phlegm. In good health, all of the humors were in balance. In women, excess blood, a warm humor, accumulated through the month, causing them to be "out of order" until menstruation temporarily restored balance. "Females ought to be exceeding cautious of what they eat or drink at the time they are out of order. Everything that is cold . . . ought to be avoided" (529). The word *cold* simultaneously meant a humoral quality, environmental temperature, and the common cold and its sequelae. To "catch a cold" meant either to miss a menstrual period or to have a respiratory infection involving congestion of bodily fluids. Drinking cold water and the "sudden stoppage of customary or necessary evacuations, as the *menses*," (382) might also lead to dropsy, a less common diagnosis in amenorrhea, but one based on similar principles.

One diagnosis in amenorrhea might be an excess of one of the cold humors: black bile or yellow bile. Thus emetics, laxatives, cathartics, and diuretics were frequently employed to reduce these cold influences. Similarly, the warm humor might simply be obstructed or repressed (in English), or hidden or lost (in German), in which case administering a bleeding or the ingestion of red-tinted herbal liquids might signal the appropriate uterine response through both sympathetic magic and expulsive herbal constituents. These medicines were designed either to stimulate the uterus specifically or to tone the body generally. Footbaths, a euphemism for a vaginal douche, would also stimulate the uterus and imitate the appropriate pattern of fluidity. Obstructions, suppressions, and lost menses might be jogged loose by carriage rides, horseback riding, dancing, jumping rope, forcible pressure to the abdomen, and other exercise. These activities were considered therapeutic in rheumatism as well as in amenorrhea (Barton 1828: 106).

Closely related to these medical conditions was the treatment of intestinal parasites. The hard, bulging bellies of the worm-infested, the inflated abdomens of the hysteric, and the swollen bodies of the dropsical could look much the same. Since small animals might seem to rumble through one's innards, causing colic and hysteria, and since intestinal worms could cause similar internal sensations, the conditions must be related, according to contemporary thought. Even though amenorrhea was not involved in cases of worms, emmenagogic medicines were often administered. Here eighteenth-century medicine came close to erasing the distinction between emmenagogues and abortifacients. If foreign creatures might be expelled by emmenagogues in cases of worms, these medicines might also be understood to work to expel the fetus. The use of many plants both as vermicides and as emmenagogues also blurred distinctions between abortifacients and emmenagogues.

Emmenagogic medicines were not confined to amenorrhea, nor amenorrhea to emmenagogic treatments; but disease and therapy overlapped with dropsy, intestinal worms, colds, rheumatism, pleurisy, and other diseases. The expulsion of foreign or dangerous fluids, the destruction of little animals, and the reduction of abdominal swelling were goals in all these conditions. Women did not need to stress their amenorrhea when utilizing emmenagogic drugs or procedures, since amenorrhea might be only one among many pathological indications. An example of this logic comes from a description of the preparations of juniper, which were alleged to "increase all secretions, but may produce hemorrhagy and abortion, acting chiefly on the uterus. Pregnant women ought never to use them; but they are very useful in dropsical complaints, menstrual suppressions, also in rheumatism, gout, worms, &c." (Rafinesque 1828–30, 2:16). Both medical writers and the general public drew a line between the symptoms of pregnancy and of disease that is by no means clear today, while disease categories and treatments overlapped in a seemingly imprecise fashion that is at odds with twentieth-century nosology. The illogic is only retrospective, for women in the eighteenth century read their mental and physical signs to distinguish between sickness and pregnancy. If ill health was determined, then the opinions of others—friends, kin, pharmacists, doctors, midwives—might help sort through reported and visible symptoms to try to pinpoint the cause. Emmenagogic medicines were applicable in cases of congestion, swelling, infestation, and anxiety, but so were diuretics, cathartics, tonics, and other drugs.

From the beginning of European settlement, women, doctors, druggists, and the scientifically minded sought out native species of emmenagogic plants. Initially seeking the familiar, they discovered red cedar or Virginia juniper, *Juniperus virginiana* L., a relative of the common European emmenagogue and abortifacient savin, *Juniperus sabina* L., as well as native species of dittany (*Cunila mariana* rather than the European *Origanum dictamnus*), madder (*Michella repens,* European *Rubia tinctorum* L.), pennyroyal (*Hedeoma pulegioides,* European *Mentha pulegioides*), artemisia and smalledge (various varieties), and hellebore (*Veratrum viride,* European *Helleborus niger* or *Veratrum album*). Later, Old World plants were naturalized in the New World. These included rosemary, rue, the mints, and feverfew, among many other herbal species. European plants were imported in bulk by druggists and were advertised in local newspapers. Savin was among the most common of these imports.

Occasionally usage changed in crossing the Atlantic. Americans began using gum guaicum as an emmenagogue, just as Europeans were discarding the drug as ineffective in the treatment of syphilis (Stuart 1979:199). Ergot of rye, commonly used in Europe, does not appear in American pharmacopoeias until the nineteenth century and then only with dire warnings about its safety. German medical botany differed from English practice in employing mosses and ferns as emmenagogues (Wilmann Wells 1980:470–75; DeBenneville [1760–79?]).

Native American and African emmenagogues were added to European traditions. The use of squaw mint, *Hedeoma pulegioides,* squaw vine, *Michella repens,* squaw bush, *Vibirnum opulus,* squaw root, *Cimicifuga racemosa* or *Caulophyllum thalictroides,* and squaw weed, *Erigon philadelphicum,* can be traced to Native American medicine (Vogel 1970: 243–44; Tantaquidgeon 1942; Fenton 1941). The snakeroots—Seneca snakeroot, *Polygala senega,* black snakeroot, *Cimicifuga racemosa,* Virginia snakeroot, *Aristolochia serpentaria* and other species of Aristolochia, button snakeroot, *Eryngium aquaticum*—and the root of the cotton plant, *Gossypii radix,* reflect West African medical classifications and practice (Goodson 1990; Simon 1976:114; Oliver-Bever 1986:232; on snake symbolism in West African medical practice, Harley 1970). One African plant, *Aloes barbadensis,* was cultivated commercially in the Caribbean and imported to the mainland, becoming an important item in emmenagogic medicines (Oliver-Bever 1986:238; Stuart 1979: 149). *Aristolochia serpentaria,* Virginia snakeroot, was called birthwort after its close relative, the ancient emmenagogue and oxytocic *Aristolochia clematitis. Asarum europeum,* another Old World aristolochiacea, was likewise called birthwort, while its American counterpart, *Asarum canadense,* wild ginger, was unusual in having a reputation solely as a contraceptive both among Native Americans and among Germans (Stuart 1979:156, 159–60; Klepp 1994:86). Certain related plants, particularly aristolochia, polygala, and lilacea, had similar reputations among people originally from three continents.

Women ascribed emmenagogic properties to various other indigenous plant species and a few mineral substances, but patent and proprietary medical compounds began to supplant these simple remedies after the middle of the eighteenth century. These substances were either imported from London or made locally in accordance with published formulae. Newspapers, almanacs, lending libraries, women's recipe books, professional advice, and word of mouth provided access to these medications, which might be taken orally as liquids or pills, rectally as enemas, vaginally as douches, or topically as applications. One of the most frequently advertised emmenagogues was Hooper's Female Pills, which included aloes, iron sulfate, hellebore, and myrrh among other ingredients (Klepp 1994:84 n.23).

Opinions were divided on the efficacy of these drugs. By the early nineteenth century some doctors, particularly the followers of William Cullen and his theory of cardiovascular overstimulation as the basic cause of disease, were arguing that emmenagogues "are a set of medicines the most unfaithful and very frequently disappoint our expectations." In part, according to Robert Allen in his survey of the medical literature, this was because there "are no medicines in the materia medica which have a specific action on the uterus by which they produce catamenial evacuation." He advocated abolishing the whole classification of emmenagogues in order to concentrate on a whole-body, tonic approach to amenorrhea (Allen 1813:5, 12). But women, botanists, and professors of materia medica persisted in asserting the specific virtues of these and other drugs well into the nineteenth century (Carson 1867:82–84).

The records of the Philadelphia Dispensary, a charitable outpatient medical service, are a unique eighteenth-century source that allows an insight into the efficacy of contemporary medicine (Griffitts et al. 1793; Estes 1980:351). From December 1786 through November 1792, a committee tabulated the outcomes of patient treatment by disease (see table 2.1). They provided annual numbers of patients cured, deceased, or relieved (but not cured), as well as figures for those who were held over for additional treatment, dismissed for disorderly behavior, or sent to charitable institutions. Their tabulations lack data on age, sex, and detailed diagnoses and do not indicate the treatment supplied, but this record does permit a measure of success and failure.

The first section of the table shows the cure rates for amenorrhea and the diseases involving amenorrhea: chlorosis, or iron-deficiency anemia; haematemesis, the bloody vomiting associated with irregular

Table 2.1 Records of the Philadelphia Dispensary, 1786–92

	A*	B†	C‡	D§	E‖	F#	Total
Diseases Associated with Amenorrhea							
Amenorrhea	66	0	4	4	2	6	82
Chlorosis	1	0	0	0	0	0	1
Haematemesis	9	1	0	1	0	0	11
Hypochondria	14	0	10	2	0	0	26
Hysteria	174	0	59	1	0	12	246
	72.2%	0.3%	19.9%	2.2%	0.5%	4.9%	100.0%
Diseases Associated with Swelling and Congestion: Dropsy, Rheumatism, Worms							
	656	19	113	7	9	51	855
	76.7%	2.2%	13.2%	0.8%	1.1%	6.0%	100.0%
Other Gynecological Conditions: Parturition, Uterine, Breast							
	184	0	13	1	1	10	209
	88.0%	0.0%	6.2%	0.5%	0.5%	4.8%	100.0%
Venereal Diseases							
	644	6	26	35	13	87	811
	79.4%	0.8%	3.2%	4.3%	1.6%	10.7%	100.0%
All Diseases Treated by the Dispensary							
	7,915	439	614	151	77	521	9,717
	81.4%	4.5%	6.3%	1.6%	0.8%	5.4%	100.0%

SOURCE: Griffitts 1793.

* Cured.
† Dead.
‡ Relieved of symptoms.
§ Discharged, disorderly person.
‖ Remanded to the hospital or to the house of employment.
Remaining under care.

menses (it was thought that the blood had been diverted upward); hypochondria; and hysteria. In this grouping of women's diseases, 72 percent of cases were cured, but 1 in 5 patients was only relieved of her symptoms. These rates are lower than overall cure rate of 81 percent at the dispensary. The figures may reveal one reason that some physicians were so critical of emmenagogues. Hysteria and hypochondria, the diseases associated with strong emotional symptoms as well as with amenorrhea, proved particularly resistant to treatment; only 69 percent were cured. However, the cure rate for amenorrhea alone was 80 percent, close to the dispensary's average. The reason for these different treatment outcomes is unclear. It may indicate that emmenagogic drugs had some effect on amenorrhea but were unable to affect tangential emotional distress. Or, it may be that many of those complaining of amenorrhea were cured simply by the passage of time and their underlying good health, while the other patients were sicker.

Dropsy, rheumatism, and worms, all linked to amenorrhea by swollen abdomens and congested bodily fluids, were only slightly more likely to be cured through medical treatment than were other diseases associated with swelling or amenorrhea. Venereal diseases had cure rates nearing the dispensary's mean. The dispensary's record on other gynecological diseases and conditions is particularly impressive, with reported cure rates approaching 90 percent even in the face of the contemporary dangers in childbirth, puerperal fever, menorrhagia, and uterine dysfunction. The gap between the experiences of women with amenorrhea and those with other gynecological problems is large. Yet a reported success rate of even 72 percent in cases of amenorrhea and related diseases in the eighteenth century seems remarkable.

How did doctors treat these diseases? Another source from the same city offers some clues. The full billing records of partners Dr. Phineas Bond and Dr. Thomas Bond of Philadelphia give some indication of the course of treatment for women with amenorrhea. When called upon to treat Richard Edward's wife on 17 October 1753, the attending physician gave her pills for pain relief. He returned 4 days later to prescribe pain relievers and 4 emmenagogic pills. Ludowic Cosser's wife had a similar course of treatment, although the doctor added 4 "Hyst[eric] Pills" of unknown composition. Thomas Bottom's wife appears to have had an adverse reaction to these emmenagogic treatments. She was subsequently treated with cordials for strength, styptics to stop bleeding, and Tincture Martis, a salt of iron used in cases of anemia. During the fall of 1753, the doctor treated shopkeeper Robert Taigart's wife with a purgative and diuretic. Ten days later she was given a drug to induce vomiting; the following day a refrigerant powder, used to reduce fever; and five days later emmenagogic pills. In the spring of 1754, she was treated with liniments, mercuric pills, and styptics, probably indicative of syphilis, but she also received two doses of emmenagogic pills. In all these cases, treatment for hysteria or other illnesses preceded emmenagogic treatment. Amenorrhea was not treated as an isolated symptom.[3] A success rate of 75 percent was achieved in these cases, roughly the same as the dispensary record (Bond 1753, 1:385; 1754–55 2:9, 347, 358). Respectably married women with symptoms of emotional and physical distress accounted for the overwhelming majority of cases.

Not all patients were married women. Widow Robeson was given two rounds of emmenagogues in March and April 1752, as well as two mercuric pills (Bond 1752, 1:210). Because she traveled some 20 miles from her small-town residence to Philadelphia for treatment, she may have sought secrecy. In 1759 Mr. John Wallace's "Negro woman" received a liniment, a bleeding, a cathartic, and an illegible dosage. Since the law did not recognize marriages among enslaved men and women, she was probably not legally married. She received an emetic two days later. The following day a combination of emmenagogues and 20 pills for hysteria were prescribed (Bond 1759, 3:62). One wonders whether she requested this treatment or it was forced upon her. A servant's productivity would be reduced by pregnancy, and a pregnant slave could not be fired. Contemporary advertisements of slave sales frequently pointed out the inconvenience of pregnant enslaved women to the master's family. The dosage this unnamed woman received was unusually large, as was the cost of £7/9/6, nearly one-third of the average price of an adult slave.

Enslaved women could also seek out treatment. Slaveholders did not consider respectability a factor in the treatment of enslaved women and assumed abortive intentions rather than health problems requiring emmenagogues (Goodson 1987:5). In 1826 a New Jersey slave owner recorded that during the night, his slave Peg, then three months' pregnant, cried out that she "would die for ad[ministering a] dose of Copperine [?, perhaps copperas, vitriol, ferri sulphas] &c. [which] Jo had Provided for her to Produce abortion. It Came near killing her" (Vail 9–10 September 1826). Despite the laconic nature of the diary, some of the circumstances of Peg's case can be pieced together. Peg had had a child in April. It had died in early July, when she must have been four to six weeks' pregnant. It is possible that her second pregnancy had left her unable to nurse her firstborn, causing its death. Perhaps she resented the pregnancy, perhaps she was exhausted by two pregnancies within 11 months. Joe and Peg were described by their master as cooperatively "Working Exsperiments to Produce abortion," not to preserve her health, although their own intentions are unknown. Their experiments indicate that they had either no knowledge of or access to more usual drugs. The attempt to abort was fruitless and Peg bore a son on 11 April 1827. The candor of this description and the absence of any comment apart from the diarist's irritated notations of the disruptions to his family and the necessity of a doctor's visit exemplify our general knowledge about the institution of slavery: Masters judged slaves in terms of cost and convenience and ascribed the worst possible motivation to their actions. Slaves were usually considered incapable of morality or honor.

For the respectably married, health issues dominate even in cases that could not be construed as menstrual regulation. Elizabeth Coates Paschall wrote in her recipe book, intended for her daughter's use, that she once had a "Violent Chollick Pain in the Bowells" when she was "three months Gone with Child." After the failure of the doctor and the midwife to terminate the pregnancy, she employed an enema of chamomile (an emmenagogue), olive oil, brown sugar, and salt. Within an hour the "Child Came from me in the after Birth all togather & with verry Little pain." She soon after used a similar recipe to cure "a Could" accompanied by "a Most Racking" joint and bowel pain that was caused by "Standing two Long in the Shop without having my meals in Due time" (Paschall 1747–66:9). Society granted a great deal of latitude to respectable married women.

Doubts regarding the morality of menstrual regulation and the distinction between emmenagogic purposes and abortive ones arose when no illness was present and married women denied their pregnancies. Elizabeth Drinker worried about her recently married daughter, who at first did not admit to her pregnancy and who did not reduce her activities or change her diet as was expected. But even though the pregnancy was confirmed, Drinker administered emmenagogues to her daughter at 3 and 5 months' gestation. First treatments were given because of "great pain in her [daughter's] bowels" due to "taking colds," while the second instance involved hysteric symptoms. The medications contained several plant and mineral items with emmenagogic reputations as well as red dye, thus combining empiric remedies with sympathetic magic. Only after the sixth month of the pregnancy did Drinker stop medicating her daughter and assist in preparing baby linen. The pregnancy went full term, but the child was stillborn (Drinker [1746–1807] 1991, 2:873–74, 878, 897, 904–34).

When Landon Carter's daughter-in-law miscarried in Virginia in 1771, he had "suspected her being with child some months ago," but she did not admit to pregnancy. Her behavior before the miscarriage led Carter to think that "there must have been some intention to forward the abortio[n]." In 1774 Winifred Carter again miscarried. She said that "she had not felt the child these 2 months; a thing she had never spoak of to one soul." She subsequently told her father-in-law that when "she told me she was not with child, . . . that [this] was intended to discover the Child was dead within her." Her statements seem both unconvincing and self-serving, at least as recorded by her suspicious and unsympathetic father-in-law. The following day she remembered a fright she had received two months earlier, sufficient to cause fetal death according to contemporary medical belief. Carter, a curmudgeonly sort, was not convinced and remarked, "It is her own fault, a woman that hardly moves when not with child, always is Jolting in a Chariot when with Child. This is the 3d destroyed this way" (Carter 1965, 2:620, 859, 861). There was some anxiety or distaste expressed in these two cases of respectably married women who denied their pregnancies, but no lasting stigma attached to their actions.

English-language medical guides carefully distinguished between the acceptable use of emmenagogic medicines in illness or in parasitic infestations, and the dangerous consequences of emmenagogic use in pregnancy. This is an indication of a desire by doctors, jurists, and patients to maintain as separate categories practices that were in fact quite blurred in actual performance. In German-language guides, however, the efficacy of emmenagogic medicines was asserted both in cases of amenorrhea and in pregnancy. One German-language herbal included instructions for the use of these medicines when the fetus had died in utero; another included the same directions for use in expelling "live fruit" as well as dead (Wilmann Wells 1980:470–75). There were cultural variations in the acceptability of both emmenagogues and abortifacients in the New World, yet the German-speaking population also made a moral distinction between amenorrhea due to a "cold" or "fright," which needed medical intervention, and amenorrhea due to "disorderly neglect," where intervention was unacceptable (470). How "disorderly neglect" was defined is not known, but the word *disorder* commonly referred to the transgression of accepted social rules.

Anglo-American legal codes did not attempt to regulate pregnancy before quickening. After this milestone occurred, British law (which might apply in British territories) considered abortion a misdemeanor. Felony murder charges could be brought only when the abortion failed and a live-born child subsequently died of the drugs or battery. No colonial legislature bothered to address the issue of abortion in its codes. Yet a handful of suspected incidents of abortion did come before the courts during the prosecution of the crimes of infanticide, rape, fornication, adultery, assault, and slander (Brown 1996:433 n.38, 306–13, 204; Horle 1991, 2:610–12, 879, passim; Norton 1996:36–37, 265–68; Olasky 1992:20–25; Spruill [1938] 1972:325–26; Thompson 1986: 25–26, 58, 107–8, 182–83). In addition, there was one abortion by surgical instrument that led to the woman's death (Dayton 1991:23–29). Where a specific substance was named in these 15 cases encompassing suspicions or accusations of abortion, savin was the agent in 9. Of these cases, only 1 involved a married woman. She swore that she only took savin as a vermifuge, not knowing that it would produce the death of the fetus she still carried. One mention each was made of steel powder, wormwood and a combination of pennyroyal, horehound, nip, and marigolds. There was one case of surgical abortion that resulted in expulsion of the fetus, but also the woman's death from septicemia. Virtually all these attempted abortions were failures, although had they succeeded there might have been little public knowledge of the activities that brought the accused into court. It is clear from the surviving trial depositions that knowledge of the abortive reputations of emmenagogic drugs was widespread.

What brought these cases into court was not only the often gruesome details of the abortions or attempted abortions in the context of criminal behavior, but the transgression of important social boundaries. Cross-racial couplings appeared in two cases, while another concerned a Jewish doctor in a predominantly Protestant colony. Several of the accused had crossed lines of social rank, authority, and deference. Servant women, some of whom had previously come before the authorities and some of whom were involved in liaisons with their masters, were often singled out as culprits, while Anne Tayloe was a wealthy woman involved with a poorer man. It was particularly gendered transgressions that were pursued. The facts in at least six cases found that men had forced emmenagogues/abortifacients on unwilling women in order to hide evidence of sexual transgression. There was little public concern about male sexual predation. The anxiety focused instead on the presumption that men were not normally supposed to meddle in gynecology or obstetrics—this was women's business. Shame, dishonor, and unruly behavior offended community norms.[4] Yet despite the scandal, social anxiety, and revulsion caused by such cases, few convictions, particularly of men, resulted. Most attempts to prosecute occurred in the late seventeenth century. From the middle of the eighteenth century until the middle decades of the nineteenth, there was little public interest in the abortive use of emmenagogic medicines, no matter what the circumstances.

Two factors served to separate emmenagogues from abortifacients and morality from immorality during the eighteenth century: the physical and emotional symptoms of disease, and the respectability of the woman reporting the symptoms. And of these two factors, respectability was far more important. Where no obvious disease was present, or when hysteria, colds, or other disease appeared even when pregnancy was obvious, then respectability was often sufficient to categorize drug usage as emmenagogic and medically necessary. Where little or no respectability existed, as masters assumed about their slaves and servants or as some found when a man administered drugs against a woman's will, then there was a tendency to see only abortive intentions.

Words as basic as *health, sickness, pregnancy, amenorrhea,* and *abortion* had very different meanings in the past. *Health* in the eighteenth century could incorporate mental symptoms such as anxiety and fear, as well as purely physical symptoms. Illnesses were largely self-diagnosed, so that the reputation of the patient was crucial in assessing her claims. This criterion gave married women a great deal of latitude and servant women virtually none. *Amenorrhea* might be symptomatic of colds, rheumatism, dropsy, intestinal worms, or gout as well as of pregnancy, but not, apparently, of infertility. Emmenagogues were used even when amenorrhea was not present but where abdominal swelling or intestinal distress existed. *Pregnancy* need not begin with conception, but might be accepted only after quickening. *Abortion* could only occur outside of marriage. Certainty was a moral goal, but a medical and real-life impossibility. Consequently, ambiguity marked eighteenth-century American women's intentions in regulating their menses.

NOTES

I wish to thank George Alter, Janet Brodie, Elise Levin, Sangeetha Madhavan, Elisha Renne, Gigi Santow, and Etienne van de Walle for their sensitive readings of earlier drafts and their many helpful suggestions.

1. This failure to make the connection between amenorrhea and sterility may be caused in part by the fact that iron-deficiency anemia or low body weight/low body fat mentioned by several conference participants in their papers was rare in early America, at least among free adult women. The exhaustive study of New England medical practice by J. Worth Estes found that chlorosis, iron-deficiency anemia, was infrequent (Estes 1980:321, 337). The sterility that might be induced by syphilis or tuberculosis, which were then common diseases, was not necessarily ac-

companied by amenorrhea. However, it is true that iron filings, iron sulfate, and other preparations of iron were still common in emmenagogic medicines, particularly in proprietary medicines imported from England.

2. Thus when Mary Summerford was indicted for murdering her newborn in 1688 and she denied being pregnant, her friend testified in her defense that 3 months earlier, "shee Could not perceive any Appearance of her being with Childe by her having tried her breasts & found shee had not milke in them" (Horle 1991, 1:611).

3. The Drs. Bond did not leave case records, but their full accounting system allows the reconstruction of much of their therapeutic practice. The bill charged to Thomas Bottom in 1755, for example, reads as follows:

Aug. 9	To xx [20] Hyst[eric] Pills	5—[shillings/pence]
	To Sp[ir]t[us]. Sal [muriate of] Ammon[ia, a diuretic, tonic]	3/6
10	To Gutt[a, liquid drops]: Emmen[agogue]:	5/—
14	To Bol[us, a pill] anod[yne, painkiller]	2/6
	To Cord[ial] Julip [a cordial, tonic]	5—
19	To 4 Stypt[ic]: Powders [to stop bleeding]	4—
20	To Tinct[ure] Martis [a salt of iron]	5—

(Bond 1755, Vol. 2:347)

4. See also Brodie (1994:38) for a contraceptive example.

REFERENCES

Allen, Robert. 1813. *An Inaugural Dissertation on Emmenagogues and their Modus Operandi.* Baltimore: Dobbin and Murphy.

Barton, William B. 1828. *Outlines of Lectures on Materia Medica and Botany Delivered in Jefferson Medical College, Philadelphia.* Philadelphia: Auner.

Bond, Thomas, and Phineas Bond. 1751–68. Co-Partnership Ledgers. 6 vols. Manuscript, College of Physicians of Philadelphia.

Brodie, Janet Farrell. 1994. *Contraception and Abortion in Nineteenth-Century America.* Ithaca, N.Y.: Cornell University Press.

Brown, Kathleen M. 1996. *Good Wives, Nasty Wenches, and Anxious Patriarchs: Gender, Race, and Power in Colonial Virginia.* Chapel Hill: University of North Carolina.

Buchan, William. 1795. *Domestic Medicine: Or, a Treatise on the Prevention and Care of Diseases by Regimen and Simple Medicines . . . Adopted to the Diseases of the United States.* Rev. ed. by Samuel Powell Griffitts. Philadelphia: Dobson.

Carson, Joseph. 1867. *Synopsis of the Course of Lectures on Materia Medica and Pharmacy Delivered in the University of Pennsylvania.* Rev. ed. Philadelphia: Henry C. Lea.

Carter, Landon. 1965. *The Diary of Colonel Landon Carter of Sabine Hall, 1752–1778.* 2 vols., ed. Jack P. Green. Charlottesville: Virginia Historical Society, University Press of Virginia.

Dayton, Cornelia Hughes. 1991. "Taking the Trade: Abortion and Gender Relations in an Eighteenth-Century New England Village." *William and Mary Quarterly,* 3d ser., 48:19–49.

DeBenneville, George. [1760–79?]. "Medicina Pensylvania, or The Pensylvania Physician." Microfilm of manuscript. American Philosophical Society.

Drinker, Elizabeth. [1746–1807] 1991. *The Diary of Elizabeth Drinker.* Ed. Elaine Forman Crane et al. Boston: Northeastern University Press.

Estes, J. Worth. 1980. "Therapeutic Practice in Colonial New England." In *Medicine in Colonial Massachusetts, 1620–1820,* vol. 57 of the *Publications of the Colonial Society of Massachusetts.* Charlottesville: University Press of Virginia.

Fenton, William N. 1941. "Contacts between Iroquois Herbalism and Colonial Medicine." In Smithsonian Institution, *Annual Report of the Board of Regents.* Washington, D.C.: Government Printing Office.

Goodson, Martia Graham. [1987] 1990. "Medical-Botanical Contributions of African Slave Women to American Medicine." *Western Journal of Black Studies.* Reprinted in *Black Women in American History: From Colonial Times through the Nineteenth Century,* ed. Darlene Clark Hine. New York: Carlson Pub.

Griffitts, Samuel P., et al. 1793. "To the President and College of Physicians of Philadelphia [A return of the Diseases of the Patients of the Philadelphia Dispensary]." *Transactions of the College of Physicians of Philadelphia,* vol. 1, pt. 1. Philadelphia: Dobson.

Harley, George Way. 1970. *Native African Medicine: With Special Reference to Its Practice in the Mano Tribe of Liberia.* London: F. Cass.

Horle, Craig W., ed. 1991. *Records of the Courts of Sussex County, Delaware, 1677–1710.* 2 vols. Philadelphia: University of Pennsylvania Press.

Jennings, Samuel K. [1808] 1972. *The Married Lady's Companion; or, Poor Man's Friend.* New York: Arno.

Klepp, Susan E. 1994. "Lost, Hidden, Obstructed, and Repressed: Contraceptive and Abortive Technology in the Early Delaware Valley." In *Early American Technology: Making and Doing Things from the Colonial Era to 1850,* ed. Judith A. McGaw. Chapel Hill: University of North Carolina Press.

Norton, Mary Beth. 1996. *Founding Mothers and Fathers: Gendered Power and the Forming of American Society.* New York: Knopf.

Olasky, Marvin. 1992. *Abortion Rites: A Social History of Abortion in America.* Washington, D.C.: Renery Pub.

Oliver-Bever, Bep. 1986. *Medicinal Plants in Tropical West Africa.* Cambridge: Cambridge University Press.

Paschall, Elizabeth Coates. 1747–66. Receipt Book. Manuscript. College of Physicians of Philadelphia.

Rafinesque, C. S. 1828, 1830. *Medical Flora; or Manual of Medical Botany of the United States of North America.* 2 vols. Philadelphia: Atkinson and Alexander.

Rosenberg, Charles E. 1982. "Medical Text and Social Context: Explaining William Buchan's *Domestic Medicine.*" *Bulletin of the History of Medicine* 57:22–42.

Shryock, Richard Harrison. 1960. *Medicine and Society in America, 1660–1860.* New York: New York University Press.

Simon, William J. 1976. "A Luso-African Formulary of the Late Eighteenth Century." *Pharmacy in History* 18:103–14.

Spruill, Julia Cherry. [1938] 1972. *Women's Life and Work in the Southern Colonies.* New York: Norton.

Stuart, Malcolm. 1979. *The Encyclopedia of Herbs and Herbalism.* London: Orbis.

Tantaquidgeon, Gladys. 1942. *A Study of Delaware Indian Medicine and Folk Belief.* Harrisburg: Pennsylvania Historical and Museum Commission.

Thompson, Roger. 1986. *Sex in Middlesex: Popular Mores in a Massachusetts County, 1649–1699.* Amherst: University of Massachusetts Press.

Vail, Stephen. [1820s–40s?] Diaries. Computer printout of diary entries related to the enslaved woman 'Peg' provided by Dorothy Truman, research associate, Historic Speedwell, Morristown, New Jersey. The diaries are the property of Historic Speedwell and are used by permission. My thanks to former and current members of the staff for help in tracking this information.

Vogel, Virgil J. 1970. *American Indian Medicine.* Norman: University of Oklahoma Press.

Wilmann Wells, Christa M. 1980. "'A Small Herbal of Little Cost', 1762–1778: A Case Study of a Colonial Herbal as a Social and Cultural Document." Ph.D. diss., University of Pennsylvania.

CHAPTER 3

Menstrual Interventions in the Nineteenth-Century United States

Janet Farrell Brodie

In nineteenth-century America, menstruation carried deeply ambiguous meanings about fecundity. Because a menstruating woman was presumed to be fertile, promoting menstruation was a means of ensuring that a woman was ready to conceive. On the other hand, inducing menstruation might end a newly conceived pregnancy. Emmenagogues—to restore or promote suppressed menstruation—constituted an especially large category of women's medicine in nineteenth-century U.S. gynecology and obstetrics, just as they had long held a firm place in folk and sectarian medical thought. Doctors and the lay public alike assumed that remedies that would "overcome obstructions" to menstruation in a nonpregnant woman might, in larger doses, sweep away the "obstruction" of pregnancy. Emmenagogues held an established place in reputable medical practice and folklore; so too did abortifacients, for physicians needed remedies to procure miscarriages if a woman could not survive childbirth. Early medical and folk beliefs tended to distinguish between the two remedies. Abortifacients connoted the termination of recognized pregnancies; the functioning of emmenagogues remained more ambiguous, however, because many nineteenth-century Americans believed that fetal life did not begin until movement could be felt—until "quickening." Therefore, women who took actions to bring on menstruation before quickening did not necessarily view themselves as procuring abortion.

   A number of factors contributed to a refashioning of social attitudes toward emmenagogues and abortifacients: from the 1840s onward, the widespread movement of middle-class and working couples to restrict the size of their families via contraception and abortion; the growth of a commercial trade in fertility control information, devices, drugs, and services; and the emergence in the second half of the nineteenth century of a crusade to change popular beliefs about when fetal life began. The campaign against what came to be termed criminal abortion escalated after 1860. It was largely orchestrated by official physicians, then known as regulars, who sought tighter regulations and control over medicine as a profession. One result of this activism was the eventual displacement of abortifacients from the licit materia medica. Although an official distinction remained between the still-respectable emmenagogues and the increasingly disreputable abortifacients, over the course of the century the lines between the two categories of menstrual regulators grew increasingly blurred (Brodie 1994; Mohr 1978).

Historians and demographers have long studied the decline in marital fertility that occurred early in the United States when the number of children born to native-born, married white couples declined almost by half between 1800 and 1900 (Wells 1985). In 1800, white women whose marriages lasted through menopause bore an average of 7.04 children. By 1900, the average had declined 49 percent, to 3.56 children. More than half of the total decline—55 percent—occurred between 1840 and 1880. Much of that fertility reduction occurred because couples chose various strategies for limiting the total number of their children, including increasing the length of time between births, stopping childbearing at younger ages (before menopause), using a variety of contraceptive methods, procuring high rates of induced abortions, and, in some cases, practicing degrees of sexual abstinence (Brodie 1994; Gordon 1990; Reed 1984; Mohr 1978).

This chapter explores the ideas and practices concerning menstrual intervention, a particularly intriguing aspect of the important issue of how and when Americans came to practice reproductive control. Women who wanted to delay pregnancy or to prevent it altogether, as well as couples who sought some control over the timing and spacing of their children, had a great stake in the monthly arrival of the menses. Americans in the nineteenth century took active means to regularize menstruation. This chapter, then, explores some of the richly layered connotations surrounding menstruation in Victorian America.

MENSTRUATION IN NINETEENTH-CENTURY U.S. MEDICAL AND LAY PRACTICE

Nineteenth-century medical literature reflects the confusion among physicians regarding the causes, effects, and physiological properties of menstruation. In medical journals, physicians debated whether menstruation marked the period of ovulation, the relationship between menstruation and conception, what constituted healthy menses, and, above all, the dangers of obstructions to menstruation (Tauszky 1879b; J. Goodman 1875; Bullough and Voght 1973). In the 1840s, American physicians throughout the country discussed the influential arguments of French scientists Félix Pouchet (1842, 1847) and Adam Raciborski (1844). Pouchet and Raciborski maintained that menstruation marked a regular and predictable ovulation, a physiologically regular period during which an ovum or ova (they disagreed on the number) descended each month from the ovaries into the fallopian tubes and then into the uterus to be fertilized. Official and sectarian U.S. physicians debated the meanings of this new "ovular theory of menstruation" (Carpenter 1846; Henke 1874; Jackson 1876; Parvin 1877; Tauszky 1879a, 1879b). It profoundly affected, among other things, practices of fertility intervention, since the theory spawned a variety of advice regarding what a later generation would understand as the rhythm method of contraception.[1]

Official and unofficial medical men and women also debated the consequences of irregular and suppressed menstruation. There was considerable consensus that women would suffer grave threats to their health if they did not menstruate with great regularity. Some physicians believed—and their female patients apparently agreed—that a healthy and normal menstrual cycle recurred not only to the day, but to the hour, every month (Engelmann 1880; Oldham 1849; Parvin 1877). Physicians encouraged women to take their monthly periods very seriously: avoid strenuous exercise just before and during their menses, shun hot or spicy foods, abandon constrictive clothing, and forego any overexertion of mind or body. They also advocated resting, sipping herbal teas, and dosing with mild emmenagogic medicines around the time their patients' periods were due each month to assure prompt arrival. Much medical literature advised women to continue taking the same medicines and teas throughout the menstrual flow to lessen cramps and staunch excessive flow. An Ohio physician wrote in *The American Druggists' Circular and Chemical Gazette* in 1859 that women should take one teaspoon of the tincture of *Sanguinaria canadensis* 3 times a day for 2 weeks before their periods were due.[2] Yet the prominent water-cure physician, Joel Shew, scolded women in his 1853 text *Midwifery and the Diseases of Women* for taking drugs to bring on a tardy menstruation. He particularly chastised mothers who gave their daughters remedies such as oil of savin to prevent amenorrhea. Shew's objections, however, stemmed more from his dislike of drugs and his preference for hydropathic remedies rather than any disagreement with prevailing medical opinion about the seriousness of a delayed menstruation. The Lydia E. Pinkham Company, one of the best-known mail-order vendors of women's medicines, always sold a variety of emmenagogues. One advertisement recommended taking the company's most famous product, the "Vegetable Compound and Uterine Tonic," in cases of delayed menstruation until "the flow was well established" (L. Pinkham n.d.).

Although gynecologists now consider the suppression of menstruation for reasons other than pregnancy to be a clinical symptom of another disease or of various other diseases,[3] nineteenth-century American physicians believed it to be a discrete disease. Not only did physicians regard amenorrhea as a serious ailment, they believed it to be increasingly common among U.S. women. Edward Bliss Foote, a regularly trained physician as well as a prolific writer and entrepreneurial popularizer of midcentury domestic medicine, believed with many that "neglected menstrual derangements" could lead to infections of the brain, liver, heart, or stomach, as well as to apoplexy, hemorrhage, and consumption (Foote 1880:460). Self-taught "new school" botanical practitioner Alfred G. Hall, traveling through Upstate New York to Ohio and south to Washington, D.C., in the late 1840s and 1850s, hawked drugs (including emmenagogues and abortifacients), products (douches and douching syringes), and his advice book, *The Mother's Own Book and Practical Guide to Health . . . Designed for Females Only* (1843). Hall devoted several chapters in the book to menstrual problems, especially that of suppressed menses. Menstruation could be brought on, he advises, by hot footbaths; applying hot bricks to the navel to induce perspiration; and drinking teas made from tansy, rue, savin, pennyroyal, or thyme (Hall 1843:52–53; 1845, chap. 6). He warns women to take prompt action if their menses were late by so much as a day. Among the book's 60 "vegetable and domestic recipes with directions," Hall included several calling for savin, black cohosh, pennyroyal, rue, and tansy to induce suppressed menstruation (1845, chap. 22, "Recipes for Common Obstructions"). Notably, he makes the ambiguous comment that his "specific emmenagogue"—pulverized bloodroot steeped in gin—might prevent conception "by relaxing the uterus" (1843:54). Whether he intended to advise or to warn readers with this remark remains unclear.

Another example of the medical entrepreneurship surrounding menstruation in midcentury came from author and lecturer Frederick Hollick. In personal consultations; in his voluminous, cheaply priced advice books and pamphlets; and in his well-attended public lectures, Hollick provided considerable counsel on menstruation. He advised women to observe their menstrual rhythms carefully so that they could learn to identify ovulation and the beginning of what he believed was a monthly sterile period—a theory he promulgated widely. At his medical lectures "for married persons" in the 1850s, couples learned how to restrict family size using Hollick's version of the rhythm method; they learned about sexual anatomy from the life-sized papier-mâché manikins and colored charts he demonstrated from the stage; and women learned about menstruation, pregnancy, childbirth, sexuality, and birth control from his advice books that in cheap paperbound, stereotyped editions sold in the hundreds of thousands from the 1840s through the 1880s (Hollick 1860, chap. 3, p. 224; Brodie 1994: 112–17).

Physicians differed on the causes of the "obstructions" resulting in amenorrhea. Charles Meigs, a prominent nineteenth-century U.S. physician, believed that amenorrhea came primarily from a lack of blood circulation in the form of anemia ("no vigor in the blood"), from blockages to blood circulation, or from viscosity of the blood. In the chapter on emmenagogues in his popular text, *Woman: Her Diseases and Remedies, a Series of Letters to His Class* (1854:62), Meigs expresses doubt about the effectiveness of botanical products, but advocates the use of footbaths and leeches to bring on a tardy or obstructed menstruation.

A generation of women from the 1840s through the late nineteenth century obtained advice about menstrual regulation from "regular" physicians, but also from those categorized as "sectarians" or "irregulars," such as botanical doctors, Thomsonians, neo-Thomsonians, Eclectics, homeopaths, and water-cure practitioners. Itinerant, self-taught practitioners peddled products, books, and advice door to door in New England and the Mid-Atlantic states, and through the Mississippi and Ohio River valleys. In their heyday in the 1840s, for example, Thomsonians provided thousands of women with gynecological and obstetrical advice and products through agents, newspapers, paperbound literature, and conferences sponsored by "the botanic brotherhood" (Thomson 1832; Numbers 1977).[4] The medical regimen that Samuel Thomson invented (and tried to patent) in the 1830s, and whose popularity flourished in urban and frontier areas across the United States in the 1840s, depended on elaborate promotional and distributional networks of itinerant agents, newspapers, and "Thomsonian physicians." Thomson organized his followers—men and women—into Thomsonian societies pledged to his medical regimen. The products agents sold included douching syringes, douching substances, and emmenagogues. Between 1825 and 1845 more than 40 Thomsonian newspapers circulated throughout the United States, some extensively.

Along with the Thomsonians, water-cure practitioners reached large audiences. Thomsonians and hydropathists alike emphasized the importance of women reading and talking freely about menstruation, ovulation, conception, and pregnancy. These sectarians, even when not focused specifically on menstruation, taught their followers to plan ahead, to take daily, even hourly actions that prevented disease and fostered health. Sectarian emphases on action and optimism encouraged their followers to intervene actively to promote health. The Thomsonians in particular encouraged women to buy and read medical guides, become licensed Thomsonian practitioners, establish Thomsonian societies, act as agents to sell Thomsonian products and botanical drugs, attend lectures, and participate in national conventions.[5] Thomsonian Thomas Hersey's *The Midwife's Practical Directory* (1834, 1836), provided fold-out, tinted plates of women's internal organs and the stages of gestation and pregnancy, and provided much practical gynecological and obstetrical advice. Hersey warned women about the dangers of suppressed menstruation and advised his readers to take herbal teas and botanical drugs to stimulate delayed menses.

The degree to which women heeded such medical advice cannot be traced with certainty, but there can be no doubt that they paid attention to their menses. Some kept careful track of their monthly cycles. Mary Poor, an educated, relatively wealthy New England woman, kept a faithful record of her menstruation for 23 years, from her marriage in 1845 through menopause in 1868. In the small pocket-sized diaries she kept for 65 years of married life, she penciled a small "+" in the margin every 28 days except the months when she was pregnant or breast-feeding. She used her menstrual record to recognize as early as possible whether she might be pregnant.[6] Following the birth of her third child, whom for health reasons she did not breast-feed, neither Mary nor her husband, Henry, wanted another child soon. Their contraceptive methods worked well and for 29 months Mary dutifully recorded the very regular monthly arrival (almost to the day) of her menstruation. Then around 17 May 1851, she missed a month. She made no other references in diary or letters to her fears, but always alert to any delay in menstruation as an early sign of pregnancy, she scrawled in pencil on 17 June, "one month" and on 17 July, "two months." On 25 July she suffered a miscarriage. She did not leave any evidence about remedies or actions she may have taken to induce menstruation, although at other times she actively intervened to promote her health by following a water-cure regimen that included sitz baths, wearing wrapping sheets, douching, and following the dietary prescriptions of reformer and vegetarian Sylvester Graham (avoidance of alcohol, meat, and coffee). Later in her life, when she believed herself pregnant and feared that she would not survive another childbirth, Mary Poor noted in her diary that she had taken long walks and carriage rides over rough country roads. She wrote to her husband, however, that in her suspected condition she did not "dare to walk or ride" (Mary Pierce Poor to Henry Varnum Poor, August 1863). If she took herbal remedies having emmenagogic or abortifacient reputations, she did not confide it, even to her diary.

Mary Poor's diary entries yield further information about one mid-Victorian woman's attentiveness to her menstruation, both because she worried about her general health and because she wanted the earliest possible sign of pregnancy. From the 1860s onward, fearful about her health and satisfied with the number of children she and Henry already cared for, Mary Poor became obsessively attuned to any twinge of nausea, to any "biliousness" or faintness, or to even a day's delay in the anticipated arrival of menstruation. In the summer of 1862 she endured a 2-month pregnancy scare, which she described elliptically in letters to Henry from her vacation in Maine. After considerable anguish day to day, fearing she might be pregnant, she finally marked a firm "+" in her diary margin and added a meaningful postscript to her letter to Henry: "Events have proved my fears to be groundless" (Mary Pierce Poor to Henry Varnum Poor, 11 June 1862).

The idea of a sterile period sometime between the end of one menstruation and the beginning of the next percolated in U.S. culture from the 1840s through 1880s, giving women even more reason to keep precise records of their menstrual cycles. Advice differed from doctor to doctor, but no matter whose recommendations a woman ended up following, all heard that they had days every month when they were unlikely to become pregnant. Some advisors urged women to begin counting from the first day of menstruation, while others urged the last day; some said to wait 8 days, while others insisted on 14 or 16 from the first day of counting. Whatever the schedule, many women believed that they had a monthly "agenetic period."[7] Hydropathic physician Russell Thacher Trall, for example, advised women patients in the late 1860s to observe carefully their "menstrual habit" so as to recognize their personal infertile period (Trall 1867:206–7). In his best-selling 1869 tome, *The Physical Life of Woman*,[8] George H. Napheys expected women to have such exact understanding of their menstrual periods that he advised scheduling the marriage night "about the tenth day after menstruation" because "the first nuptial relations should be fruitless" (Napheys 1869:69–137). Amherst, Massachusetts, doyenne Mabel Loomis Todd kept track of her menstruation as a way to regulate sexual intercourse during what she believed to be her fertile period. She and her husband, David Todd, also relied upon coitus interruptus to prevent conception. Their preventive methods apparently worked, since Mabel had only one pregnancy—one she unhappily attributed to her experimentation with a variant of the ancient idea of avoiding conception by avoiding simultaneous orgasm. Whatever Todd and her long-time lover, Austin Dickinson (also a prominent Amherst citizen and brother of the reclusive poet Emily Dickinson), practiced as birth control also proved reliable, because she recorded no further pregnancies.[9]

Emmenagogues

Official, sectarian, and folk medicine in the nineteenth century attributed to a number of botanical products widely known and available in the United States the power to induce menstruation. The 1880 edition of *Index Medicus* (then called the *Index-Catalogue of the Library of the Surgeon-General's Office*) listed 17 botanical emmenagogues, including (in nineteenth-century taxonomy) ergot, *Polygonum* (buckwheat family), *Guaiacum* (caltrop family), *Anthemis* (camomile) and *Achillea millefolium* (yarrow, of the composite family), *Aconite* (crowfoot Family), *Digitalis* (figwort family), *Chenopodium odidum* (goosefoot family), quinine and madder root (madder family), *Gossypium herbaceum* (cotton root, of the mallow family), Apiol (parsley family), *Juniperus virginiana* (savin, of the pine family), "le ciposse usate" (cherries) and "Petioli cerasorum acid" (rose family), *Ruta graveolens* (rue, of the rue family), and *Polytrichum ricinus* (probably castor bean, of the spurge family).[10]

Many of the remedies associated in folk medicine with menstruation induction came from official materia medica categories of drugs to induce sweating and blood circulation. Within the logic of a medical system that attributed many diseases, including amenorrhea, to sluggishness of the blood or an obstruction to circulation, cures were to be found by inducing sweating, sitting over steam, taking hot baths, or breathing the vapors of emmenagogic herbs. By midcentury, domestic medical manuals put oral traditions and folklore into print. *The Cherokee Physician, or Indian Guide to Health* told women to drink tea of tansy, dittany, balm, rattle-root, pennyroyal, or some other "sweating tea" the day before they expected their periods and to continue the doses until menstruation actually arrived (Foreman 1845). The book also suggested that women sit over the steam of pine tops or cedar—an interesting variant, since pine products such as savin, cedar berries, juniper berries, and turpentine were long associated with abortion. Two New England physicians wrote in 1848 that "the best and most powerful medicines for the regulation of retained or obstructed menses may be found upon almost any farm in New England," recommending in particular 14 different kinds of herbal teas, including hot tea of wild gingerroot 3 times a day, or teas made of fennel seed, wintergreen leaves, pennyroyal mixed with black pepper, juniper berries, or "Seneca Snakeroot." Tea made from the tops and flowers of tansy they recommended "for *any* reason the flow is retarded." Their special remedy to bring on a delayed menstruation "in four out of every five cases" consisted of savin tea with one scruple of powdered savin added, to be taken 3 times a day (Capron and Slack [1848], cited in Meyer [1973]).

Abortifacients

Abortion-inducing remedies had their own accepted and respectable place in official and domestic American medicine up through the second half of the nineteenth century. In contrast with the modern medical opinion that it is difficult to self-induce abortion, nineteenth-century Americans believed that any woman could relatively easily induce an abortion early in pregnancy. Folkloric beliefs held that miscarriages were most likely to occur at the times when a woman would have been menstruating if she were not pregnant. This lore was repeated in official and popular medical literature well into the late decades of the century, as illustrated by an advertisement for Lydia E. Pinkham's Vegetable Compound and Uterine Tonic:

> Their generative functions are at this time [the days when, if not pregnant, a woman would have been menstruating] in a state of unstable equilibrium which very slight circumstances may disturb. The action of a cathartic or emmenagogue or anything which determines blood to the pelvis, may easily cause the insecurely attached ovum to be loosened and expelled (Pinkham Papers, advertisements).

Nineteenth-century Americans believed not only in the ease of procuring abortion, but that a wide variety of methods would, in the euphemism of the era, "produce the desired effect." Women did not weigh abortion options equally, preferring to try exercise and mild drugs before they turned to the harsher ecbolics and abortifacients, before using probing instruments, and before seeking out an abortionist. For centuries, women and men in preindustrial cultures of eastern and western Europe, and among the native tribes of North America, credited certain botanical products with the ability to induce miscarriage, particularly early in a pregnancy. The sub-rosa reputations of the botanicals had a longevity and power such that mid-Victorian women were likely to know both the respectable and the clandestine reputations of some dozen products whose names mean little to us today. In some isolated pockets of the United States, however, the connotations remained well into the twentieth century. For example, women in the Ozarks during the 1930s took care not to be seen ingesting certain "character sp'ilin'herbs" (Randolph 1947).

Women who drank tansy tea (or pennyroyal or rue) as a mild emmenagogue in the case of amenorrhea, and who took small quantities of the same remedy throughout menstruation as a relaxant, sometimes turned to stronger doses of these botanicals to induce abortion.[11] A physician noted a case in 1870 of a 28-year-old married woman, who, "accustomed to taking five-drop doses [of oil of tansy] without inconvenience" for her menstrual periods, took 15 to 20 drops, hoping to procure abortion. She went into severe convulsions, but, unlike many women who overdosed with toxic drugs, did not die. The physician did not report the impact of the drugs on the pregnancy (*Medical and Surgical Reporter* 1870:588).

By the second half of the nineteenth century, U.S. physicians regularly warned one another to beware of duplicitous female patients who pretended to want remedies for amenorrhea but actually wanted to rid themselves of an unwanted pregnancy. Gynecologist Charles Meigs wrote, "Many have been the occasions of my being consulted for catamenial obstruction with a design to entrap me into the administration of drugs that might remove the difficulty by procuring abortion" (Meigs 1852:155). Similarly, a Massachusetts physician wrote in 1870 that emmenagogues had caused more miscarriages than any other remedy. The U.S. public, according to Joseph G. Pinkham (unrelated to Lydia E. Pinkham of patent-medicine fame), regarded abortifacient drugs as harmless and effectual. He believed that women with unplanned pregnancies who would never have used an instrumental abortion or the services of an abortionist, had no qualms about taking emmenagogues whenever their periods were due in hopes of inducing miscarriage. Pinkham's article illustrates the problems facing the opponents of abortion in the second half of the century, for he published it in the prestigious *Journal of the Gynecological Society of Boston*—an organ of the regular medical establishment that opposed abortion; yet in spite of his opposition, Pinkham provides a prescription for an emmenagogue made of aloes, guaiacum, and ergot that he claims never failed to induce menstruation (Pinkham 1870).

Nineteenth-century American women turned to 3 categories of drugs from the reputable materia medica when they wanted to induce abortion. As noted earlier, they frequently turned to emmenagogues. They also tried purgatives, the largest category of remedies in official and folk medical arsenals; or they turned to a category of medicines known in official medicine as oxytocics: remedies to stimulate uterine contractions as a means of speeding labor, delivering the placenta, and staunching postpartum hemorrhage. In modern medical practice, oxytocic drugs are rarely used because of their dangers and unpredictability. The severe and sustained uterine contractions induced by these drugs can cause laceration of the cervix, rupture of the uterus, and fatal embolisms to the pregnant woman. The drugs' effects are not easily controlled, for oxytocics are not specific to the uterus and can affect other smooth muscles of the body, including the heart (Goodman 1970). In nineteenth-century practice, however, a number of botanical products received wide recognition and use as obstetrical aids in childbirth. Such products appear to have worked as abortives, especially in late pregnancy, although their dangers were manifold. Medical authority today holds that such drugs are generally less effective in early pregnancy because most oxytocics affect only a gravid uterus during the final trimester.

The most common substances used in nineteenth-century medicine as oxytocics to aid in childbirth and, less licitly, as abortifacients, are discussed more fully below.

Ergot

The best-known parturient and illicit abortive was ergot. Also known as *secale cornutum, pulvens parturiens,* "spurred rye," and the German *mutterkorn,* ergot comes from a poisonous parasitic fungus that grows on rye. First used in U.S. medicine in 1807 to expedite a woman's labor, officially trained and domestic physicians alike used it for a wide variety of gynecological and obstetrical purposes: to cure intrauterine polypi, staunch uterine hemorrhage, and check postpartum hemorrhaging via uterine contractions, employ as an agent to dry up the milk of lactating women, and, above all, cause uterine contractions in pregnancy, speed delivery, or induce abortion late in pregnancy.[12]

Nineteenth-century physicians did not always agree about ergot's abortifacient properties, but many reported that women believed it to be effective.[13] Gynecologist and author Augustus K. Gardner, an outspoken opponent of abortion and contraception, wrote in his "Essay on Ergot" in 1853, "Every physician knows that in conjunction with tansy, pennyroyal, and other herbs, 'spurred rye' enjoys a reputation along the common people and is frequently tried for the purposes of inducing abortion and yet among the thousands of cases where it is taken every year, how few can be found to be recorded" (Gardner 1853).

Cotton Root

After ergot, the botanical most commonly debated in U.S. gynecological and obstetrical medicine between the 1840s and the 1870s came from the root of the cotton plant, *Gossipium herbaceum*. Physicians reported that the seeds increased lactation in women, while a strong decoction of the roots would staunch hemorrhage. During the Civil War, some physicians substituted cotton root for the scarcer ergot. It quickly gained a reputation as a clandestine abortifacient.[14] In 1871, New York gynecologist Ely Van de Warker reported that the sale of cotton root had quadrupled in the preceding 5 years, particularly among "small miscellaneous country merchants" who sold it exclusively as an abortive preparation (Van de Warker 1871a:241). In 1876 John U. Lloyd, a respected pharmacist and collector of a noted library of folk medicine, investigated the reputed abortifacient properties of cotton root. He found preparations of the dried root unreliably effective, but decoctions of the fresh plant, he believed, would work as abortifacients if taken in large doses. Naively, Lloyd concluded that commercial preparations of cotton root were not likely to be effective abortives because their alcohol content would preclude women from drinking them in large enough quantities to cause abortion (Lloyd 1876).[15]

Blue and Black Cohosh

When physicians could not obtain ergot, they turned to other folk drugs having purported oxytocic powers—botanicals that also had reputations as abortifacients. These included Native American remedies such as black cohosh (*Cimicifuga racemosa* of the crowfoot family), known colloquially as squaw root or black snakeroot; blue cohosh (*Caulophylum thalictroides* of the barberry family), drunk by Indian women as a tea for up to 2 weeks before childbirth to lessen the duration of labor; and *Senecio* of the composite family, also known as ragwort and female regulator (Vogel 1970).[16] The herbs most commonly associated with menstrual intervention in the nineteenth-century United States, either as emmenagogues or abortives, held well-established places in American folk medicine. Some individual species had been associated with fertility regulation for centuries. Ten genera of composites had special associations with menstrual regulation in American folk medicine, including *Achillea millefolium* (common yarrow, milfoil), *Anthemis* (camomile), *Artemisia vulgaris* (common mugwort), *Senecio* (ragwort, life root), and *Tanacetum* (tansy).

In the 1870s Ely Van de Warker, one of the founders of the Syracuse, New York, Hospital for Women and Children and for 25 years its surgeon-in-chief, wrote a series on the commercial trade in abortion.

His investigation into "criminal abortion" focused on the chemical and botanical composition of the era's most popular abortifacient drugs, which Van de Warker subjected to chemical and laboratory tests. Although he opposed abortion and warned repeatedly of the dangers of abortive drugs, he explains how and why the drugs worked. Aloes, one of the most widely used drugs of the century for its effectiveness as a purgative, proved to be an effective abortive, Van de Warker explains, because women overdosed, taking aloetic pills 2 and 3 times a day for up to 2 weeks to bring on menstruation. He concludes, "I attribute then to aloes great power as an abortifacient, when used with a determination to accomplish a criminal object. . . . Notwithstanding the fact that the profession are disposed to regard aloes as comparatively innocent, still from the large use made popularly of female pills composed chiefly of aloes, I believe people give due credit to the drugs" (Van de Warker 1871b:353).

Van de Warker found that commercial abortifacients came in two varieties: pills, generally consisting of aloes, hellebore, powdered savin, ergot, iron, and solid extracts of tansy and rue; and fluid extracts, most commonly made of oil of savin, oil of tansy, or oil of rue dissolved in alcohol and improved in taste by the addition of wintergreen (Van de Warker 1873). Women, he explains, bought commercial abortifacients and washed them down with tansy tea or other teas recognized as emmenagogues. Tansy too worked as an abortive, according to Van de Warker: "women will mention case after case among their acquaintances whom tansy 'relieved.' I have no hesitation in ascribing to tansy abortifacient powers. . . . Tansy is a tradition among American women for its certainty as an abortifacient" (1871b:363). In addition to analyzing the contents, Van de Warker tested a number of the drugs to determine their physiological effects. He injected a dog with a lethal dose of oil of tansy and he personally tried small doses of cotton root, ergot, oil of tansy, and oil of savin. He found that they caused various symptoms, from drowsiness, increased salivation, and increased heart rate to delusions, convulsions, vomiting, loss of consciousness, and, in the case of the dog—death.

Effectiveness

It is difficult to assess the actual effectiveness of nineteenth-century menstrual regulators. The colloquial names associated with folk medicine often make it impossible to identify precisely any botanical product. Snakeroot was long associated with abortion, but consider even a few of the plants with that name: *Aristolochia serpentaria* (birthwort),

also known as virginia snakeroot; Asarum (wild ginger), known as
Canada snakeroot; and Liatris (blazing star), known as button-
snakeroot. *Cimefuga racemosa* (black cohosh) was known as black
snakeroot, while *Polygala senega* (Seneca snakeroot), the most famous
of the snakeroots, came from the milkwort family and had several
other folk names. Dozens of other snakeroots known in Native American and early American materia medica included the well-known *Tril-
lium erectum* of the lily family, also known as rattlesnake root, wake-
robin, and squaw-root—widely believed to be effective in stimulating
parturition.

The chemical effectiveness of any plant varies greatly, owing to many
factors. The active principles are affected by age, habitat, preparation
method, the constituent parts used, and time of use. For example, the
potency of toxic glucosides in the leaves of *Digitalis purpurea* varies according to the amount of sun and moisture the plant received while
growing. The toxicity of *Conium maculatum* (hemlock) is altered by age,
so that 1-ounce plant extracts killed laboratory rabbits in less than
1 hour, but 8 ounces had no effect at all 1 year later (Newman 1948).
Further complicating any assessment of these menstrual regulator is
the fact that many of the commercial preparations of the midnineteenth century contained several ingredients, since drugs exhibit internal pharmaceutical reactions in the presence of other chemical principles. In other words, the complex compounds within each plant
ingredient may be affected by the other compounds in a single remedy.

The final complication in assessing effectiveness of nineteenth-
century drugs revolves around fraud and adulteration. It is unlikely
that the patent medicines, including abortifacients, actually contained
in pure form all of the drugs the vendors claimed. Quinine, for example, had a reputation as an abortive, but it is improbable that all of the
medicines sold as "cinchona" or "quinine" were pure. Costly quinine
had to be imported, and it was relatively easy to fool a consumer by
supplementing or even exchanging the drug with any bitter bark or
cinnamon-colored bark plus a bitter-tasting additive. We have no way
of knowing—nor did the customers themselves—whether the quinine
preparations women believed they were ingesting to produce abortion
actually contained quinine at all.

Given the problems inherent in assessing effectiveness of the
nineteenth-century menstrual regulators, it is nevertheless clear from
the medical literature, even writings from physicians vehemently opposed to abortion, that the professional and lay public firmly believed
in the efficacy of many of the remedies. Charles Millspaugh, the late
nineteenth-century physician and folk-medical encyclopedist, wrote

of pennyroyal *(Hedeoma pulegioides)* that if taken as a hot infusion for amenorrhea, "it will often bring on the menses nicely, and, combined with a gill of brewer's yeast, it frequently acts well as an abortivant, should the intender be not too late with her prescription" (Millspaugh 1887:118). Ely Van de Warker, whose study of abortives has been discussed earlier, concluded his investigation by noting the extensiveness of the trade and the comparative rarity of fatal cases:

> I know many married women who have gone years without the birth of mature children, who resort habitually to some one of the many advertised nostrums with as much confidence of 'coming around' as if they repaired to the shop of the professional abortionist. (Van de Warker 1873:26)

The placebo effect, in which drugs with no known curative properties actually work in some cases, may help account for some of the beliefs in the efficacy of abortives and emmenagogues. Placebos are not well understood medically, but a woman who feared either pregnancy or the medical consequences of a delayed menstruation might have been sufficiently anxious every month to actually delay the menses. Simply by taking a medicine which she believed would induce menstruation may have relieved enough of her anxiety to start the menstrual flow. Thus pennyroyal tea and its ilk, while having no real chemical or medicinal properties as abortifacients, may have worked as emmenagogues because they were relaxants; they only seemed to work as abortives because the user was not pregnant in the first place. In addition, some abortifacients may have seemed to work when the actual explanation was a natural "spontaneous abortion," or miscarriage, for which there exist high estimates relative to full-term pregnancies.[17]

It is also likely that some of the remedies women took as emmenagogues and abortives did work, although the short- and long-term effects on health are incalculable. Scientists have identified scores of plant species containing antifertility substances—plants that inhibited fertility in laboratory animals (de Laszlo and Henshaw 1954; Swyer 1970; Jackson 1966; Segal 1974; Kreig 1964). Ingested botanicals containing estrogen or progesterone may have produced chemical interference at an early stage of pregnancy or hormonal imbalances that blocked fertilization of an ovum or the uterine implantation of an embryo. In addition, changes in a woman's progesterone balance can cause menstruation in spite of fertilization of an ovum. Naturally occurring folic acid antagonists can cause early abortions (Thiersch 1952). Some of the active principles in plants with folk medical reputations as abortives—*Podophyllum peltatum* and savin, for example—

contain proven antineoplastic agents, meaning they are capable of destroying tumors or new growths of abnormal human tissue and possibly, therefore, interfering with a newly conceived pregnancy.

COMMERCIAL TRADE IN EMMENAGOGUES AND ABORTIFACIENTS IN THE NINETEENTH-CENTURY UNITED STATES

By the second quarter of the nineteenth century, products purporting to affect menstruation flourished in ever greater quantity in an escalating commercial trade. Americans who wanted emmenagogic drugs to stimulate menstruation or abortives to end an unwanted pregnancy had access to scores of commercial pills, fluids, and extracts marketed innocuously as Woman's Friend, Female Regulator, Menstrual Regulator, and Periodical Drops. The Boston drug firm Goodwin and Company offered seven brands of "female pills" in 1874, along with Belcher's Female Cure, Hardy's Woman's Friend, The Samaritan's Gift for Females, and Lyons's Periodical Drops (Goodwin & Co. 1874). Although state and federal laws against advertising birth control information limited such ads, Chicago druggists in the mid-1880s still advertised Chichester's Pennyroyal Pills, Colchester's Pennyroyal and Tansy Pills, Cook's Cotton Root Compound, and Dr. Caton's Tansy Regulator (Fuller & Fuller Drug Co. 1885).

Entrepreneurs marketed the remedies as emmenagogues, but many labels carried blatant abortifacient instructions. The label on Graves Pills for Amenorrhea, for example, gave the following warning:

> These pills . . . [are] a never-failing remedy for producing the catamenial or monthly flow. Though perfectly harmless to the most delicate, yet ladies are earnestly requested not to mistake their condition (if pregnant) as *miscarriage would certainly ensue*. One dollar per box by mail. ("Criminal Abortion" 1858)

In the early 1860s, at their New York City Lying-In Institute, H. D. and Julia Grindle offered rooms for nursing and unwed mothers as well as provided abortions. They also sold H. D. Grindle's book, *The Female Sexual System; or The Ladies Medical Guide,* and, for two dollars a bottle, a remedy that

> when taken according to directions will remove all obstructions of the womb and bring on the menstrual periods, from whatever cause

produced. . . . [C]aution: If this medicine is taken during the early
months of pregnancy it will be sure to produce a miscarriage. However, if any should make a mistake and a miscarriage be the result, it
will not in the least injure their health. (Grindle 1864)[18]

Even when the abortifacient warnings were not present, the connotations were. In June 1870, *Day's Doings*—a "racy" New York newspaper
carrying sensationalist articles and theatrical and sporting news—advertised 7 medicines, using language some women had long associated
with abortion, including "Madame Van Buskirk's Regulating Medicine," "Dr. Richau's Female Remedy," and "Dr. Harrison's Female Antidote . . . certain to have the desired effect in twenty-four hours without
any injurious results" (*Day's Doings* 1870).

Peddlers, druggists, itinerant physicians, traveling vendors of patent
nostrums, and scores of mail-order sources offered such preparations
widely across the United States from the 1840s through 1880s, advertising them extensively in circulars, flyers, and newspapers. Anyone inter-
ested in ergot preparations, for example, could readily obtain pills,
fluid extracts, and powders in varying strengths and at varying costs.
A Detroit druggist in 1880 even advertised a "pocket mill for powder-
ing ergot" available wholesale or retail. Domestic health advice literature included ergot in prescriptions for the well-stocked family medical cabinet, as did Luther M. Gilbert's *The Home Physician* ("for people
far from doctors"), which in 1883 listed fluid extract of ergot among
the 37 medicines every family should possess in quantities of at least
1 ounce (Gilbert 1883).

Customers for menstrual drugs also could obtain them from druggists in towns and villages throughout the East, Middle Atlantic, and
Midwest, from peddlers and "jobbers" who hawked goods, and by mail
order. Downing's Drug Store in Hanover, New Hampshire, bought
from jobbers and wholesale drug companies more than 3,000 dollars'
worth of drugs in 1883 alone, including numerous ergot preparations,
"Woman's Friend," bottles of "Pierce's Douche," tannic acid troches, and
"toilet vinegars" (useful for contraceptive douching) (Downing's Drug
Store 1883–84). In the 1860s, "Chapman's Old Established Drug House"
in New York offered its goods by mail, including abortifacient pills,
condoms, female syringes (for douching), and an advice tract called
A Confidential Circular for the Married (Chapman 1860). In the midnineteenth century, then, even farmers and rural villagers throughout the
Midwest, and Middle-Atlantic, and New England clearly found themselves bound up in thriving U.S. commercial markets. They did not lack
access to even such intimate medical information and products as em-

menagogues and abortifacients. Wherever freethinkers or botanical practitioners traveled, rural men and women could obtain books, gynecological and obstetrical supplies, and drugs. They could buy products by mail too. In the late 1840s, farmers and villagers in the Sugar Creek, Illinois, area could pick up packets of mail delivered by mail stage to the postmaster every day except Sunday (Faragher 1986:177; Brown 1989). The extraordinary financial success of the mail-order "medicinal herb industry" of the Shaker religious sect largely rested on its business in dried herbs, including herbal emmenagogues such as pennyroyal, rue, blue cohosh, black cohosh, and cotton root bark (Andrews 1933; *The American Druggists' Circular and Chemical Gazette Advertising Pages* 1880).

Advertisements for emmenagogues and abortives peppered health reform newspapers, but they were also sold by druggists and apothecaries, doctors and peddlers in towns and cities across the nation. Urban newspapers from the 1830s through the 1860s routinely carried advertisements for sexual, gynecological, and other medical products including abortion drugs, cures for venereal disease, and aphrodisiacs, and even for surgical abortions. Respectable health journals carried emmenagogue ads, but so did the more common genre of "medical newspapers," which were actually vehicles to promote an entrepreneur's products. Harmon Knox Root's *The Medical Advertiser,* in the early 1850s, included medical advice on scores of "female complaints" and offered drawings of male and female anatomy, but principally advertised Root's vegetable medicines, his book *The People's Medical Lighthouse,* and condoms. Frederick Hollick's *People's Medical Journal and Home Doctor,* published between July 1853 and December 1854, functioned as a similar advertising vehicle. Druggists inserted ads for abortion drugs and procedures into almanacs and cookbooks distributed free to customers.[19]

🖎

Over the course of the nineteenth century, American women and men turned to a growing repertoire of methods for fertility intervention. They wanted control over pregnancy, and they sought such control by intervening with the regularity and duration of menstruation. If they did not yet have twentieth-century concepts of "family planning" or expectations of 100-percent effective birth control, couples and individuals nevertheless sought some method for spacing pregnancies at desired intervals and/or restricting the total number of children born to them. Of course, infertility too caused anguish, and affected couples also sought methods to promote menstruation. Menstrual regulation held promise for both fertility promotion and control. As this chapter has argued, however, the medical discourse over such interventions, and the emergence of an entrepreneurial, commercial trade in fertility-intervening drugs, advice literature, and services, complicated earlier cultural understandings and deepened the ambiguous nature of the principal categories of drugs affecting menstruation—emmenagogues and abortifacients.

NOTES

1. For the influence of Pouchet on American gynecology, see Smith (1858), chap. 3 "Ovulation." Brodie (1994:79–86) analyzes the medical debate about a monthly infertile period.

2. An example of this belief can be seen in druggists' advertisements. See, for example, The Luyties Homeopathic Pharmacy Company's (n.d.) recommendations on a package of amenorrhea tablets. The company advised women to take 3 tablets every 2 hours for 3 days before the period was due and to continue taking the pills through the menstrual flow. The pills consisted of savin and ergotin.

3. Novak (1970) notes that a woman not menstruating by age 18 was diagnosed as having primary amenorrhea; women who had menstruated but who had ceased for the equivalent of 3 to 4 menstrual cycles for reasons other than pregnancy had secondary amenorrhea, which could be caused by any number of diseases involving the cervix, ovaries, or uterus.

4. For discussions of the size, geographical spread, and class appeal of Thomsonians, see Rothstein 1972:125–51; Kett 1987:106–107; and Morantz-Sanchez 1984:346–58.

5. *The Independent Botanic Register* contains scattered information about Thomsonian physicians, drugstores, peddler/agents, conventions, and various types of publications.

6. In addition to the menstrual record, Mary Poor kept a record of the times she and her husband had sexual intercourse. Brodie (1994:10–13) analyzes the diary records. Evidence of women keeping menstrual records can be found in Tauszky (1879b:307–11).

7. The terms *agenesis* or *agenetic period* were in common usage in mid-nineteenth-century medicine. See, for example, "Agenesis in France," from the *British Medical Journal*, cited without author in the *Medical and Surgical Reporter* (Philadelphia) (1867:177).

8. Napheys's book went through at least 19 editions between 1869 and 1889, many of them stereotyped, which meant a printing in the tens of thousands.

9. Mabel Loomis Todd kept her menstrual record in part to calculate some variant of the rhythm method. See Gay (1984:258).

10. *Index Medicus* also recognized nonbotanical emmenagogues, including external applications of electricity, leeches, or mustard plasters to the breast, or products such as chloroform, iodine, or phosphorus.

11. Millspaugh (1887) discusses the uses of botanicals for abortion, including tansy (86) and savin (166–73); Mulheron (1874:385–91) cites a case of a woman taking oil of tansy to procure abortion.

12. John Stearns (1807:308) provided the first official U.S. medical recognition of the obstetrical properties of ergot. Druggists' catalogues illustrate the variety and quantity of ergot pills, powders, oils, extracts, and other compounds available in the last third of the nineteenth century. Boston druggist Charles C. Goodwin, for example, sold Richard's Extract of Rye for 1 dollar a bottle in 1874, and 13 varieties of ergotine and ergot products in 1885.

13. Van de Warker (1871a:236) notes that ergot was the principal drug women used for abortion. He believed it worked as an abortifacient only occasionally in early pregnancy. See "Does Ergot Tend to Produce Abortion?" (1877:422).

14. Porcher (1849:677) notes that decoctions of the plant had emmenagogic properties, with specific action on the uterine organs. See also Seeds (1875:211–13), who criticized its effectiveness. Eckler (1920) reviews efforts to identify the chemically active constituents. William Henry Wetherly (1861) doubted its abortifacient but not its emmenagogic properties.

15. Weiner (1972) lists cotton root as one of 8 abortifacient botanicals used by Native Americans and cites laboratory studies in which it caused ergotlike uterine contractions in animals.

16. Millspaugh (1887) lists *Cimicifuga racemosa* as an oxytocic and abortifacient, noting that it caused abortion by rapid dilation of the cervix and uterine contractions (no. 11). He notes that Indians used *Senecio* for general uterine problems and specifically as an antihemorrhagic, abortifacient, and wound healer (no. 91). Cheney (1900) lists 3 abortifacients: bark of cotton plant, rue, and spurred rye. As parturients Cheney cites cotton, ergot, and blue cohosh.

17. Simpson and Carson (1993:287) estimate that 10 to 15 percent of recognized pregnancies are lost in the first trimester, and many more "are lost before they are even recognized clinically." Their chapter examines recent studies of fetal wastage during various stages of gestation.

18. A copy of the advertising notice can be found pasted in the back of the copy of Grindle (1864) in the Rare Book Room at the Harvard Medical School Library.

19. John Todd (1867) complained about this practice.

REFERENCES

The American Druggists' Circular and Chemical Gazette. 1857–65. New York.
Andrews, Edward D. 1933. *The Community Industries of the Shakers*. New York State Museum Handbook no. 15.

Anthony, Milton. 1838. "On Menstruation." *Southern Medical and Surgical Journal* 2:135–56.

The Boston Medical and Surgical Journal. 1839.

Brodie, Janet Farrell. 1994. *Contraception and Abortion in Nineteenth-Century America.* Ithaca, N.Y.: Cornell University Press.

Brown, Richard D. 1989. *Knowledge Is Power: The Diffusion of Information in Early America, 1700–1865.* New York: Oxford University Press.

Buchan, William. 1820. *Domestic Medicine.* London: W. Lewis, p. 329.

Bullough, Vera, and Martha Voght. 1973. "Women, Menstruation and Nineteenth-Century Medicine." *Bulletin of the History of Medicine* 47: 66–82.

Capron, George, and David Slack. 1848. *New England Popular Medicine.* N.p. In *American Folk Medicine,* by Clarence Meyer. New York: Thomas Y. Crowell Company, 1973.

Carpenter, W. M. 1846. "Remarks on the Periodical Maturation and Discharge of Ova in Man and Other Mammiferae and the Practical Bearings of This Theory." *The New Orleans Medical and Surgical Journal* 2: 563–72.

Chapman, Thomas C. 1860. *Chapman's Old Established Drug House.* N.p.

Cheney, G. S. Co. 1900. *Druggists Handbook of Medicinal Roots, Barks, Herbs, and Flowers.* Boston: n.p.

"Criminal Abortion." 1858. *The American Druggists' Circular and Chemical Gazette* 2:139.

Day's Doings. 1870. June. New York: "Published at 535 Pearl Street."

"Does Ergot Tend to Produce Abortion?" 1877. *Medical and Surgical Reporter* 36:422.

Downing's Drug Store. 1883–84. Records. Bills for Goods to L. B. Downing. Baker Library Special Collections. Harvard Business School.

Drinker, Cecil K. 1937. *Not So Long Ago: A Chronicle of Medicine and Doctors in Colonial Philadelphia.* New York: Oxford University Press.

Eckler, Charles E. 1920. "Contribution to the Pharmacology of Cotton Root Bark." *Lilly Scientific Bulletin* July, ser. 1, no. 10 (July).

Engelmann, George J. 1880. "Time of Conception and Duration of Pregnancy." *St. Louis Courier of Medicine and Collateral Sciences* 3:441.

Faragher, John Mack. 1986. *Sugar Creek: Life on the Illinois Prairie.* New Haven, Conn.: Yale University Press.

Foote, Edward Bliss. 1880. *Plain Home Talk About the Human System and Habits of Men and Women.* New York: Murray Hill Publishing Company.

Foreman, Richard. 1845. *The Cherokee Physician, or Indian Guide to Health.* Chattanooga, Tenn.: James W. Mahoney newspaper office.

Fuller & Fuller Drug Co. 1885. *Trade Catalogue.* Chicago.

Gardner, Augustus K. 1853. "Essay on Ergot." *New York Medicine,* n.s., 11.

Gay, Peter. 1984. *The Bourgeois Experience, Victoria to Freud.* Vol. 1, *Education of the Senses.* New York: Oxford University Press.

Gilbert, Luther M. 1883. *The Home Physician.* New York: G. P. Putnam's Sons.

Goodman, J. 1875. "Menstruation and the Law of Monthly Periodicity." *Richmond and Louisville Medical Journal* 20:553–67.

Goodman, Louis S., and Alfred Gilman. 1970. "Drugs Affecting Uterine Motility." Section 9 in *The Pharmacological Basis of Therapeutics.* 4th ed. New York: The Macmillan Company.

George C. Goodwin & Co. 1874, 1885. *Catalogue of Patent Medicines, Druggists' Sundries, Perfumery, Toilet Articles, & Etc..* Boston: Horace Partridge & Co., Printers.

Gordon, Linda. 1990. *Woman's Body, Woman's Right: A Social History of Birth Control in America.* New York: Penguin.

Grindle, H. D. 1864. *The Female Sexual System.* New York: n.p.

Hall, Alfred G. 1845. *Womanhood: Causes of Its Premature Decline, Respectfully Illustrated . . .* 2d ed. Rochester, N.Y.: E. Shepard.

———. 1843. *The Mother's Own Book and Practical Guide to Health . . . Designed For Females Only.* Rochester, N.Y.: n.p.

Henke, Emil. 1874. "Ovulation and Menstruation." *Medical and Surgical Reporter* 30:305–308.

Hersey, Thomas. 1834. *The Midwife's Practical Directory: or, Woman's Confidential Friend; Comprising Extensive Remarks on the Various Casualties and Forms of Disease.* Columbus, Ohio: Clapp, Gillett & Co.

———. 1836. *The Midwife's Practical Directory . . .* 2d ed. Baltimore: self-published.

Hollick, Frederick. 1849. *The Matron's Manual of Midwifery . . .* 47th ed. New York: T. W. Strong.

———. [1852?] 1860. *The Marriage Guide, or Natural History of Generation . . .* 200th ed. New York: T. W. Strong.

———. 1853–54. *The People's Medical Journal and Home Doctor.* New York: T. W. Strong.

The Independent Botanic Register. 1834–35. Columbus, Ohio: Thomas Hersey, editor and publisher.

Index-Catalogue of the Library of the Surgeon-General's Office. 1880–1961. Ser. 5. Washington, D.C.: Government Printing Office. Entries under "Abortifacients," and "Amenorrhea." [Later titled *Index Medicus.*]

Jackson, A. Reeves. 1876. "The Ovulation Theory of Menstruation: Will It Stand?" *Transactions of the Illinois State Medical Society,* pp. 128–61.

Jackson, Harold. 1966. *Antifertility Compounds in the Male and Female: Development, Actions, and Applications of Chemicals Affecting the Reproductive Processes of Animals, Insects, and Man.* Springfield, Ill.: Charles C. Thomas, Publisher.

Kett, Joseph K. 1987. *The Formation of the American Medical Profession: The Role of Institutions, 1780–1860.* New Haven, Conn.: Yale University Press.

Kreig, Margaret B. 1964. *Green Medicine: The Search for Plants That Heal.* Chicago: Rand McNally & Company.

Laszlo, Henry de, and Paul S. Henshaw. 1954. "Plant Materials Used by Primitive Peoples to Affect Fertility." *Science* 119:626–30.

Lloyd, John U. 1876. "Cotton-Root Bark." *Proceedings of the American Pharmaceutical Association* 24:518–26.

The Luyties Homeopathic Pharmacy Company. n.d. *A Practical Treatise & Repertory on the Treatment of Disease by Homeopathic Remedies.* St. Louis.

Meigs, Charles D. 1852. *Obstetrics: The Science and the Art.* 2d ed. rev. Philadelphia: Blanchard and Lea.

———. 1854. *Woman: Her Diseases and Remedies.* 3d ed. Philadelphia: Lea and Blanchard.

Meyer, Clarence. 1973. *American Folk Medicine.* New York: Thomas Y. Crowell Company.

Millspaugh, Charles F. 1887. *Medicinal Plants.* New York and Philadelphia: Boericke & Tofel.

Mohr, James C. 1978. *Abortion in America: The Origins and Evolution of National Policy, 1800–1900.* New York: Oxford University Press.

Morantz-Sanchez, Regina. 1984. "Making Women Modern: Middle-Class Women and Health Reform in Nineteenth-Century America." In *Women and Health in America,* ed. Judith Walzer Leavitt, 346–58. Madison: University of Wisconsin Press.

Mulheron, S. J. 1874. "Foeticide." *The Peninsular Journal of Medicine* 10: 385–91.

Napheys, George H. 1869. *The Physical Life of Woman.* Philadelphia: George Maclean.

Newman, Leslie F. 1948. "Some Notes on the Pharmacology and Therapeutic Value of Folk Medicines, I." *Folk-Lore* 59:118–35.

Novak, Edmund R. 1970. *Novak's Textbook of Gynecology.* 8th ed. Baltimore: The Williams & Wilkins Company.

Numbers, Ronald L. 1977. "Do-It-Yourself the Sectarian Way." In *Medicine Without Doctors: Home Health Care in American History,* ed. Guenter B. Risse et al. New York: Science History Publications.

Oldham, Henry. 1849. "Clinical Lecture on the Induction of Abortion in a Case of Contracted Vagina From Cicatrization," *London Medical Gazette* ser. 54:45–52.

Parvin, Theophilus. 1877. "A Brief Study of One Hundred Cases of Menstruation." *The American Practitioner* (Louisville, Ky.) 16:65–69.

Pinkham, Joseph G. 1870. "The Very Frequent and Inexcusable Destruction of Foetal Life in Its Earliest Stages by Medical Men in Honorable Standing." *Journal of the Gynecological Society of Boston* 3:374–77.

Pinkham, Lydia E. n.d. Papers. Vol. 379, Advertisements. The Schlesinger Library, Radcliffe College.

Poor, Mary Pierce. 1842–1880s. The Poor Family Papers. The Schlesinger Library, Radcliffe College.

Porcher, Francis P. 1849. "Report on the Indigenous Medical Plants of South Carolina." *Transactions of the American Medical Association* 2:677.

Pouchet, Félix. 1842. *Théorie positive de la fécondation des mammifères.* Paris: Librairie encyclopédique de Roret.

———. 1847. *Théorie positive de l'ovulation spontanée et de la fécondation des mammifères.* Paris: J.-B. Baillière.

Raciborski, Adam. 1844. *De la puberté et de l'âge critique chez la femme.* Paris: J.-B. Baillière.

Randolph, Vance. 1947. *Ozark Superstitions.* New York: Columbia University Press.

Reed, James W. 1984. *The Birth Control Movement and American Society: From Private Vice to Public Virtue.* Princeton, N.J.: Princeton University Press.

Root, Harmon Knox. 1854. *The People's Medical Lighthouse . . .* New York: Published by Adolphus Ranney; Cincinnati: H. M. Rulison.

Rothstein, William G. 1972. *American Physicians in the Nineteenth Century: From Sects to Science.* Baltimore: Johns Hopkins University Press.

Seeds, O. H. 1875. "The Therapeutic Use and Abuse of *Gossypium herbaceum.*" *Transactions of the Texas Medical Association* 7:211–13.

Segal, Sheldon. 1974. "The Physiology of Human Reproduction." *Scientific American* (August):53–62.

Shew, Joel. 1853. *Midwifery and the Diseases of Women.* New York: Fowlers & Wells, Publishers.

Simpson, Joe Leigh, and Sandra Carson. 1993. "Biological Causes of Foetal Loss." In *Biomedical and Demographic Determinants of Reproduction,* ed. Ronald Gray, Henri Leridon, and Alfred Spira. Oxford: Clarendon Press.

Smith, William Tyler. 1858. *The Modern Practice of Midwifery, a Course of Lectures on Obstetrics.* New York: Robert M. DeWitt.

Stearns, John. 1807. "Account of the Pulvis Purturiens, a Remedy for Quickening Childbirth." *New York Medical Repository* 2:308.

Swyer, G. I. M. 1970. "The Scientific Basis of Contraception." *Population Studies Supplement* (May):44–47.

Tauszky, Rudolph. 1879a. "Ovulation and Other Theories of Menstruation." *The Physician and Pharmacist and Bulletin of the Medico-Legal Society* 12:8–24.

———. 1879b. "The Anomalies of Menstruation." *The Physician and Pharmacist* 12:307–11.

Thiersch, John B. 1952. "Therapeutic Abortion with a Folic Acid Antagonist." *American Journal of Obstetrics and Gynecology* 63:1298–1304.

Thomson, Samuel. [1822?] 1832. *New Guide to Health; or Botanic Family Physician.* 3d ed. Boston: n.p.

Todd, John. 1867. *Serpents in the Dove's Nest.* Boston: Lee and Shepard.

Trall, Russell Thacher. 1867. *Sexual Physiology.* 5th ed. New York: Miller, Wood & Co.; London: J. Burns.

Van de Warker, Ely. 1871a. "Detection of Criminal Abortion, Part II." *The Journal of the Gynecological Society of Boston* 5 (October):229–45.

———. 1871b. "The Detection of Criminal Abortion, Part III." *The Journal of the Gynecological Society of Boston* 5 (December):350–70.

———. 1873. "The Criminal Use of Proprietary or Advertised Nostrums." *New York Medical Journal* 17:23–35.

Vogel, Virgil. 1970. *American Indian Medicine.* Norman: University of Oklahoma Press.

Weiner, Michael A. 1972. *Earth Medicine—Earth Food: Plant Remedies, Drugs, and Natural Foods of the North American Indians.* New York: The MacMillan Co.

Wells, Robert V. 1985. *Uncle Sam's Family: Issues in and Perspectives on American Demographic History.* Albany: State University of New York Press.

Wetherly, William Henry. 1861. "Oleum gossypii (Cotton-Seed Oil)." American Druggists' Circular, June. N.p.

CHAPTER 4

Emmenagogues and Abortifacients in the Twentieth Century: An Issue of Ambiguity

Gigi Santow

16 January 1924, Surrey: Mr. L. E. to Marie
Stopes: . . . I am a working man with 5 children
the oldest 10 to the youngest 16 months. my wife
is three weeks over her time she is worrying
herself so that she as made herself quite ill she as
been taking difference kinds of pills people have
told her about but of no use.

—Ruth Hall, *Dear Dr. Stopes*

Like so many other aspects of the human experience, reproductive behavior, medical knowledge and practice, and popular attitudes toward reproduction, reproductive physiology, contraception, and abortion changed more during the twentieth century than any previous one. The course of this reproductive revolution is exemplified by shifts throughout the century in the ways that professionals and lay people viewed menstruation and its disorders, and in the ways that growing desires for control over childbearing were met. These shifts, and the ambiguities they reveal, are the subject of this chapter.

The movement of information, people, and drugs makes it extremely difficult to construct distinct national histories of the use of emmenagogues and abortifacients during the twentieth century. My edition of *The People's Home Medical Book,* for example, written by T. J. Ritter, M.D., "formerly" of the University of Michigan, is a reprint of the 1910 edition that was published simultaneously in Toronto, Sydney, and Cape Town in 1928 and bought in a second-hand shop in an Australian country town in 1972. Similarly, take the case of Thomas Neill Cream, who received his medical training in Montreal, gave strychnine to women who were seeking abortion in Canada and the United States, and was finally executed for murder in 1892 when he repeated such behavior in England (McLaren 1994). Patent medicines were similarly unconfined by national borders, with emmenagogues produced in the United States, for example, being sold early in the century in Australia (Royal Commission into Secret Drugs, Cures and Foods 1907: 23–24). I have therefore chosen to address the English-speaking world as a whole, with occasional forays onto the Continent.

As with geography, so too with time frame. Despite my focus on the twentieth century, it has proved necessary to delve briefly into the nineteenth, to trace continuity with past beliefs and practices and identify modern shifts in behavior. In addition, not only did popular writing tend to lag behind the professional literature, especially in the early decades of the century; but some source material published after 1900 consists of later editions of earlier works.

REGULATING THE MENSES

Medical Knowledge and Professional Texts

Although "[i]n the maze of eighteenth century medical theorization, gynaecology as a specialty did not exist" and "the causes of menstruation remained baffling and unexplainable" (Ricci 1943:540), the nineteenth century, especially toward its end, was characterized by remarkable progress (Ricci 1945). Embryology made great advances and physiology some; the speculum, the uterine sound, and the curette gained more acceptance; anesthetization first with ether in 1846, and later with chloroform, made surgery a matter more of routine than heroics; and the midcentury introduction, thanks to Semmelweis and Lister, of antiseptic procedures made it a matter more of life than of death. Thereafter, operative successes "slowly guided the profession into surgical channels, and were largely responsible for the new specialty—gynaecology" (46).

Nevertheless, this triumphal progress was neither uniform nor unimpeded. New discoveries came slowly, as did their acceptance. Although the interdependence of ovulation and menstruation was established in 1840, no attempt was made to correlate data on these events until 1863. Not until 1896 did an experiment showing that the ovaries governed menstruation remove the nervous system from consideration and lead to the idea that the ovaries acted by means of a secretion carried in the blood (Ricci 1945:525–29). Moreover, with many older theories of menstruation and ovulation having been revived in the first half of the nineteenth century and proving remarkably persistent, the closing decades of the century were a time of great diversity of opinion and of treatment, with surgery's "meteoric rise" being paralleled by "non-surgical innovations and crazes in gynaecological therapy" (47).

This variety of gynecological theories and practices is reflected in the writings of 3 near-contemporaneous American gynecologists. The first, Henry Garrigues (1900), an "outstanding gynaecologist of his time" (Ricci 1945:250), despite considerable prowess as a modern surgeon was a follower of the old, medical approach toward menstruation, exemplified in such works as Marc Colombat de l'Isère's *Diseases of Women,* which was translated by the eminent Philadelphian Charles Meigs in 1845 (Ricci 1945; Castiglioni 1941:726). Garrigues distinguishes between suppression of the menses, "the condition in which the flow after having begun is suddenly arrested" (1900:255), and amenorrhea proper, "the condition in which the menstrual flow fails to appear, although the patient has reached the proper age and feels as if she would be relieved by its coming, or where it does not reappear at the usual period in persons who have already menstruated" (256). Garrigues reserves the use of emmenagogues for the treatment of this latter condition, which may be caused by overwork, insufficient food, or change of climate and habits, or associated with debilitating disease (anemia, phthisis, malaria, typhoid, diabetes), poisoning, narcotic addiction, insanity, or obesity. Having cautioned that no treatment is required for an otherwise healthy girl whose initial menstrual periods are irregular, and that if the cause is anemia, then that is what should be treated, Garrigues lists treatments unspecific to the underlying cause. Aloes is the aperient "most credited with emmenagogue power" (257). Quinine and arsenic may be used in the case of malaria. Bromides, antipyrin, or phenacetin are useful in the case of nervous upset. Baths and injections as in the case of suppressed menstruation may also be helpful. It is daunting to learn that Garrigues also recommends electricity as "a powerful remedy," specifically "bipolar intra-uterine faradization, with secondary current, or, best of all, galvanism, with the negative pole in the uterus" (257).[1]

Yet at the same time that Garrigues was looking back to midcentury works such as Colombat's, some of his younger colleagues were resolutely looking ahead. In particular, they placed far less emphasis on the importance of regular menstruation. Edward Montgomery (1900), for example, one of a new group of U.S. gynecologists who came to prominence at the end of the century (Ricci 1945:39), merely observes in his own textbook that although most women menstruate every 28 days, intervals may vary from 21 days to 5 or 6 weeks, and the precise timing cannot be predicted for an individual woman. Moreover, in noting popular euphemisms for menstruation, Montgomery appears to relegate respect for it to the past. Somewhat later, William Graves lists many of the causes of amenorrhea that had been identified by Garrigues, concluding with "functional amenorrhea," under which he classes "such cases of temporary cessation of the menses or delayed menarche as are not related to any definite pathologic condition" (Graves 1918:572). The causes are "sudden psychic emotion, especially that of fear or anger . . . chilling of the body from cold baths, exposure to the weather, wet feet, etc.," or "change of climate or occupation, as seen commonly among domestics" (573). Graves, therefore, has more to say on this subject than Montgomery, but considerably less than Garrigues. Like Montgomery, but unlike Garrigues, Graves does not recommend treatment.

Biology, biochemistry, and endocrinology made major advances during the 1920s and 1930s (Siegler 1944). The most significant for the demystification of the phenomena of menstruation was the independent discovery by Ogino and Knaus that ovulation does not coincide with menstruation but occurs approximately 2 weeks before the next episode of bleeding (Ross and Piotrow 1974). Apart from placing the practice of the rhythm method on firmer scientific ground, this finding had the effect of drawing medical attention toward ovulation, and away from menstruation, as a critical determinant of the capacity to conceive. Once the hormonal determinants of ovulation were understood, the development of hormonal means of suppressing ovulation was only a matter of time. The oral contraceptive pill, which created painless, less copious, regular bleeds mimicking menstruation, was released in the early 1960s (see Potter, this volume) and did irreparable damage to the dignity of menstruation. Thus, for example, the most recent edition of Hatcher et al.'s (1998) *Contraceptive Technology,* for 30 years the bible of contraceptive providers in the United States, does not even comment on menstrual irregularity. Investigation is recommended in the case of amenorrhea—defined, among women who have ever menstruated, as at least 3 months of missed periods in previously regular women, and 6 to 12 months of no menses in women who previously had irregular cycles—because it may reflect underlying pathology.

Popular Texts

A bestseller when it was first published in London in 1856, *Enquire Within Upon Everything* reached its 43rd edition in 1871 ("four hundred

and ninety thousand copies have been published"), its 78th in 1888
("one million and thirty-nine thousand copies"), its 115th in 1925
("completing one and a half million copies"), and its 126th in 1976,
when it claimed, as it was doing by 1925, to be "the most famous book
of domestic reference in the world" (Bremner 1988:vi). Treatment for
"scanty menstruation" was already being recommended in the first edition:

> In strong patients, cupping the loins, exercise in the open air, the feet
> in warm water before the expected period, the pills No. 45;[2] in weak
> subjects, No. 46. Gentle and regular exercise. Avoid hot rooms, and
> too much sleep. (1856:153)

By 1871 it is additionally recommended that strong patients take ergot
of rye (1871:105), although by 1888 the book advises that ergot
"should only be taken under medical advice and sanction" (1888:117).
Moreover, the text after "sleep" in the preceding extract continues in
this edition as follows:

> In cases of this description it is desirable to apply to a medical man
> for advice. It may be useful to many to point out that pennyroyal tea
> is a simple and useful medicine for inducing the desired result. (1888:
> 114).

Emmenagogues first rate an entry somewhere between 1871 and
1888, being described as "medicines which exercise a direct action on
the uterus or womb, provoking the natural periodical secretion, such
as castor, asafoetida, galbanum, iron, mercury, aloes, hellebore, savine,
ergot of rye, juniper, and pennyroyal" (1888:142). An identical entry
appears in 1925, although the entry on scanty menstruation differs
slightly from that of 1888 in referring neither to cupping, which presumably had gone out of fashion, nor to pennyroyal tea.

Greater differences exist between the editions of 1871 and 1888, with
the inclusion of an entry on emmenagogues and the recommendations
to seek medical advice, than between those of 1888 and 1925, a period
twice as long. Nevertheless, over the latter period there were major
changes in the seriousness with which menstrual disturbances were
viewed and the rigor with which they were treated, and considerable
diversity of opinion and treatment existed side by side.

In her *Discourses to Women on Medical Subjects,* Mrs. Longshore-Potts,
M.D. (1896) distinguishes between voluntary and involuntary suppressed menstruation. The former occurs when women take action to
prevent a menstrual period that "would have been an obstacle to some
enjoyment, some proposed visit, party, wedding, or other engage-

ment" (77) by drinking vinegar or alum water; eating a lemon, cinnamon, nutmegs, or cloves; or—shades of the older medical texts—placing their feet in cold water for up to half an hour, "any of which
improprieties may jeopardize life, or at least ruin the health and make
life miserable." Involuntary suppression comes from wearing wet un-
derwear, walking through streams, sitting in cold water, "sitting upon
damp grass, or spending the day in a school-room in damp garments"
(78). The primary remedy involves warmth, whether applied in warm
footbaths or by sitting over warm water; but frequent draughts of hot
pennyroyal tea, tea of motherwort, or hot milk are also helpful. If these
remedies fail, Mrs. Longshore-Potts advises that "more radical treatment" (unspecified) should be followed, since suppression of the menses will lead to serious illness.

Contemporaneous with this work is the *Ladies' Guide* of J. H. Kellogg
(1895), physician and surgeon, Seventh-Day Adventist and vegetarian,
author of works on the injurious effects of corsets (Ricci 1945:546,
550), and pioneer of the development of dry breakfast cereals. Unlike
Longshore-Potts (1896), Kellogg stresses repeatedly (for example, Kellogg 1895:57, 512, 515) that failure to menstruate at the expected time
is not a cause but a symptom of disease. When amenorrhea exists because of weakness or anemia, attention should be given to improving
the sufferer's general health by nutritious food; daily exercise in the
open air; massage; "the local application of electricity by a competent
person" (515), à la Garrigues; warm baths; and so on. Kellogg warns,
however, that "it will be of no advantage to restore the function while
the cause remains, since its suspension is simply a means adopted by
nature for economizing her resources; and to force her to perform a
function for which she is unprepared, will be the means of injury."
Moreover, he warns against the use of emmenagogues:

> There is quite a long list of these remedies, none of which, however,
> are [sic] reliable. Those which are the most efficient as stimulants of
> the uterus are so poisonous and potent for evil that much more harm
> than good is likely to come from their use, and hence none of them
> are to be recommended. If used at all, they can do good only when
> discreetly used by an experienced physician. (Ibid.)

Emmenagogues are not even mentioned in Richards and Richards's
(1912) *Ladies Handbook of Home Treatment,* which was simultaneously
published, like Kellogg's book, in London, Cape Town, and Lucknow.
The Edinburgh-trained authors declare that the "doctors of the old
school depended almost entirely upon the administration of drugs in
the treatment of disease; but the modern practitioner regards drugging

with growing disfavour" (Richards and Richards 1912:412) and, instead, advocate "water treatments and other rational remedies" (413). Their descriptions of suppression and absence of menstruation are strongly reminiscent of Kellogg's, although briefer. For the patient who does not respond to a regime of enemas, douches, baths, exercise, and improved diet they recommend that medical assistance should be sought to detect the underlying cause.

The advice given by authors of other popular medical works was sometimes not so disinterested. A particularly unsubtle example is provided by Law and Law (1906), who, pronouncing that "under all circumstances amenorrhea is a very serious condition, and if neglected will lead to detrimental or fatal results" (174), recommend their system of Viavi Hygiene in order to "restore the normal physiologic balance, and to equalize waste and repair" (177). No constituents are listed, but a complex regimen of treatment is proposed for "suppression (amenorrhoea)," including nightly use of Viavi capsules, daily application of the Viavi "cerate," and the Viavi laxative (178–79, 490–93). The authors warn that "menstruation may not be restored for some time after beginning the Viavi treatment, but the sufferer may be assured . . . that important benefits are being secured" (179)—at least by the Viavi Company.

Another such self-promoter is R. V. Pierce, whose *Common Sense Medical Adviser* allegedly sold 3,188,000 copies by the time of its 99th edition in 1926. Pierce declares that retention and suppression of the menses can result from morbid conditions of the blood, especially among "robust, plethoric females" (Pierce 1926:717) who may be accustomed to "luxurious living" and predisposed to "abnormal activity of the alimentary functions." The prescribed treatment is vigorous exercise; a reduced, light diet; Dr. Pierce's Pellets; and Dr. Pierce's Favorite Prescription. When retention and suppression result from anemia, Pierce advises nutritious diet, increased activity (including "amusing exercises, walking, swinging, riding, games of croquet, traveling, singing" [729]), cleanliness, hard beds, useful employment, and Dr. Pierce's Favorite Prescription, which is proclaimed, perhaps with strictures such as Kellogg's in mind, "not a strong emmenagogue" (719).[3] When there are symptoms of returning menses, "their visitation may be encouraged by the use of hot foot and sitz-baths, and frequent doses of Dr. Pierce's Compound Extract of Smart-Weed" (720). When acute suppression results from strong emotions, violent excitement, or sudden exposure to cold, Pierce encourages the use of a hot footbath, warm sitz bath, Dr. Pierce's Extract of Smart-Weed, and, should this treatment not be productive, Dr. Pierce's Favorite Prescription.

A concern with disorders of the blood in general and of menstruation in particular, and a desire to bestow on sufferers the benefits of one's own patent remedies, were not restricted to North American medical practitioners. Narodetzki's *La Médecine Végétale Illustrée* [1935?] clearly represents the survival of a considerably older work, not simply because this edition claims to be the 132nd, but because of the author's disquiet over the slightest indication of menstrual disturbance. Variations in the duration of the flow, the regularity of its commencement, and the quantity and color of blood—details left unmentioned by his more fastidious trans-Atlantic confrères, although of interest to his European ones at least since the 1840s (Ricci 1945:528)—should all be treated with as much seriousness as if menstruation had never appeared at all, because they could stem from a serious cause (Narodetzki [1935?]: 469–70). Narodetzki runs through the now-familiar list of causes and recommends treatment with various patented compounds that should be taken before ("Vitalgine Stam") and after ("Elixir Spark") each meal. In a section on plants and medicines, he singles out rue and savin as warranting particular care because a very weak dose of the former, a potentially lethal poison, is an "energetic" emmenagogue, and because the latter has a strong effect on the uterus and can cause abortion. Similarly, Dr. Dehaut (1910), in the 28th edition of his *Manuel,* declares that whereas women's health depends on the regularity of their menses, his own purgatives are generally sufficient so that "the following month, everything will be in order" (724). Yet, far from recommending other emmenagogues, he cautions against their use: rue and savin can be dangerous; and while ergot is a powerful and useful drug, especially in difficult confinements, its use should be directed by a doctor or midwife. More trenchantly, Galtier-Boissière (1924) designates plants such as absinthe, armoise, cerfeuil, rosemary, rue, savin and saffron not as emmenagogues, but very dangerous abortifacients (441).

In contrast with these works, the tone of T. J. Ritter's *The People's Home Medical Book* of 1928 is refreshingly matter-of-fact. Ritter's aim was to facilitate the home nursing of various ills while providing a clear guide to cases in which a physician should be consulted. In addition, "in treating of the diseases of women" (Ritter 1928:i), he acknowledges a particular debt to the work of C. B. Penrose, a leading light (with Montgomery and others) of Philadelphia gynecology at the turn of the century (Ricci 1945). Although Ritter advocates that treatment of amenorrhea be dictated by its cause and lists the familiar remedies, he maintains that most cases "demand general toning treatment" (Ritter 1928:364). He advises that girls be kept out of school when they are menstruating, and avoid study ("Good health is of even more importance than a book education" [1928:365]), avoid catching cold, and refuse invitations to dances. The proper treatment is bed rest, hot footbaths or sitz baths, and hot drinks made from hops, tansy, pennyroyal, ginger, or motherwort, taken until they cause sweating.

A profound departure from previous advice manuals is apparent in *The Marriage Book* (1935?), which instructs not only on cooking, home decoration, sewing, and knitting, but also on basic reproductive physiology and the sexual adjustment of newlyweds. In a section on how to answer the "awkward questions of children"—surely not a topic that would have warranted attention a generation earlier—parents are given factual, model answers to questions about puberty.

The normalcy of menstruation is stressed in a section on questions from daughters. Thus:

> To speak of the need for care of health, or any restrictions on normal life, at the same time as one is trying to show that menstruation is something connected with growing up and health, will make needless difficulty. . . . Nothing should be said that will cause a girl to regard menstruation as an illness. (*The Marriage Book* [1935?]:243)

Nevertheless, older views and practices did not disappear all at once, so the old and the new sometimes coexist confusingly in the one manual. Thus, for example, Robinson (1943) advocates the use of electricity in medicine not just in uncontroversial applications, such as to remove metallic foreign bodies from the eye, but also in the treatment of diverse ailments including "difficult and painful menstruation" (249). Yet elsewhere he provides accurate information on the physiology of menstruation and the causes of amenorrhea, and declares the following:

> Although a woman who is menstruating commonly refers to herself as "unwell," this is not to be taken literally, as formerly it very often was. Menstruation is a physiological process and calls for no great change in ordinary habits. (465)

All catamenial drama has been lost by the time we come to Derek Llewellyn-Jones's *Everywoman: A Gynaecological Guide for Life*, a present-day descendant of works such as Kellogg's *Ladies' Guide* of 1895. First published in 1971, *Everywoman* remains in print, has been frequently revised, and at its sixth edition in 1993 ("completely updated edition with new material") had allegedly sold more than two million copies. Llewellyn-Jones ascribes "less frequent periods" primarily to "the effect of the emotions, which in turn alter the sequence of hormonal release" (1978:325); his failure to comment on the deleterious effects of the sorts of debilitating diseases listed by earlier authors testifies to the epidemiological transition through which we have passed since their time. Amenorrhea may occur "if a girl leaves home to take up a job in a different environment, or if she is under great emotional stress," with examples being provided of amenorrhea after the death of a loved one, and during wartime internment. Additional predisposing factors cited in the 1993 edition are excessive exercise or strict dieting. Medical help should be sought if a woman has less frequent periods over an interval of 6 months, or is completely amenorrheic. But "infrequent periods are generally of no concern and what a woman needs is to be reassured that she is normal. . . . Treatment using hormones is not indicated" (1978:325). Similarly, "provided the amenorrhoea is not due to disease (and usually it is not), and provided the woman does not want to become pregnant, there is no indication for giving hormones to produce a menstrual bleed" (ibid).

The disappearance of anxiety over irregular menstruation is highlighted in Bremner's (1988) encyclopedic tribute to the old *Enquire Within*. Noting that cycle lengths vary both among and within women, Bremner explains that "[w]e aren't machines. Our body reacts to every aspect of our lives. . . . When deeply upset, for example, periods may suddenly stop for a while, or become very heavy. In fact, doctors are only just realizing just how much emotions affect a woman's rhythm" (1988:576). She is wrong in this regard, of course, because if there is one point on which all our authors agree, it is in the influence of the emotions. Bremner takes the rest of the entry on menstruation to dispel myths about periods, some of which echo the recommendations of earlier writers (that one should not engage in active sports or swim, for example); discuss period pain; and provide an account of the newly defined pathologies of premenstrual tension and premenstrual syndrome.

Today, respectful mention of emmenagogues is confined to the world of alternative, herbal, holistic, or New Age medicine. According to one such author, "most uterine tonics are also emmenagogues. There are even emmenagogues that work by stimulation that verges on irritation, which can be of benefit in some cases, but is also the action of herbal abortifacients" (Hoffmann 1997:99). He cites as the most useful emmenagogues blue cohosh, false unicorn root, life root, motherwort, parsley, pennyroyal, rue, southernwood, squaw vine, and yarrow. As herbs to avoid during pregnancy, Hoffman lists autumn crocus (colchicum), barberry, goldenseal, juniper, male fern, mandrake, pennyroyal, poke root, rue, sage, southernwood, tansy, thuja, and wormwood (102), using their familiar names. In a pleasing conjunc-

tion of ancient and modern, he describes how women can tone up
their systems after going off the Pill, and accelerate the process of re-
gaining their "natural harmonic functions," by using herbal remedies
"that act as endocrine balancers and uterine tonics" (101). The mixture
he recommends contains derivatives of four plants, two of which
(black cohosh and motherwort) are reputed emmenagogues.

THE RISE OF ABORTION

The rise of abortion toward the end of the nineteenth century was by
no means confined to Australia, but the situation in that country is
particularly well documented because of a number of Royal Commis-
sions that examined the causes of the decline in the birthrate and the
means by which this might have been achieved. The first volume of
the first Royal Commission's report was tabled in the New South Wales
Legislative Assembly in 1904.[4] One of the original commission's
tasks—"to examine into the trade in secret nostrums, in proprietary
child-foods, and in secret preparations for the prevention of conception, and for the destruction of the human embryo"—proved to be
impossible to execute within the given time frame, so Octavius Beale, a
member of the original commission, was commissioned a second time.

Beale's 1907 report, *Royal Commission into Secret Drugs, Cures and
Foods* (hereafter *Secret Drugs and Cures*) is an idiosyncratic mélange of
opinion and observation. Among the former are his general abhor-
rence of birth control and specific disapproval of Annie Besant, Mal-
thus, and Mill. Among the latter are detailed and authoritative accounts of proprietary drugs:

> No attempt will be made to give a comprehensive statement of the
> means adopted to induce miscarriage. The unnatural practice is as-
> sisted by the free sale of drugs, often at exorbitant prices, under pro-
> prietary names. These are openly advertised in Anglo-Saxon coun-
> tries, which differ therein from one another only in degree, the names
> and descriptions of the drugs being well understood by dealers and
> users. Windows of drug stores exhibit an assortment of these danger-
> ous compounds, the packages usually, but not always, bearing names
> of real or fictitious makers. "Steel and Pennyroyal Pills," "Tansy
> Packet," "Amenorrhoea Mixture," "Ladies' Regularity Pills Nos. I, II,
> and III—ordinary, strong, and extra strong, warranted effectual,"
> "Apiol Pills, better than Pennyroyal," in much variety . . . the pregnant

woman who . . . seeks the destruction of her unborn child, first tries some or several reputedly abortifacient drugs. A method much resorted to is to combine the administration of simple or compound poisons with the use of local violence. (*Secret Drugs and Cures* 1907:14)

Beale then lists "some reputed abortifacients," drawing information from a number of English and American textbooks; he also describes "lead-poisoning to procure miscarriage," a "newly-noted practice which has already attained a vogue in certain districts of Great Britain" (16). Although pennyroyal seemed to be the most common abortifacient, Beale pronounces it ineffective as an infusion and poisonous as an oil. Oil of tansy, popular in the United States, is likewise deemed poisonous. Beale is convinced that "Reliable Female Regulating Pills" (23) containing tansy, pennyroyal, and cotton root, manufactured by the New York and London Drug Co., were actually an abortifacient advertised as an emmenagogue, he suspects, to "dodge 'the law.'" Later commentators also interpret the herbal and chemical remedies mentioned in *Secret Drugs and Cures* as abortifacient in intent if not in effect, although many were strong purgatives and some were fatally poisonous (Siedlecky and Wyndham 1990:69).

The prevalence of abortion in Australia, and the pharmacist's referring role, is documented in other sources. In his memoirs, a surgeon in Sydney during the period just before the First World War describes the following:

Just down the road an old abortionist practised flagrantly, though she made some pretence of doing midwifery. Such self-named "nurses" were then to be found in every suburb, so hard was it to get a conviction against them. The monetary reward was high, so they were ready and willing to take any risk. Sometimes one of the less reputable chemists would act as an agent. There is one thing which has always amazed me: that certain women should be willing, even anxious, to pour out their troubles over the counter to a man who knows how to mix drugs but has never seen disease except in his own home. This rarely seems to prevent him, however, from giving the most explicit advice. (Moran 1939:100–101)

The abortifacient trade was by no means confined to this particular Australian city; indeed, the period from 1896 to 1914 has been called the abortion age in Britain (Francome 1986:19–21). As women began to die (as Beale recounts) from lead poisoning, *Lancet* campaigned in 1898 against advertisements for abortifacients. In articles published in the *British Medical Journal* in 1900 and 1902, it was reported that when a woman's menstrual period was overdue, her first step was often to take "pills or potions 'to bring the period on'" (Brookes 1986:160), and that poisoning with lead or oil of absinthe (wormwood) had had serious or fatal results.

Cases of lead poisoning continued to be described in both the *British Medical Journal* and the *Lancet* until at least 1913, when Ethel Elderton (1914) completed her investigation of the decline in the birthrate in the north of England. In her *Report,* published by the Galton Laboratory, statistics on the decline of the total marital fertility rate within each county and registration district between 1851 and 1911 are supplemented with residents' reports of "the extent of propagandism by advertisement or otherwise for the limitation of the family," along with their opinions on whether "deliberate limitation has been . . . a factor in the reduction of the birthrate" (Elderton 1914:9).

For us the primary value of the *Report* lies in these verbatim statements, of which the responsibility for publishing was bravely assumed by Karl Pearson, the laboratory's director. More information was reported about abortion than contraception. "'Quite a lot of drugs'" were taken by women in Croston (Elderton 1914:43); abortion was sought more by drugs than instruments in Middleton (46); by drugs and operations alike in Bolton (53); and less by drugs (lead preparations) than instruments in Bradford with North Bierley (98). Newspaper advertisements for pills to prevent or remove irregularities or to remove obstructions were collected in Burnley (38), Ashton-under-Lyne (51), Brighouse (96–97), and York (137–39). Popular abortifacients were diachylon (lead) in Colne (38); colocynth (bitter apple) in Bolton (54); "female pills" in Warrington (64); bitter apple, lead plasters, and nutmegs in Birkenhead (80); colocynth, pennyroyal, Widow Welch's Female Pills,[5] apiol and steel, borax, gin and gunpowder, and diachylon in York (136); pennyroyal and lead plaster in Chester-le-Street (188); "steel pills for female irregularities" and lead plaster in Sunderland (190); and diachylon plasters and pills, as well as "the ordinary 'remedies,' pennyroyal, iron and aloes, colocynth and ipecacuanha" in Newcastle (199).

In addition to the usual professional men, mainly doctors, from whom Elderton sought information, she obtained "shrewd expressions of opinion from one or two wives of York working men" (136). One, "a keen but uneducated observer," made the following remarks:

> Six out of ten working women take something, if it is only paltry stuff. . . . One tells another. There's no hawking here; its all done in secrecy. . . . One woman said to me, 'I'd rather swallow the druggist shop and

the man in't than have another kid.' She used to boil ten herbs together, I forget the names on 'em now, mixed up with gin and salts
. . . and take a glass every morning before breakfast . . . nauseous stuff
it was. . . . And the kid came in the end. . . .
    . . . most women goes on taking pennyworths here and there. . . .
Or they'll try as many as twenty different kinds one after the other.
. . . (Ibid.)

Elderton goes on to report that two other working women "of most
respectable type, put the proportion of working women who take
drugs, etc., as at least seven and probably eight in ten" (137).

People who could not afford to call in a doctor were accustomed to
buying all sorts of proprietary drugs, and not necessarily from a pharmacy. Robert Roberts (1980), whose mother ran a small shop in the
early decades of the century in Salford, the world's first industrial slum,
describes the end-of-week ritual of purging with massive amounts of
laxatives, and the colorful pills and general tonics supplied by the corner shop. Medical announcements in the local newspaper "offered as-
surances to 'Ladies', 'Women' and 'Females' of their ability to remove
'obstructions' of all kinds, 'no matter how obstinate or long-standing.'
. . . But most of our women in need of such treatment relied on prayer,
massive doses of pennyroyal syrup, and the right application of hot,
very soapy water" (Roberts 1980:127). Some women took veterinary
abortifacients, others favored aloes and turpentine, and "the controlled fall downstairs also had its advocates. But if all else failed someone always knew a woman who knew a woman who . . ." (ibid.; Roberts's punctuation).

In her follow-up report of the first 300 cases registered at the Cambridge Clinic between August 1925 and May 1927, Lella Florence reports that many patients had occasionally taken drugs "in an effort to
bring on a delayed period." In the case of a mother whose ninth baby
had died: "The mother was 'glad when it died.' She has often taken
drugs to try to bring about a miscarriage" (Florence 1930:87). No Cambridge patient told Florence that she had lost a pregnancy through mechanical means, but many told her "fearful tales of abortions produced
amongst their friends by the use of a knitting-needle or a similar im-
plement" (122). Nevertheless, Florence "often felt convinced that a
fall from a chair or a sudden fright (the reasons they gave) had occurred at a moment when a timely explanation for a miscarriage was
needed."[6] Some patients confessed that they had exercised strenuously
in order to miscarry, or taken large doses of gin and quinine or patent
pills, but without success. Many went to their chemist for "medicine"

which, despite its claims to the contrary, usually "didn't do no good" (123).

Florence believed that, despite women's willingness to talk about other aspects of their reproductive lives, self-induced abortion was underreported;[7] that it was increasing, especially in industrial areas; and that it was contributing to the increasing rate of maternal mortality. She thought, of course, that acceptable contraception was the answer, but observes that the misinformed thought that contraception and abortion were the same thing (145).

It is impossible to quantify accurately the extent of illegal abortion in past generations, let alone the means used. Only 9 percent of such abortions reported in a large American study of reproductively active women during the first half of the century were reported to have been induced by drugs rather than a mechanical procedure. Nevertheless, since drug-induced abortions were much more likely to be self-induced—and self-induced abortions were more underreported than operative ones, as Florence believed—the figure of 9 percent may be too low. Other American and European studies published between 1931 and 1955 report an impressive variety of herbal and metallic substances that were used to procure abortion, but do not indicate the prevalence of their use (Gebhard et al. 1958:193–99; Sutter 1950). Gebhard et al. (1958:194–95) note that although drug-induced abortions were only a small minority of the induced abortions reported by their sample, they were reported the most frequently by poor black women. By this time, the affluent were more likely to seek a surgical rather than a medical solution.

The pharmacist retained an important role in pregnancy termination until at least the 1960s. When she was working with the Birmingham Family Planning Association about 1950, Lella Florence inferred from the way in which some patients "talked freely about 'taking everything in the chemist's shop'" (1956:131)—shades of Elderton's (1914:136) informant of 40 years earlier—that attempts to procure an abortion in this way were made frequently and openly. Writing of Britain's "Swinging Sixties" before the legalization of abortion in 1968, Hordern (1971: 2–3) describes the by-now-familiar process whereby women try to terminate an unwanted pregnancy first by vigorous exercise, hot baths, and self-medication. Although it was illegal to advertise or supply abortifacients in England and Wales, chemists or rubber-goods shops sold "female pills" for "irregularity," whose constituents, apart from iron salts, were purgatives or emmenagogues. Pennyroyal continued to be a recommended abortifacient in twentieth-century Norfolk (McLaren 1984:104), and "apiol and steel" and ergot compounds were still available in Australia in the 1960s (Siedlecky and Wyndham 1990:69).

AN ISSUE OF AMBIGUITY

In referring to the issue of the twentieth-century use of emmenagogues and abortifacients as one of ambiguity, I do not mean that this ambiguity derives from only one source, for indeed there are many. The first question is, was there a connection between the home medical texts advocating the use of emmenagogues and the commercialization of abortifacients? Second, are the various emmenagogues and abortifacients mentioned earlier actually effective? Third, what were the motivations of the women who took such substances?

The Motivations of Popular Authors

With our superior knowledge of reproductive physiology, and our awareness of the former popular concern with menstrual regularity, the rise of patent medicine during the nineteenth century, and the epidemic of abortion that began toward its close, it is all too easy to find instances of deliberate abortion, or attempts to procure abortion, wherever we look. For example, of the 12 gynecological operations performed in the Royal Adelaide Hospital in 1880 and 1881, Sumerling (1985:117) believes that one was abortion-related, since it was performed on a 19-year-old woman for "retained menses." Yet since this condition had a real pathology at the time, the diagnosis may well have been formed honestly, however fanciful or even sinister it may seem today.

Even contemporaneous popular works about gynecological matters vary considerably in the degree of alarm with which they view menstrual disorders, and in the nature and extent of the treatment they recommend. About the turn of the century, some medical writers (e.g., Kellogg 1895; Longshore-Potts 1896; Richards and Richards 1912) still regarded such disorders with concern, but advocated general toning treatment rather than the strenuous application of herbal or metallic compounds. Other authors did advocate such treatment (e.g., Pierce 1891, 1926; Ritter 1928), but in so doing were in line with a medical tradition that, although in the process of being abandoned in the early 1900s (e.g., Montgomery 1900), was still followed by an older generation of practitioners (e.g., Garrigues 1900) who remained impressed by European works of half a century earlier.

Altruism is unlikely to be the sole motivation of any author, but an additional interpretational difficulty arises in the case of those writers who recommended their own patented products. Law and Law (1906) of Viavi Hygiene fame are obviously commercial charlatans, but others who promoted their own wares (e.g., Narodetzki [1935?]; Dehaut 1910; Pierce 1891, 1926), by echoing earlier medical writings, however archaic, and by providing botanical information, reveal themselves as not just practical businessmen but genuine purveyors of health-enhancing information—at least as they understood it. Narodetzki, Dehaut, and Galtier-Boissière (1924) warn explicitly that certain plants are dangerous abortifacients, although the first two authors may also have intended thereby to promote the sales of their own, safer products. Pierce, who held a seat in Congress until 1880—if this can be taken as evidence of respectability—openly condemns induced abortion for reasons other than the safeguarding of the mother's health, although he expresses considerable approval of the woman who knowingly sacrifices her health, or even her life, to produce a child (1891: 218–19).

Nevertheless, the home medical texts detailing problems of amenorrhea and suppressed menstruation, and that branch of the patent-medicine industry that fairly openly advertised its wares as abortifacient in effect, did not flourish independently. The former provided the latter with not just the recipes but the respectable nomenclature of the older art of menstrual regulation. The word *obstruction,* for example, is used straightforwardly by writers such as Kellogg (1895) and Ritter (1928), but more sinisterly in advertisements for abortifacients. Similarly, the "irregularity" and "suppression" that are of concern to many of the medical writers are transformed into euphemisms for pregnancy in many advertisements.

Such borrowing did not go unnoticed by the general public: even as advertisements were being disseminated in newspapers and handbills, outraged readers declared them to be unashamedly abortifacient in intent. It is likely that the writers of the home medical texts, even if not under specific attack, became anxious lest their integrity be impugned by association. The removal of the reference to pennyroyal from the eminently respectable *Enquire Within* somewhere between the editions of 1888 and 1925 suggests such apprehension. So does the appearance, between the 1891 and 1926 editions of Pierce's *Common Sense Medical Adviser,* of testimonials to not only the benefits but the safety of taking his proprietary tonics during pregnancy. Mrs. Geo. Souders, for example, writes that she "took three bottles of the 'Favorite Prescription' this summer and a healthy baby was born to us the eighth of September"; Mrs. Chas. Jones "took Doctor Pierce's Favorite Prescription while in a delicate condition," and has a "fine healthy daughter" (Pierce 1926:751); and Mrs. R. F. Redford "had taken six bottles of 'Favorite Prescription' and three of 'Golden Medical Discovery,' when there was a fine baby girl born to us" (764). In addition, in 1891 Pierce reveals a cautious liberality—for the time—in discussing both induced abortion and the prevention of conception. By 1926, however, he is silent on the means of prevention, and mentions abortion only to declare that it is murder, that abortionists are murderers, and "[w]e wish to have it distinctly understood that we will not under any circumstances prescribe medicines or perform any operation to relieve women of pregnancy" (685). With the reading public's growing tendency, as was increasingly advocated by the home medical books, to seek professional help; with the modernization of medical knowledge and practice that eventually led to the modernization of popular texts; and with the increasing efficiency and acceptability of contraception, such sensitivities may well have contributed to the ultimate decline of popular texts that recommended herbal remedies for disorders of menstruation.

Efficacy

A constant refrain that runs through even the earliest literature I have cited is that substances said to be emmenagogic or abortifacient are dangerous, ineffective, or both. This judgment was made by medical men such as J. H. Kellogg and activists such as Octavius Beale. The question is, was this judgment sound?

Some substances that were used are indeed extremely dangerous. From the paint factories of the Midlands came the epidemic of lead poisoning to which Beale and others referred: perhaps, in some hideous sort of natural experiment, the dangerous properties of lead were recognized by women exposed to what Potts, Diggory and Peel (1977: 257) dub, with some understatement, "poorly regulated hazards facing female factory workers." Similarly, in the last quarter of the nineteenth century, phosphorus poisoning was implicated in the vast majority of abortion-related deaths in Sweden, then the major manufacturer of phosphorus matches. Some herbal preparations too are highly toxic when prepared in concentrated form. Both Beale (*Secret Drugs and Cures* 1907) and Ritter (1928) accurately pronounced oil of pennyroyal poisonous. Indeed, death or serious illness from taking pennyroyal oil to induce an abortion occasionally still occurs (Riddle 1991:19).

Claims have recently been made—although not without challenge (e.g., van de Walle 1994)—for the historical efficacy of a great variety of herbal contraceptives and abortifacients (Riddle 1991, 1997). But there are serious problems with the evidence. One is that pharmacological research on the properties of herbs is invariably conducted not on human females, who have menstrual cycles, but on rodents, who do not. Another problem is that a fine line exists between inducing abortion in either a woman or a rat by means of an emmenagogue or abortifacient, and poisoning her.

As for substances being ineffective, even some of their advocates were not confident that they would act in the desired manner. Garrigues, for example, a staunch advocate of the old, medical approach to menstrual regulation, recommended the combination of several drugs in one prescription, since the effect of any individual drug was "very uncertain" (Garrigues 1900:257). This said, he goes on to recommend backup treatment with "other remedial agents" ranging from "proper alimentation," and "moderate exercise in the open air, horseback riding" to "hot vaginal and rectal injections, warm hip-baths, warm foot-baths with or without mustard," noting, in addition, that "electricity in all its forms is a powerful remedy." Even the purveyors of abortifacients generally did not guarantee the effectiveness of their products. Rather, they claimed that they were the "finest" or "most reliable." One advertisement collected by Elderton (1914:96) claimed to "cure 25 per cent. more cases than any other advertised remedy."

Most significantly, the judgment that emmenagogues and abortifacients were useless or dangerous was made by users themselves. A number of the women answering the Women's Co-operative Guild questionnaire mentioned that they or others had used "drugs" but often with no other effect than damage to their own or the child's health. One wrote, "I have resorted to drugs, trying to prevent or bring about a slip. I believe I and others have caused bad health to ourselves and our children. But what has one to do?" (Women's Co-operative Guild 1916:38). Similarly,

> Knowing that it is mostly women and girls who are working in these factories gives you the feeling that their bodies are going round with the machinery. The mother wonders what she has to live for, and if there is another baby coming she hopes it will be dead when it is born. The result is she begins to take drugs, I need hardly tell you the pain and suffering she goes through if the baby survives, or the shock it is to the mother when she is told there is something wrong with the baby. (42)

On a more personal level, another woman wrote the following:

> I confess without shame that when well-meaning friends said: "You cannot afford another baby; take this drug," I took their strong concoctions to purge me of the little life that might be mine. They failed, as such things generally do, and the third baby came. (45)

Lella Florence documents both failures, and side effects affecting either mother or child. The woman mentioned earlier who was glad when her ninth baby died "once . . . was blind and deaf for three days as the result of taking too much quinine" (Florence 1930:87).[8] Another woman, with 10 live confinements and 2 miscarriages, had often taken gin and Beecham's pills to bring about a miscarriage, and thought that some of her children "were born frail and weakly for this reason" (88).

If nonlethal emmenagogues or abortifacients are largely ineffective, then how did they achieve their reputation to the contrary? There are a number of explanations. First, the woman who fears she is pregnant, intervenes, and bleeds may not have been pregnant at all: amenorrhea almost invariably follows pregnancy but is by no means an infallible guide, especially in the very early stages. The possibility that not all women who seek abortion are pregnant used to be legally recognized in the United States. In 18 states attempted abortion was punishable only if the woman were actually pregnant, whereas in most of the others, soliciting or consenting to the procedure was punishable regardless of pregnancy status (Gebhard et al., 1958:192).

The question of abortion without pregnancy was discussed in some detail at a conference on abortion held in 1942 at the New York Academy of Medicine. One participant reported that in about one-eighth of a sample of curettings, pathological analysis detected no sign of pregnancy (Taylor 1944:34).[9] Pascal Whelpton described how some of the respondents to the Indianapolis study in 1941 reportedly induced an abortion by taking quinine. Nevertheless, according to the physicians he had consulted, if such women had not experienced "considerable bleeding, great discomfort, or some type of sickness" (35), then they had probably not been pregnant in the first place. Whelpton believed that one of the survey's problems was not that pregnancies were underreported, but that they were overreported, citing the case of a woman who reported 1 live birth and an extraordinary 26 induced abortions: as far as the woman was concerned, these were abortions, since she had paid for prompt intervention and subsequently not been pregnant (16).

Another explanation for the emmenagogues' reputation of effectiveness is that abortions also occur spontaneously. Thus a certain proportion of pregnant women who abort after ingesting some compound would anyhow not have carried their pregnancy to term. In light of the prevalent medical opinion that abortifacients were either useless or highly dangerous, Gebhard et al. (1958:195) believed that "if induced abortions by herbs or natural drugs are reported, there is a likelihood that a spontaneous abortion would have resulted in any case" (see also Hordern 1971:3).

In the absence of induced abortion, about 15 percent of recognized pregnancies can be expected to abort spontaneously, primarily between the second and fourth months of gestation. Thus, the earlier in a pregnancy an abortifacient is taken, the greater will be its apparent success. In a study of women who had applied for legal abortion, 12 percent aborted spontaneously between the sixth and twentieth weeks of pregnancy while they were waiting for a decision or after their application had been refused (Pettersson 1968:61–64); the naive interpretation is that making an application for abortion had an abortifacient effect in about 1 case out of 8.

A third explanation for the reputation of emmenagogues is simply that women wanted them to be effective. The strongest message of Riddle's (1997) detailed cataloguing of sometimes ancient herbal recipes is not that women controlled their childbearing, but that they sometimes wished to. Elderton came to a similar conclusion when analyzing a set of abortifacient advertisements:

> Till the pills, etc. have been fully analysed, it would be idle to assert that they are a source of grave danger to prospective motherhood, but the daily appearance in provincial papers of scores of such advertisements demonstrates that there is a widespread feeling against childbirth and that many persons are willing to pay quite considerable sums in the hope of purchasing "remedies." (Elderton 1914:139)

The Motivations of Users

Writing of the long-disappeared Oxfordshire hamlet in which she grew up during the 1880s, Flora Thompson (1973) pronounced with characteristic assurance on the contents of women's herb gardens:

> As well as their flower garden, the women cultivated a herb corner, stocked with thyme and parsley and sage for cooking, rosemary to flavour the home-made lard, lavender to scent the best clothes, and peppermint, pennyroyal, horehound, camomile, tansy, balm, and rue for physic . . . the women had a private use for the pennyroyal, though, judging from appearances, it was not very effective. (115)

Hamlet families of the time were, it is true, rather large. But was Flora really implying that women were using pennyroyal in an apparently vain attempt to reduce their fertility?

The Thompson family felt socially superior to the rest of the little population, and Flora left the hamlet in her early teens to begin her ascent into the town-dwelling (and bestseller-writing) middle class. Perhaps this is why, on this point at least, she seems out of touch.[10] She does not seem to appreciate that emmenagogue use suited the popular notion that regularity in general was desirable, which in the case of the digestive system led to the consumption of large quantities of laxatives; in addition, many of the treatments for amenorrhea and suppressed menstruation recommended that the bowels be kept open. Emmenagogues also fitted in well with the regular taking of nonspecific tonics. Indeed, many emmenagogic substances had multiple purposes: for example, pennyroyal tea, which promoted sweating, was recommended also for whooping cough, colds, and colic; tansy was recommended also for hysteria, urinary troubles, stomach troubles, flatulence, jaundice, and worms; and the American smartweed could be used also for sprains, bruises, rheumatism, and bladder stones (Ritter 1928).

The use of emmenagogues also conformed with the popular view of contraception and abortion:

> The hamlet women's attitude towards the unmarried mother was contradictory. If one of them brought her baby on a visit to the hamlet they all went out of their way to pet and fuss over them. "The pretty dear!" they would cry. "How ever can anybody say such a one as him ought not to be born. Ain't he a beauty! Ain't he a size! . . . An' don't you go mindin' what folks says about you, me dear. It's only the good girls, like you, that has 'em; the others is too artful!" (Thompson 1973: 139)

In contrast, there was nothing "artful" about the regular use of emmenagogues. They could be taken before a menstrual period was obviously overdue, let alone before it was so long overdue that a woman had begun to suspect that she was pregnant. Certainly, the user would not need to interrogate her own motives, nor would an onlooker: she was merely "keeping herself regular."

What happened, though, when emmenagogues failed to produce the desired result within a few months? Some women would have resigned themselves to having another baby, perhaps thinking of it as a baby rather than a pregnancy once they had felt it move (McLaren 1990: 228–29); some of Flora Thompson's hamlet women may have thought this way. Others would have decided after a few months of attempting to restore regularity that they really did not want to carry the pregnancy to term, or would have used that time to pluck up the necessary courage to seek an abortion by mechanical means. Others would have been immediately sure that the pregnancy was unwelcome, and after attempts to dislodge it by emmenagogues, abortifacients, hot baths, poisons, and vigorous exercise, would have turned to an abortionist.

Thus there is a process. It is reported numerous times in the literature I have examined, from *Secret Drugs and Cures* (1907:14, quoted earlier) onward. The horror stories of death and disability resulting from a botched or septic surgical abortion undoubtedly deterred many women from seeking this way out of their difficulty—at least at the outset. If there was a chance that emmenagogues would work, or any of the other nonsurgical means, then women would be willing, on the grounds of safety, comparative cheapness, and privacy, to try them first.

But this is probably only part of the story. A woman may dose herself with pennyroyal tea made from herbs gathered from her own garden— or even with Towles's Pennyroyal and Steel Pills "to correct all irregularities, all obstructions, and relieve all distressing symptoms" (*Secret Drugs and Cures* 1907:33)—without admitting to herself that she would like to abort, or even without having come to that decision at all. Such ambiguity of intention is lost to the woman who seeks surgical intervention. By doing so she signals her intention to interfere with nature, and to participate in an act that throughout history has generally been judged to be immoral, illegal, or both. In light of this judgment, she understandably might wish to avoid taking such a step if at all possible, or she might need a few weeks or months to pluck up the necessary courage while she exhausts all the other possibilities. After all, one of them might just work.

Finally, just as the woman who seeks surgical abortion leaves no doubt as to her intention, so too does the "artful" woman who uses contraception. Of the 160 women (out of a total of 368) whose letters were published by the Women's Co-operative Guild, only 7, by my count, reveal that they had deliberately limited the size of their families. One of these, who in 1915 had been married for 32 years and had only 3 children, reports both that she and her husband "were quite agreed on the point of restricting our family to our means" and that she had "disgusted some of our Guild members by advocating restrictions" (Women's Co-operative Guild 1916:115). Another respondent—not one who admitted taking precautions herself—ventured the following:

I feel that I must write and explain why I advocate educating women to the idea that they should not bring children into the world without the means to provide for them. I know that it is a most delicate subject, and very great care must be used in introducing it, but still, a word spoken sometimes does good. Someone has said that most of the trouble with delicate children were [sic] caused by women trying to destroy life in the early days of pregnancy. I do not, of course, recommend that sort of thing. It is absolutely wrong. But it is terrible to see how women suffer, even those that are in better conditions of life. (59)

Contraception was thus a shocking matter, yet all the respondents who mentioned women's taking "drugs" to abort did so with considerable sympathy. To women who were undecided about the morality of contraception, douching (if they had easy access to water) may have been acceptable on the grounds of "hygiene"; the safe period (rhythm) might have been another acceptable method, because it involved the avoidance of intercourse rather than the taking of explicit steps to avoid its outcome. But the pessaries, sponges, caps, and diaphragms that were the female contraceptives of the pre-Pill era had to be used at each act of sexual intercourse—no room for ambiguity there.

The advent and mass adoption of the Pill affected attitudes toward not only contraception but also menstruation. As a retired Australian doctor reports, "The pill has changed things around a bit. My patients talked about 'my friends,' now it's 'the curse'" (Siedlecky 1998). This term attests to a subtle shift during the twentieth century in the popular perception of menstruation, because a menstrual period can be viewed primarily as a "curse" only if it is not interpreted as a sign of health, or if the woman involved does not wish to conceive and is confident that she hasn't.

Irregular menses were initially thought to bring ill health; next they were believed to result from ill health; today we believe that they may reflect ill health, or they may not. The damage done to the mystery of menstruation in the 1930s when Ogino and Knaus broke the temporal identification of menstruation with ovulation, and in the 1960s when the mass adoption of oral contraceptives placed regular monthly bleeding under the user's personal control, is probably irreversible. Further demystification has ensued from the increasing affordability of professional medical help. The recommendation of herbs to promote regular menstrual bleeding, or alleviate general menstrual symptoms, is now relegated to books on alternative medicine and to the suppliers of herbal "nutritional supplements" (Riddle 1997: 258), as they must be known for legal reasons in the United States. That this situation does not yet prevail in other parts of the world is evidenced by the second part of this volume.

NOTES

I am grateful to Suzanne Falkiner for information, advice, and succor.

1. The use of electricity in gynecological therapy was one of the end-of-century American crazes to which Ricci (1945) refers, noting, however, that "[t]he English gynaecologists, always steadier in their approach to innovations, remained indifferent to the enthusiasm of the American practitioners for this form of treatment" (547).

2. The number of prescriptions, which are described elsewhere in each volume, fell from 64 to 49 between the editions of 1871 and 1888 but remained constant until at least 1925.

3. Independent chemical analysis showed its major constituents to be quinine and savin (Ritter 1928:298).

4. Material thought too shocking for general distribution was relegated to a second volume, of which only 12 copies were printed, 3 were released, and 2 have survived. Norman Himes ([1936] 1970), the doyen of the history of contraception, includes a substantial digression concerning the Royal Commission in his discussion of the "commercialization of contraceptive instruction," remarking that although "there is more opinion than science in the verbose, bulky report, . . . it is of great interest for this subject" (326–27).

5. These are either the same as, or trade on the reputation of, Kearsley's Original Widow Welch's Female Pills, which were advertised in the Australasian newspapers as early as 1866 (Quiggin 1988:108).

6. Similarly, one respondent to the Women's Co-operative Guild inquiry on pregnancy, childbearing, and child survival reported 3 miscarriages, "one caused through carelessness in jumping up to take some clothes off the line when it commenced to rain, instead of getting a chair to stand on, another through taking some pills which were delivered as samples at the door, and a third through a fright by a cow whilst on holidays" (Women's Co-operative Guild 1916:86–87).

7. This is the evidence also of Britain's postwar Royal Commission on Population (Lewis-Faning 1949:171).

8. Such side effects are well documented (Potts, Diggory and Peel 1977: 203).

9. See also Rongy (1933:168–69).

10. Hence also, perhaps, her failure to comment on the rue and the tansy.

REFERENCES

Bremner, Moyra. 1988. *Enquire Within Upon Everything.* London: Guild Publishing.

Brookes, Barbara. 1986. "Women and Reproduction, 1860–1939." In *Labour and Love: Women's Experience of Home and Family, 1850–1940,* ed. Jane Lewis, 149–171. Oxford: Basil Blackwell.

Castiglioni, Arturo. 1941. *A History of Medicine,* ed. and trans. E. B. Krumbhaar. New York: Alfred A. Knopf.

Dehaut. 1910. *Manuel de Médecine, d'Hygiène et de Pharmacie Domestiques par Dehaut, Docteur en Médecine de la Faculté de Paris.* 28th ed. Paris, n.p.

Dixon-Mueller, Ruth. 1988. "Innovations in Reproductive Health Care: Menstrual Regulation Policies and Programs in Bangladesh." *Studies in Family Planning* 19:129–40.

Elderton, Ethel M. 1914. *Report on the English Birthrate. Part I. England, North of the Humber.* London: Dulau and Co.

Enquire Within Upon Everything. 1856. 1st ed. London: Houlston and Sons.

———. 1871. 43d ed., revised and enlarged. London: Houlston and Sons.

———. 1888. 78th ed., revised. London: Houlston and Sons.

———. [1925?]. 115th ed., revised and enlarged. London: Herbert Jenkins Limited.

Florence, Lella Secor. 1930. *Birth Control on Trial.* London: George Allen and Unwin.

———. 1956. *Progress Report on Birth Control.* London: William Heinemann Medical Books.

Francome, Colin. 1986. *Abortion Practice in Britain and the United States.* London: Allen and Unwin.

Galtier-Boissière, J. 1924. *Larousse Médical Illustré.* Paris: Librairie Larousse.

Garrigues, Henry J. [1894] 1900. *A Text-Book of the Diseases of Women.* 3d rev. ed. Philadelphia: W. B. Saunders & Company.

Gebhard, Paul H., Wardell B. Pomeroy, Clyde E. Martin, and Cornelia V. Christenson. 1958. *Pregnancy, Birth and Abortion.* New York: Harper and Brothers.

Graves, William P. 1918. *Gynecology.* Philadelphia: W. B. Saunders Company.

Hall, Ruth, ed. 1981. *Dear Dr Stopes: Sex in the 1920s.* Harmondsworth: Penguin.

Hatcher, Robert A., et al. 1998. *Contraceptive Technology.* 17th rev. ed. New York: Irvington.

Himes, Norman E. [1936] 1970. *Medical History of Contraception.* New York: Schocken.

Hoffmann, David. 1997. *The New Holistic Herbal.* 3d ed. Shaftesbury, Dorset: Element.

Hordern, Anthony. 1971. *Legal Abortion: The English Experience*. Oxford: Pergamon Press.

Kellogg, J. H. 1895. *Ladies' Guide in Health and Disease. Girlhood, Maidenhood, Wifehood, Motherhood*. London: International Tract Society.

Law, Hartland, and Herbert E. Law. 1906. *Viavi Hygiene for Women, Men and Children*. San Francisco: The Viavi Company.

Lewis-Faning, E. 1949. *Report on an Enquiry into Family Limitation and Its Influence on Human Fertility during the Past Fifty Years*. Vol. 1 of *Papers of the Royal Commission on Population*. London: His Majesty's Stationery Office.

Llewellyn-Jones, Derek. 1978. *Everywoman. A Gynaecological Guide for Life*. 2d ed. London: Faber and Faber.

———. 1993. *Everywoman. A Gynaecological Guide for Life*. 6th ed. Ringwood, Victoria: Penguin.

Longshore-Potts, A. M. 1896. *Discourses to Women on Medical Subjects*. San Diego and London: self-published.

McLaren, Angus. 1984. *Reproductive Rituals*. London: Methuen.

———. 1990. *A History of Contraception from Antiquity to the Present Day*. Oxford: Basil Blackwell.

———. 1994. " 'Not a Stranger: A Doctor': Medical Men and Sexual Matters in the Late Nineteenth Century." In *Sexual Knowledge, Sexual Science: The History of Attitudes to Sexuality*, ed. Roy Porter and Mikulás Teich, 267–83. Cambridge: Cambridge University Press.

The Marriage Book: For Husbands and Wives—and All Who Love Children. [1935?] London: The Amalgamated Press.

Montgomery, Edward E. 1900. *Practical Gynecology. A Comprehensive Text-Book for Students and Physicians*. Philadelphia: P. Blakiston's Son & Co.

Moran, H. M. 1939. *Viewless Winds. Being the Recollections and Digressions of an Australian Surgeon*. London: Peter Davies.

Narodetzki, A. [1935?] *La Médecine Végétale Illustrée*. 132d ed. [Paris?]:n.p.

Pettersson, Folke. 1968. *Epidemiology of Early Pregnancy Wastage*. Uppsala: Medical Faculty, Uppsala University.

Pierce, R. V. 1891. *The People's Common Sense Medical Adviser in Plain English; or, Medicine Simplified*. 25th ed. Buffalo, N.Y.: World's Dispensary Medical Association.

———. 1926. *The People's Common Sense Medical Adviser in Plain English; or, Medicine Simplified*. 99th ed. Buffalo, N.Y.: World's Dispensary Medical Association.

Potts, Malcolm, Peter Diggory, and John Peel. 1977. *Abortion*. Cambridge: Cambridge University Press.

Quiggin, Pat. 1988. *No Rising Generation: Women and Fertility in Late Nineteenth-Century Australia*. Australian Family Formation Monograph Series, no. 10. Canberra: Department of Demography, The Australian National University.

Ricci, James V. 1943. *The Genealogy of Gynaecology: History of the Development of Gynaecology throughout the Ages, 2000 b.c.–1800 a.d.* Philadelphia: The Blakiston Company.

———. 1945. *One Hundred Years of Gynaecology, 1800–1900.* Philadelphia:
The Blakiston Company.

Richards, F. C., and Eulalia S. Richards. 1912. *Ladies' Handbook of Home
Treatment.* Melbourne: Signs Publishing Company.

Riddle, John M. 1991. "Oral Contraceptives and Early-Term Abortifacients during Classical Antiquity and the Middle Ages." *Past and Present* 132:3–32.

———. 1997. *Eve's Herbs: A History of Contraception and Abortion in the
West.* Cambridge, Mass: Harvard University Press.

Ritter, T. J. [1910] 1928. *The People's Home Medical Book. Book I of the People's Home Library.* Reprint, Toronto, Sydney, and Cape Town: The Oce-
anic Publishing Company.

Roberts, Robert. [1971] 1980. *The Classic Slum: Salford Life in the First
Quarter of the Century.* Reprint, Harmondsworth: Penguin.

Robinson, Victor, ed. 1943. *The Modern Home Physician.* New York: International Readers League.

Rongy, A. J. 1933. *Abortion: Legal or Illegal?* New York: The Vanguard
Press.

Ross, Clara, and P. T. Piotrow. 1974. "Birth Control without Contraceptives." *Population Reports,* ser. 1, no. 1.

Royal Commission into Secret Drugs, Cures and Foods. 1907. Report. In *Com-
monwealth Parliamentary Papers* 29, no. 4 (1907–8):61–527.

Siedlecky, Stefania. 1998. Personal communication, 27 May.

Siedlecky, Stefania, and Diana Wyndham. 1990. *Populate and Perish:
Australian Women's Fight for Birth Control.* Sydney: Allen and
Unwin.

Siegler, Samuel L. 1944. *Fertility in Women: Causes, Diagnosis and Treatment of Impaired Fertility.* Philadelphia: J. B. Lippincott Company.

Sumerling, Patricia. 1985. "The Darker Side of Motherhood: Abortion
and Infanticide in South Australia 1870–1910." *Journal of the Historical
Society of South Australia* 13:111–27.

Sutter, Jean. 1950. "Résultats d'une enquête sur l'avortement dans la ré-
gion Parisienne." *Population* 5:77–102.

Taylor, Howard C. 1944. *The Abortion Problem. Proceedings of the Conference Held under the Auspices of the National Committee on Maternal
Health at the New York Academy of Medicine, June 19th and 20th, 1942.*
Baltimore: The Williams and Wilkins Company for National Committee on Maternal Health.

Thompson, Flora. [1939] 1973. *Lark Rise to Candleford.* Harmondsworth:
Penguin.

Vlugt, Theresa van der, and P. T. Piotrow. 1973. "Menstrual Regulation—
What Is It?" *Population Reports,* ser. F, no. 2, 9–23.

Walle, Etienne van de. 1994. Review of *Contraception and Abortion from the Ancient World to the Renaissance,* by John M. Riddle. *Population and Development Review* 20:221–24.

Women's Co-operative Guild. 1916. *Maternity: Letters from Working Women.* London: G. Bell and Sons.

CHAPTER 5

Pharmacological Properties of Emmenagogues: A Biomedical View

Stefania Siedlecky

In real life, a spade is not always called a spade,
and in human affairs, the power of language over
the idea may be overwhelming.
—Egon Diczfalusy, "The History of Steroidal
    Contraception"

Early oral contraceptives were initially approved for the indication of "menstrual regulation," not contraception (Diczfalusy 1987:4). And because of the strong religious, moral, and legal sanctions that have been applied to attempts at controlling human reproduction, the use of evasive and even misleading language characterizes the history of birth control. Accordingly, although many women have been prepared to risk their lives either to achieve a desired pregnancy or to terminate an unwanted one, they have often disguised the real reason for their concern over missed periods.

The use of herbal remedies or physical interference to induce menstrual bleeding or control pregnancy is a practice that has been found in every quarter of the globe dating to prehistoric times (Himes 1936, pts. 1–4). Indeed, writers in antiquity recorded centuries of accumulated knowledge of the medicinal qualities of local plants (as described by Himes [1936], Riddle [1992], and others), but this information was already ancient by the time it was written down. The widespread use of folk medicines to bring on periods persists to this day, as other chapters in this volume can attest. This chapter discusses the use of some of these remedies from a biomedical view.

WHY DID WOMEN FEAR PREGNANCY?

To investigate the origins of emmenagogues and abortifacients, we need to consider how women living under primitive conditions dealt with obstetrical emergencies that could result in the death of mother and/or baby, or in long-term morbidity. These crises include incomplete miscarriage, dead fetus, placenta previa, uterine inertia (cessation of labor), failed delivery, retained placenta, ante- and postpartum hemorrhage, and eclampsia. Each of these conditions might require assisting the uterus to empty itself. Before the advent of Western medicine, and still in some remote areas, women have had to face these situations with minimal understanding of what was happening, with access only to folk medicine and none of the drugs, techniques, and treatment facilities we now take for granted.

As a young medical graduate in 1948, I worked for a time in Darwin in the north of Australia, then very much a frontier town recovering from wartime bombing by the Japanese. In Aboriginal culture, sex and reproduction were and still are very much "women's business" (see also Reid 1979). Aboriginal women had their babies under primitive conditions, and at that time even those living around Darwin "went bush" for their confinements.

One Sunday I received an emergency call from a mission station 4 hours away by boat. A young Aboriginal woman in her first pregnancy had been brought on foot to the mission. Her waters had broken and the baby's umbilical cord had fallen out, but her labor pains had ceased. She was a tribal woman who spoke little English. The Aborigines realized the baby was dead, and they accepted that she too would die. I found her squatting in the dirt, with the baby's cord hanging out of the vagina, but having no uterine contractions. The first and simplest rule in dealing with uterine inertia is to ensure an empty bladder. I catheterized the woman and got 56 ounces of urine (about 1.7 liters). The bush is no place to try heroic intervention, so we brought her to the hospital. During the trip her contractions started again, which she bore without a murmur. We got her into a hospital bed just in time for her to deliver a dead baby, and she had an uneventful recovery.

What alternatives might have been available for a woman in such a situation? If someone had recognized the full bladder, she might have been given a plant extract having some diuretic property; in addition, she might have been exposed to heat, massaged, or given some herbal purgative or oxytocic such as ergot or cinchona bark (quinine), if one were locally available, to try to stimulate uterine contractions. In cases such as this, where the cervix was not dilated, a ruptured uterus could have resulted, causing massive internal hemorrhage and death. Or, as the situation deteriorated, there might have been an attempt to cut open the cervix or to dilate it with the fingers and pull the dead fetus out piecemeal (indeed, some of the earliest obstetrical instruments were developed for this purpose). Alternatively, other tribal women might have tried to force the delivery of the baby by vigorously massaging the mother or by rolling a log down her abdomen, causing extensive damage to her uterus, bladder, and pelvic floor. And by then, with a prolapsed cord of several days' duration, she would have certainly become infected. Traumatic though these actions may have been, the only other alternative was that she would have probably died undelivered.

Since the beginning of time, women have faced obstetrical emergencies such as this, where recognition of the medicinal properties of local herbs may have come to practical use. Shorter (1983) has detailed the difficulties women have suffered in childbirth throughout history, hardships still being faced in West Africa in 1992 (PMMN 1992:284). It is no wonder, then, that many women have dreaded pregnancy.

With only a rudimentary understanding of physiology, the ancients were astute enough to eventually recognize various properties in plants and their effects on people and their domestic animals. They learned that some plants had therapeutic effects in small doses, yet were toxic in larger amounts. They came to recognize that plant extracts could produce hallucinations, vomiting, diuresis, pain relief, muscle stimulation, purging, and uterine contractions. They also could see a similarity between straining at stool and the straining at birth.

Some of the herbal drugs referred to in the classical writings were recommended to expel the afterbirth or a dead fetus, or to overcome uterine inertia. The knowledge acquired in dealing with obstetrical emergencies could be taken a step further, to try to bring on the bleeding that would indicate no pregnancy or end the "little bit pregnant" in the weeks before quickening. Oxytocic drugs such as ergot and quinine would have been recognized for their effects on the parturient uterus well before they were tried earlier in pregnancy as abortifacients. The next and more sophisticated step would be to try to prevent pregnancy itself. Shorter (1983:182) makes the same point.

In Western society, maternal death is rare, but in the less-developed countries in Africa and central Asia, the death rate can be even more than 1,200 per 100,000 live births (UNICEF 1998:118–19). WHO estimates that some 500,000 women die each year from pregnancy-related causes worldwide, and between one-fourth and one-third of these stem from unsafe abortion. Of abortion-related deaths, 98 percent occur in Third World countries. Thousands of other women suffer serious ill health from the complications of unsafe abortion (IPPF 1992:1). There should be no complacency, therefore, regarding the safety and reliability of folk remedies.

The writings cited by Himes, Riddle, and others list a myriad of herbs, to be taken separately or together, often over days or weeks, thereby suggesting that none was particularly reliable either as an emmenagogue or an abortifacient. Himes quotes advice from Rhazes to women in the tenth century A.D., starting with action to be taken at the time of intercourse to prevent the sperm from entering the womb (coitus interruptus and spermicides), then the use of drugs (emmenagogues), and, finally, "if the semen has become lodged, there is no help for it but that she insert into her womb a probe or a stick cut into the shape of a probe, especially good being the root of the mallow," to be left in all night and one full day as well. The stick was to be tied to the thigh "so that it may go in no further." The woman must be patient and not use force, and in 1 or 2 weeks the menses would appear and the "whole thing will become open and clean" (Himes 1936:137). If not successful, the procedure could be repeated. There was "no better operation than this . . . and it did no harm." Meanwhile, the woman was to have hot baths, massage the abdomen and uterus, and take an herb diet accompanied by violent movements and vigorous sexual intercourse. Such advice suggests that emmenagogues and abortifacients were unreliable; that women tried the simplest remedies first and when these failed, tried to initiate abortion by passing various foreign bodies into the uterus. Given the risks of these procedures, it would seem doubtful that Rhazes himself had any actual experience.

Such techniques have persisted, in many cases successfully, but also with a great risk of incomplete abortion, hemorrhage, and infection. We recognize the more modern use of sea-tangle tents (seaweed) and slippery elm bark to dilate the cervix as an adjunct to abortion. Until relatively recent times and still in some parts of the world, abortionists inserted a probe or a catheter through the cervix or syringed soapy water into the uterus and sent the woman home to await the subsequent abortion. The Higginson's syringe and the "invisible traveling enema," widely advertised in Australia from the late nineteenth century for vaginal douching (see Smyth 1893:ix) were used for this purpose even by women themselves. Its use required a deal of skill, and many women consequently suffered damage or death from bleeding or infection, or from perforation of the vaginal wall, uterus, or bowel.

Even if the woman recovered, there was a risk of pelvic infection and subsequent infertility. In Australia in 1909, a doctor called for restrictions on the sale of gum elastic catheters because of the number of women who had injured themselves trying to produce an abortion (Meyer 1909:825–30).

Many women did succeed in producing abortions. At a Melbourne hospital in 1882, among 500 married women outpatients, 262 had had 1 or more abortions, 8 had had 6 or more, and 1 patient reported 13 abortions and 8 full-term births (Jamieson 1888:103). There was no comment on how these abortions had been achieved. At the 1903–4 Royal Commission into the Decline of the Birthrate and the Mortality of Infants in New South Wales, evidence was given of the use of foreign bodies to bring on abortions, and of 1 woman who had induced 9 abortions by passing a catheter into her uterus (Armstrong 1904:102).[1]

THE EMMENAGOGUES

Early herbal emmenagogues were made from local plants. The potency and pharmacological properties of herbal extracts vary with seasons, type of soil, the part of the plant used, and the method of extraction, so the effective and toxic doses and the presence of other constituents are also variable. The wide variety of herbal extracts used as emmenagogues and abortifacients suggests that they were mostly ineffective. What most had in common was a strong purgative action, the idea being that anything that stimulated the bowel would have a similar effect on the uterus. It is also possible that many of the old recipes have been lost, which could explain why the results do not appear to justify their reputation.

With the growth of urban populations and the pharmaceutical industry during the nineteenth century, these drugs came to be prepared and sold by pharmacists and by the new drug manufacturers. Better-quality drugs may have resulted from this development, but it also meant a shift of knowledge and control regarding their use to the pharmaceutical and medical professions. It encouraged a brisk trade among the unofficial peddlers, who were prepared to take advantage of the gap in the informal market and supply what were often inadequate and falsely represented remedies to women desperately seeking to avoid an unwanted pregnancy (see *The Lancet* series).

Doctors hardly offered better solutions. David Davis, professor of midwifery at the University of London, noted in his textbook, "The proximate cause of amenorrhea is in [sic] a great mystery to us; nor can this be a matter which should excite our surprise, when we consider the fact, that we are also equally ignorant both of proximate and occasional causes of the function itself, of which the non-performance constitutes the essence of the disease" (Davis 1836:296). Recognizing suppression of menses to be a result, not a cause, of illness, he outlined a multitude of reasons for amenorrhea ranging from poor nutrition in early life, "early depravities," and febrile illness, to exposure to cold, lifestyle changes, and sudden loss (297–98). He also noted a "connexion [sic] between amenorrhoea and phthisis pulmonalis [tuberculosis] as cause and effect."

The treatments Davis suggested reflect the state of medical knowledge at the time; lucky was the woman who could be treated simply by domestic herbs. In the case of "suppressed" menses, the bleeding could be established in a few hours, provided the doctor was consulted "immediately upon the suppression taking place" (310). Treatment consisted of an emetic of tartarized antimony (tartar emetic) and ipecacuanha, followed by bleeding if necessary. If, however, there was a delay of several weeks, treatment consisted of cupping and purging with calomel, colocynth, and aloes. During the next month the woman would be given several purges along with doses of blue pill (mercury), and at the time of the expected period, leeches to the vulva and even to the vagina performed by a "modest and intelligent female" (312). When these interventions failed, the practitioner might feel "compelled" to resort to emmenagogues, which Davis refers to as "supposed" stimulants of the uterine system. His list includes madder, rue, savin, arnica, myrrh, ergot of rye and cantharides.

Davis described how women in one locality used decoctions of the leaves of the "notorious savin tree" to induce abortions, often attended by "alarming consequences" (314). He questioned the "pretensions" of ergoted rye except in a parturient uterus (316), instead favoring treatment with mercury salts to the level of toxicity, and also electricity (320). He reported a fatal case in which autopsy revealed that the woman had suffered a massive internal hemorrhage, "eighty pounds of very black blood," and a greatly distended fallopian tube, suggesting a ruptured ectopic pregnancy (306). Like other medical writers, Davis warned of young women who went to extraordinary lengths of deception to obtain abortifacients (307).

During the nineteenth century, laws were introduced in most countries that made abortion illegal. While pharmacists could admit to selling emmenagogues, they denied selling abortifacients, although they knew that women bought and used emmenagogues as such. Yet the considerable reticence among pharmacists regarding the nature of this part of their trade was not solely confined to their profession. Thomas Beecham, of Beecham's Pills fame, started in 1842 by selling pills called Female's Friend, made from his own secret formula, in the market-place in Wigan, England (Francis 1962). In time he became a respect-able and wealthy pharmacist, and Beecham's Pills became internation-ally known and aggressively marketed; at one time Beecham's was the largest advertiser in the United Kingdom. One famous Beecham's Pills advertisement made the following claims:

> Their fame has reached to the uttermost ends of the earth. Their cur-ative power is universally acknowledged to a degree unprecedented in the annals of physical science and it is echoed from shore to shore that for Bilious and Nervous Disorders, Indigestion with its dreaded allies, *and for assisting nature in her wondrous functions,* they are WORTH A GUINEA A BOX. (Davis 1974:frontispiece; italics mine.)

The italicized words were omitted in the version reproduced in the bi-ography of Thomas Beecham written by his great-granddaughter (Fran-cis 1962:81).

The Royal Commission on the Decline of the Birth-rate and on the Mortality of Infants in New South Wales heard evidence of widespread advertising in the local press for drugs to "remove obstructions." Many of these advertisements were thinly disguised claims for abortifacients. Beecham's Pills were not listed in the evidence, although it was re-ported that women took the product to induce abortion (Stevens 1904: 44). An employee of the pharmaceutical company Parke Davis, when questioned about abortifacients, stated, "From my knowledge I know that the average pill that is used for procuring abortion is a pill called the emmenagogue pill. The base is of course, ergot, iron and aloes" (Sharland 1904:24).

PHARMACOLOGY OF EMMENAGOGUES

Some information is available from the various official pharmaceutical publications about the drugs used as emmenagogues and abortifacients in the first half of this century. In Britain, *The Lancet* (1898, vol. 2 and 1899, vol. 1) published a series titled "Quacks and Abortion" that ex-posed fraudulent claims made for emmenagogues being widely adver-tised and sold at the time "to relieve obstructions." The medical journal commented, "The action of emmenagogues and ecbolics is a difficult thing to decide, and one upon which very little experimental work has so far been done. The conclusions as to the action of certain drugs rest almost entirely upon clinical evidence of very doubtful value" (1898, 2:182).

The 1910 edition of Taylor's *Principles and Practice of Medical Jurisprudence* includes a section on drug-induced abortion (Taylor 1910:157–77). The opening paragraph states:

> The following generalization, which is strictly warranted by facts, conveys a warning to would-be abortionists, whether professional and habitual, or lay and occasional —THERE IS NO DRUG AND NO COMBINATION OF DRUGS WHICH WILL, WHEN TAKEN BY THE MOUTH, CAUSE A HEALTHY UTERUS TO EMPTY ITSELF, UNLESS IT BE GIVEN IN DOSES SUFFICIENTLY LARGE TO SERIOUSLY ENDANGER, BY POISONING, THE LIFE OF THE WOMAN WHO TAKES IT OR THEM. [Capitals in the original.]

Taylor listed the emmenagogues in use at the turn of the century in Great Britain (abstracted from *The Lancet* series above). He categorized emmenagogues as being either direct (acting on the uterus or the related nervous system) or indirect (restoring the health of the body as a whole).

- Indirect emmenagogues included
  - tonics such as iron and arsenic;
  - hematinics, especially iron; and
  - purgatives, especially of the stronger kind, such as colocynth, gamboge, sodium and magnesium sulphate, and aloes, croton oil, elaterium, *hiera picra* (a mixture of aloes and canella bark), and *pilacotia* (a mixture of aloes and colocynth).
- Direct emmenagogues included
  - aloes, cantharides, caulophyllin, borax, apiol, *cimicifuga racemosa*, potassium permanganate, manganese dioxide, myrrh, anemone pulsatilla, *polygala senega*, sanguinarin, pennyroyal, grains of paradise, tansy, white and black hellebore, squills, broom, male fern, *laburnum*, and *asarum arabicum*.
- Taylor defined ecbolics as drugs increasing the expulsive power of the uterine muscle. They included
  - ergot, *hydrastis canadensis, ruta, juniper sabina* (oil of savin), quinine, sodium salicylate and
  - metals such as lead and mercury.

The Martindale *Extra Pharmacopoeia* (hereafter MEP) is issued as a companion volume to the British Pharmacopoeia. The 1941 edition lists 13 herbal and chemical preparations for the treatment of amenor-rhea, as well as estrogens, progestogens, and pituitary and thyroid ex-tract (1152–53). The text cautiously deals with these drugs by listing properties attributed to each (e.g., diuretic, diaphoretic, anthelmintic, spasmodic, emmenagogic, etc.). Describing a drug as having emmena-gogic properties, however, does not mean it will be effective in every-day use. More recent editions limit these drugs to the category of herbal preparations. Some of the best known emmenagogues are as follows.

Aloes (MEP 1941:168)

Aloes is obtained from the leaves of various species of Aloe (e.g., Cape aloes and Curacao or Barbados aloes, etc). It contains about 25 percent aloin, its principal ingredient. Taylor quotes from *The Lancet* (1889: 182) in reporting that aloes was said to have a direct effect on the uterus, but there was no evidence of this.

MEP 1941 lists 24 laxative preparations in which aloes was the major ingredient. Aloes and aloin act chiefly on the lower bowel and were used in combination with soap, iron, and strychnine in treating habit-ual constipation. MEP 1941 warns that at a dose of 10 grains, or twice the maximum recommended daily dosage, aloes is very unsafe for preg-nant women, since it is likely to cause abortion. Aloes and aloin are still available in herbal and proprietary medicines and in laxatives such as Beecham's Pills, Carter's Pills, and Agarol. MEP 1993 makes no men-tion of its possible emmenagogic or abortifacient properties. The 1996 edition of the *British Herbal Pharmacopoeia* lists aloin only as a laxative, contraindicated in pregnancy and lactation.

Apiol (MEP 1941:200–201)

MEP 1941 describes apiol (oil of parsley) as a drug obtained by alcoholic extraction from the fruit of *Carum Petrosilenum* (syn. *Petrosilenum sati-vum*, or common parsley). Other publications refer to apiol as extract of parsley seed. MEP 1941 states that "apiol is claimed to be efficaceous in primary amenorrhoea (i.e., failure to start menstruating), deficiency of secretion and dysmenorrhoea (painful periods)." Dosage was twice daily for 4 to 5 days at the time of the menstrual period, often com-bined with other drugs such as the proprietary preparation Ergoapiol (ergot extract, aloin, oil of savin, and apiol). MEP 1941 reports a fatal case of poisoning in a young woman who took 17 capsules of Ergoapiol to induce abortion. Apiol and steel was another potentially dangerous combination of apiol with ferrous (iron) sulfate. In the late 1940s, one

of my own patients died from the toxic effects of apiol and steel purchased from a local pharmacist.

MEP 1941 lists reports of toxic polyneuritis in the early 1930s following the use of apiol as an abortifacient, due to the presence of the sol-
vent tri-ortho-cresyl phosphoric acid. Apiol was recommended for inclusion in the Fourth Schedule of Poisons in the 1939 U.K. Report of
the Inter-Departmental Committee on Abortion, which meant that it
was to be provided on a doctor's prescription only. It was deleted from
the British Pharmacopoeia in 1949 and from the United States Pharmacopoeia in 1955. In the *Merck Index* of 1989, apiol is listed as synergistic
with insecticides and given no therapeutic category (*Merck* 1989:773).
Apiol has been omitted from MEP 1993.

Herbal Drugs and Phytopharmaceuticals (Wechel 1994) lists apiol as a
powerful diuretic used in folk medicine as an emmenagogue and for
the treatment of dysmenorrhea and menstrual disorders,. It was also
used as an abortifacient, and in large doses caused kidney, liver, and
cardiac damage. Wechel concludes that since the activity of parsley
seed (sic) and its preparations have not been substantiated, in view of
the risks, "their therapeutic use cannot be endorsed" (370).

Ergot (MEP 1941:503–14)

Ergot is a mixture of alkaloids obtained from the sclerotium of the fungus *Claviceps purpurea,* which grows on rye grain. MEP 1941 states, "Ergot stimulates plain muscle throughout the body but its use is confined
almost entirely to obstetrics, owing to its action in exciting uterine
contractions." Its main use was to control postpartum bleeding after
delivery. Its action as an abortifacient was doubtful.

Ergot and its derivatives can produce uterine spasm lasting up to several hours, and even rupture of the uterus. For this reason, MEP 1941
warns against their use prior to delivery. Prolonged use produces ergot-
ism, originally observed following the ingestion of infected grain. This
condition manifests as pain and gangrene of the extremities (caused
by constriction of blood vessels) even to the extent of needing amputa-
tion, convulsions and death. Taylor reports the death of a woman who
had taken ergot 3 times a day for 11 weeks without abortion occurring
(Taylor 1910:161).

Ergot is best known as the source of the alkaloids ergotoxine and
ergometrine used in modern obstetrics, and ergotamine, used in the
treatment of migraine. Ergometrine is used to stimulate uterine contractions in postpartum hemorrhage and following cesarean section,
but its effectiveness in the treatment of incomplete and inevitable
abortion is uncertain.

Cotton Root (MEP 1941:559–61)

From the root bark of *Gossypium herbaceum* and other cultivated species, cotton root *(Gossypii cortex)* has been used as an emmenagogue and abortifacient and to relieve dysmenorrhea.[2] MEP 1941 lists similar herbal drugs under the same heading (559):

- Edestine, from cotton root and also from linseed.
- Aletris (star grass, ague root, colic root) from *Aletridis farinosa,* used as a "so-called uterine tonic."
- Caulophyllum (blue cohosh, papoose or squaw root), a diuretic and emmenagogue. Its derivative Caulophyllin had "diuretic, diaphoretic, anthelmintic, spasmodic, and emmenagogue properties" (560). Paradoxically, other compounds containing caulophyllin were stated to be "sedative in dysmenorrhea and uterine disorders" (560).
- Helonias, from false unicorn root, used in colic and in "atony of the generative organs," which is not defined (560); also used as an emmenagogue.
- Piscidia, or Jamaica dogwood. This herb apparently was an analgesic: useful in neuralgia, toothache, bronchitis, pertussis, insomnia, and dysmenorrhea.
- Pulsatilla, or Pasque flower, from *Anemone pulsatilla,* used in dysmenorrhea and amenorrhea.

Oil of Pennyroyal (MEP 1941:746)

Pennyroyal is an essential oil distilled from fresh pennyroyal herb, *Mentha pulegium* (a variety of mint). Its name is derived from *puliol real* (OED 1992). MEP 1941 states that pennyroyal is mildly irritant to the kidneys, and stimulates uterine contractions. It has been used as an emmenagogue and reputedly causes abortion; other plants of the mint family have similar properties. Pennyroyal was recommended for inclusion in the Fourth Schedule of Poisons in the Report of the Inter-Departmental Committee on Abortion. Severe toxic effects have followed its use as an abortifacient, leading to convulsions, liver damage, and sometimes death (MEP 1993:2240).

Oil of Rue (MEP 1941:746–47)

Oleum Rutae was distilled from *Ruta graveolens,* rue, or herbygrass (also known as herb of repentance or herb of grace), and was once used to ward off witches (Grieve 1984:695). Rue was used in an infusion as an emmenagogue and as an antispasmodic, usually in combination with other herbs. MEP 1993:1410 reports that it is a powerful bowel irritant.

Oil of Savin (MEP 1941:747)

Oil of savin *(Oleum sabinae)* was distilled from the shoots of *Juniper sabina*. It is a violent irritant with emmenagogic and abortifacient properties. In large doses it reputedly causes abortion, usually accompanied by serious poisoning. Taylor notes that the leaves of savin were readily obtained in gardens. Tincture of savin was expunged from the British Pharmacopeia (Taylor:164), but oil of savin continued to be used. MEP 1941 reports 2 fatal cases in which there was damage to the lungs, liver, and kidneys; death occurred without the abortion taking place. The same edition also states that oil of savin was recommended for inclusion in the Fourth Schedule of Poisons in the 1939 Report of the Inter-Departmental Committee on Abortion, and was considered to have no legitimate use of any importance.

Savin was replaced in proprietary preparations by extract of *Juniper communis* (MEP 1993:1379). In the more recent publications, references to juniper and oil of juniper mean this extract. MEP 1972 lists 10 ingredients in Beecham's Pills, including rosemary, juniper, aniseed, capsicum, and ginger. In the 1993 edition, Beecham's Pills are listed only as a laxative containing aloin, and there is no mention of an emmenagogic effect.

Oil of Juniper (MEP 1941:743)

Distilled from the berries of *Juniper communis,* MEP 1941 lists oil of juniper *(Oleum juniperi, essence de genièvre)* as a diuretic and urinary antiseptic, not to be used in the presence of renal disease. Its main use was in veterinary practice, and MEP 1941 gives no mention of its use as an emmenagogue.

The extract of *Juniper communis* (also known as *Juniper fructus*) contains more than 70 components that vary considerably in concentration (Wechel 1994:283–85). Its quality depends on its origin, mode of extraction, and the ripeness of the berries. Juniper oil is used as a flavoring in gin and liqueurs and as a diuretic in veterinary medicine. Its modern use in herbal therapies is as a diuretic and urinary antiseptic, although its usefulness has been disputed because of its toxic effects on the kidneys. It must not be used in pregnancy or if kidney damage is present.

The name *gin* is derived from the various translations of *juniper (genièvre, genever,* or *geneva)*. Gin has had a long anecdotal association with abortion.

Quinine (MEP 1941:873–98)

An extract from cinchona bark, quinine and its derivatives have many uses as tonics and bitters, but have been used most in the treatment of malaria. Moderate doses stimulate, but high doses depress uterine activity in the late stages of pregnancy. The main obstetrical use of quinine has been to strengthen labor pains, and it was sometimes given late in pregnancy to prepare the uterus for the induction of labor or to prevent uterine inertia (MEP 1941:874; not mentioned in MEP 1993). Quinine also has been used as an abortifacient, either alone or in combination with other emmenagogues, but the effect was doubtful. The well-known QES tablets, used to control uterine bleeding, contained quinine, ergot, and strychnine.

MEP 1941 notes the death of a woman who took 16 quinine pills to induce abortion. Large doses were said to cause abortion and also fetal abnormalities, but the World Health Organization regards therapeutic doses in the treatment of malaria as safe for pregnant women (MEP 1993:408–11).[3] Overdosing with quinine may produce cinchonism, with ringing in the ears, deafness, headache, and nausea, leading to vomiting, pain, diarrhea, cardiac damage, and heart failure.

Lead (Diachylon) (MEP 1941:87–88)

Diachylon paste, an adhesive plaster for external use, was made from lead oxide and olive or arachis oil. The paste was also formed into balls to be taken internally as an abortifacient. This use could result in lead poisoning or plumbism, characterized by anorexia, colic, vomiting, anemia, nerve and brain damage, wrist-drop and foot-drop, coma, and possibly death (MEP 1993:1381). Lead is a cumulative poison and takes years to clear. It acquired its reputation as an abortifacient from the observed frequency of spontaneous abortion among women working in lead processing factories. Taylor reports cases of lead poisoning following the use of diachylon at the turn of the century.

Wechel (1994) warns of the risk to pregnancy of a number of herbs, including rhubarb, salvia (red sage), aloes, parsley seed (apiol), and cinchona (quinine). Pennyroyal, rue, and tansy had been excluded from this edition.

Information about reputed emmenagogues and abortifacients was circulated among women mainly by word of mouth. These preparations have passed out of use in developed countries not on the basis of clinical trials, but because they were found to be unreliable and cause very severe side effects, and because surgical abortion has become more accessible. Shorter (1983:210) comments that "the ineffectiveness of patent medicines helped ultimately to discredit—both among doctors and among women—the whole notion of drugs as an alternative to surgery." This may be true in developed countries, but Third World women still rely on herbal preparations.

RESEARCH INTO PLANT EMMENAGOGUES AND ABORTIFACIENTS

Modern medicines have their origins in herbal remedies, with the active components separated out, tested, refined, synthesized, and modified to increase efficacy and specificity and to reduce side effects. The original hormonal contraceptives, for example, were derived from plants but are now made synthetically. The foreword to the 1994 English edition of Wechel states, "We are constantly aware that the majority of the world's population relies almost entirely on the traditional medicines which are mainly plant-based" (v).

Few of the herbal emmenagogues have been subjected to the rigid testing required for new pharmaceuticals, although there are now restrictions on their promotion and use. In the United Kingdom, the Pharmacy and Medicines Act of 1941 prohibited the advertising of any article in terms calculated to lead to its use as an abortifacient. In 1972 the Council of the Pharmaceutical Society of Great Britain listed preparations not to be supplied over the counter (MEP 1972:2054). Drugs for the relief of menstrual irregularities could be supplied by prescription only. In Third World countries, however, controls over dangerous drugs are not always enforced, so women can buy preparations that may be restricted elsewhere.

In the past, some drugs were tested in ways that now would be deemed ethically unacceptable. Current drug trials are carried out in strictly controlled conditions upon volunteer subjects. But in everyday use, in a noncontrolled environment, the results may not be the same, due to the different physical conditions under which the drug is used, the different behavioral and physiological responses of the user, varying adherence to the treatment regime, and unexpected, sometimes serious, side effects. In addition, trial subjects may not be representative of the general population. Thus theoretical effectiveness confirmed by laboratory testing (in vitro) is not always translated into use effectiveness (in vivo).

Test animals may differ from humans in their physiological responses, and they and their offspring are considered disposable, as opposed to human trial subjects. It does not follow that an herbal extract that exhibits an oxytocic effect in animals will be a safe, reliable uterine stimulant in women. Nor can we assume that because an herbal drug has not been tested, it has no antifertility effects.

Also to be considered are reversibility and whether the drug has teratogenic or cytotoxic effects. Indeed, one of the anxieties women have after an unsuccessful abortion is that the fetus may have been harmed. Women are inclined, wisely enough, to blame any birth defects on drugs taken or illness occurring during pregnancy. It was women themselves who drew the attention of the Australian ophthalmologist Norman McAlister Gregg to the link between German measles during early pregnancy and the occurrence of congenital blindness and other fetal deformities following an epidemic in Sydney in 1940 (Burgess 1991: 355–56).

The discovery that thalidomide taken during early pregnancy can have teratogenic effects on the fetus led to stricter controls on new drugs. The possible effects on pregnancy and the fetus must now be included in drug research.[4] All drug information must now carry a warning of any possible side effects in pregnancy, particularly teratogenic or abortifacient properties. In the past, such a warning might have encouraged women to conclude that the drug would be useful as an abortifacient. During the late nineteenth and early twentieth centuries, many advertisements for "quack" and even proprietary preparations for the "restoration of menses" and other benefits included such a warning, thus protecting the product from legal repercussions, yet at the same time suggesting that their main use was as an emmenagogue or abortifacient (see *The Lancet* 1898 and 1899).

In 1975, Farnsworth et al. reviewed the then-current literature on research into plants having a folkloric reputation as antifertility agents. They emphasized the potential value of plants as a source of new antifertility drugs (535), and distinguished between plants having contraceptive properties, including interceptives (interfering with implantation), and those having emmenagogic and abortifacient properties, including ecbolics and oxytocics (uterine stimulants). The researchers found that the terms *emmenagogue* and *abortifacient* were often used synonymously (547). They also found that many reports had not demonstrated the mechanism for the antifertility effect, lacked adequate controls, or did not allow for species variability. They ruled out drugs that act through direct cytotoxic effects on the fetus, unless they could be shown to be 100 percent effective, completely nontoxic, and nonteratogenic (739).

Farnsworth et al. found little information in the literature on the proven abortifacient properties of the herbs widely used in folk medicine as abortifacients and emmenagogues: tansy, pennyroyal, rue, apiol, and savin. The use of these drugs as abortifacients had been deleted from standard pharmacology textbooks (582). Tests had not shown that pennyroyal, savin, or tansy could stimulate the uterus; if abortion did occur, it was only after toxic doses, and even fatal doses were not always abortifacient. The researchers concluded that apiol and its combinations were "not consistently effective as abortifacients in humans" and carried high risks of toxicity and even death (583). Quinine did stimulate the uterus once contractions had started, but it did not act to expel the premature fetus. Of the 565 species of plants having a folkloric reputation for use as emmenagogues, ecbolics, or abortifacients, 225 showed uterine-muscle-stimulating properties, but only about a dozen had been tested in humans (583). Farnsworth et al. proposed a standard regime for systematic testing of folkloric antifertility drugs for contraceptive, interceptive, or abortifacient effects, involving a proper dosing schedule, adequate controls, and the use of more than one type of extract (744).

The WHO Special Program of Research, Development and Research Training in Human Reproduction (HRP) was set up in the early 1970s. It commented in 1984 that only 1 percent of higher plant species had been investigated biochemically. Few of these had been studied for bioactivity and potential therapeutic effects, although 25 percent of marketed drugs were derived from plants or plant-derived compounds (WHO 1984:66). No systematic evaluation of fertility regulating plants had been carried out.

The HRP established a university-based global network with a mandate "to identify plant-derived compounds that might be developed into new drugs that are capable of preventing or disrupting implantation in women or of inhibiting spermatogenesis or interfering with sperm maturation in men" (Griffin 1988:230). Plants whose mode of action could not be confirmed or which produced untoward side effects were excluded. The HRP found a need to separate antifertility effects of plant extracts from toxic ones, such as liver toxicity. Of the 10,908 written articles that were collected, only 386 were found to have relevance (ibid.:235). The Task Force was phased out in 1987, although the work on promising leads continued in individual centers. It is difficult for the WHO Human Reproduction Program to maintain its level of funding, because some governments are reluctant to be associated with research that might be related to abortion.

One must wonder whether the strong disapproval of contraception and abortion in medical circles has led to some drugs being wrongly labeled as ineffective or inadequately investigated in the past. During my medical course in the early 1940s, and for several generations of students, there was minimal information on birth control and abortion, and none on the use of emmenagogues and abortifacients.

Investigation of any drug having abortifacient or interceptive properties provokes strong resistance from antiabortion activists and threatens funding for contraceptive research. The threat of boycott of other products delayed the introduction of mifepristone (RU486) for medical abortion in Europe (Hunt 1992:13–24) and Australia (Siracusa 1995: 19–24). Restrictive legislation has been introduced into the Australian Parliament requiring special approval by the Minister for Health before any abortifacient drug can be imported into Australia.

We might conclude that throughout history, women have sought the means to "bring on the periods" or to control their fertility for very good medical and social reasons. Given the irregularity of menstruation even in normal women, probably few herbal drugs were effective as emmenagogues. Any success was probably fortuitous: the late period or early abortion would have occurred in any case. Taken at levels for inducing abortion, they were probably only effective in toxic doses or when accompanied by mechanical interference, which continues to cause high levels of maternal death and morbidity.

Research into emmenagogues and abortifacients has been burdened with moralistic and restrictive attitudes on the part of the churches, governments, and the medical profession. The advent of the contraceptive pill brought democratization and medicalization of contraceptive practice, facilitated by the rise of concerns of overpopulation. But as the chapters in this volume show, many women wishing to control their fertility—particularly if they live in developing countries—still lack access to cheap, safe, and reliable emmenagogues and abortifacients, are still prey to misinformation, and still have to rely on traditional remedies of dubious effectiveness.

NOTES

1. As recently as the 1940s–50s, more than one of my own patients confided to me that they regularly passed a knitting needle into the uterus each month to make sure the period would come, thus anticipating the practice of menstrual regulation. It should always be recognized that abortion not only saves a woman from an unwanted pregnancy, but also benefits other members of the family: it conserves the family income and protects family honor; conceals illicit love affairs; and protects men from the responsibilities of paternity.

2. Cottonseed oil (Gossypol) has been investigated as a male contraceptive following its folkloric reputation in China that it reduced fertility in men (WHO 1984:74–76). Although effective in reducing spermatogenesis, it had major side effects, which make it unacceptable for use as a contraceptive (Waites 1988:215). Gossypol remains experimental.

3. Quinine was widely used in spermicidal vaginal pessaries (e.g., Rendell's Pessaries) often made up by women themselves. MEP 1941 quotes a 1935 article in *The Lancet* which recommended that as more effective spermicides with less irritant side effects were now available, the time had come for the abandonment of quinine for contraceptive purposes.

4. Thalidomide, promoted in the 1950s for the relief of morning sickness in early pregnancy, was later found to have teratogenic effects resulting in gross limb deformities in the baby (McBride 1961:1358; Lenz 1962:45). The United States, which had escaped the thalidomide tragedy because it had not approved the drug, has only recently approved the use of thalidomide for leprosy treatment, but with strict warnings (Kettle 1998:29).

REFERENCES

Armstrong, G. 1904. "Evidence." In *Royal Commission on the Decline of the Birth-rate and on the Mortality of Infants in New South Wales,* vol. 2. Sydney: William Applegate Gullick, Government Printer.

Burgess, Margaret A. 1991. "Gregg's Rubella Legacy." *The Medical Journal of Australia* 155.

Davis, David. 1836. *The Principles and Practice of Obstetric Medicine in a Series of Systematic Dissertations on Midwifery, and on the Diseases of Women and Children,* vol. 1. London: Taylor and Walton.

Davis, G. 1974. *Interception of Pregnancy. Post-conceptive Fertility Control.* Sydney: Angus and Robertson.

Diczfalusy, Egon. 1987. "The History of Steroidal Contraception: What Is Past and What Is Present?" In *Safety Requirements for Contraceptive Steroids,* ed. F. Michal. Proceedings, Symposium on Improving Safety Requirements of Contraceptive Steroids, World Health Organization. Cambridge: Cambridge University Press.

Farnsworth, Norman R., Audrey S. Bingel, and Geoffrey A. Cordell, et al. 1975. "Potential Value of Plants as Sources of New Anti-fertility Agents." *Journal of Pharmaceutical Sciences,* pt. 1, vol. 64, no. 4:535–98; pt. 2, vol. 64, no. 5:717–54.

Francis, Anne. 1962. *A Guinea a Box.* London: Hale. Plate facing p. 81. Cited in Davis 1974:frontispiece.

Grieve, M. [1931] 1984. *A Modern Herbal.* Harmondsworth: Penguin.

Griffin, P. D. 1988. "Plants for Fertility Regulation." Chapter 13 in *Research in Human Reproduction: Biennial Report 1986–87,* edited by E. Diczfalusy, P. D. Griffin, and J. Khanna. Geneva: World Health Organization, pp. 229–39.

Himes, Norman E. 1936. *Medical History of Contraception.* Baltimore: Williams and Wilkins Company.

Hunt, Mary E. 1992. "RU 486/PG and Ethics." *Bioethics News,* 12:1. Reprinted from *Conscience* 13, no. 1.

IPPF (International Family Planning Federation). 1992. "Statement on Unsafe Abortion and Reproductive Health." *IPPF Medical Bulletin* 26(1).

Jamieson, J. 1888. "On the Frequency of Abortion in Victoria." *Australasian Medical Gazette* 1.

Jeffcoate, T.N.A. 1972. *Principles of Gynaecology.* 3d ed. London: Butterworth's.

Kettle, Martin. 1998. "Thalidomide Back on Sale, 35 Years On." *Sydney Morning Herald,* 18 July.

The Lancet. 1898, vol. 2; 1899, vol. 1. "Quacks and Abortion."

Lenz, W. 1962. "Thalidomide and Congenital Deformities." Letter, *The Lancet,* 6 January.

McBride, William. 1961. "Thalidomide and Congenital Deformities." Letter, *The Lancet,* 16 December.

MEP (Martindale *Extra Pharmacopeia*). 1941, 1972, 1993. London: Pharmaceutical Society of Great Britain.

Merck Index. 1989. 11th ed. Rahway, N.J.: Merck and Co.

Meyer, F. 1909. "Some Aspects of the Question of the Artificial Termination of Gestation." *Medical Journal of Australia* 14, no. 4:175–84.

Park, W. S. 1904. "Evidence." In *The Royal Commission on the Decline of the Birth-rate and on the Mortality of Infants in New South Wales,* vol. 2. Sydney: William Applegate Gullick, Government Printer.

PMMN (The Prevention of Maternal Mortality Network). 1992. "Barriers to Treatment of Obstetric Emergencies in Rural Communities of West Africa." *Studies in Family Planning* 23, no. 5:279–91.

Reid, J. 1979. " 'Women's Business,' Cultural Factors Affecting the Use of Family Planning Services in an Aboriginal Community." *Medical Journal of Australia,* vol. 1, no. 2; special supplement no. 11:1–4.

Riddle, John M. 1992. *Contraception and Abortion from the Ancient World to the Renaissance.* Cambridge, Mass: Harvard University Press.

Sharland, William. 1904. "Evidence." In *Royal Commission on the Decline of the Birth-rate and on the Mortality of Infants in New South Wales,* vol. 2. Sydney: William Applegate Gullick, Government Printer.

Shorter, Edward. 1983. *A History of Women's Bodies.* London: Allen Lane.

OED *(The Shorter Oxford English Dictionary on Historical Principles).* 1992. Ed. C. T. Onions. Oxford: Clarendon Press.

Siracusa, Joseph A. 1995. "Too Much Responsibility?" *Monash Bioethics Review* 14, no. 1, suppl.

Smyth, Brettena. 1893. *The Limitation of Offspring: Being the Substance of a Lecture Delivered in the North Melbourne Town Hall and Elsewhere, to a Large Audience of Women Only.* 8th ed. Melbourne: Rae Brothers.

Stevens, G. 1904. "Evidence." *Royal Commission on the Decline of the Birthrate and on the Mortality of Infants in New South Wales,* vol. 2. Sydney: William Applegate Gullick, Government Printer.

Taylor, Alfred Swaine. 1910. *The Principles and Practice of Medical Jurisprudence,* updated by Fred J. Smith. London: J. A. Churchill.

UNICEF (United Nations Children's Fund). 1998. *The State of the World's Children.* Oxford: Oxford University Press.

Waites, G. M. H. 1988. "Male Fertility Regulation." Chapter 2 in *Research in Human Reproduction: Biennial Report 1986–87,* edited by E. Diczfalusy, P. D. Griffin, and J. Khanna. Geneva: World Health Organization, pp. 199–223.

Wechel, Max, ed. 1994. *Herbal Drugs and Phytochemicals.* English version ed. Norman Grainger Bisset. Ann Arbor: CRC Press.

WHO (World Health Organization). 1984. Special Programme of Research, Development and Research Training in Human Reproduction. *Thirteenth Annual Report* (Draft). Geneva: WHO.

CHAPTER 6

Demography, Amenorrhea, and Fertility

Ina Warriner

We know nothing whatsoever about
interpopulation variation [in menstruation]
in the fertile period.

—James W. Wood, *Dynamics of Human
Reproduction*

The study of the relationship between irregular menstruation and fertility has attracted scholars from not only the field of medicine, but also a variety of other backgrounds, including demography, history, and anthropology. Historical medical texts of women's diseases devote substantial attention to what was then known as suppressed menses or menstrual retention, with a concomitant concern for fertility. Demographers' interest has traditionally focused on the debate surrounding the fertility outcomes of amenorrhea resulting from poor nutrition. Nonetheless, studies in demography have largely dismissed or trivialized the impact of secondary amenorrhea on fertility, unless it was caused by breast-feeding, and have generally excluded it from their models. A closer look at the prevalence of menstrual irregularity in populations before the discovery of oral contraceptives in 1960 and in developing countries today suggests that amenorrhea may be more widespread than is generally assumed and consequently should not be ignored when assessing variations in fertility.

In this chapter, I review the literature and data on secondary amenorrhea and consider the impact of this condition on fertility. Pathological secondary amenorrhea, shortened here to secondary amenorrhea, refers to the pathological absence of menstruation in women who previously experienced regular menstrual cycles; it is unrelated to lactational amenorrhea or postpartum amenorrhea.[1] Although studies indicate that a significant number of nonpregnant women experience delayed menses for a few days to a few weeks,[2] there is little, if any, quantification of the prevalence of menstrual irregularity in populations. Knowledge of the prevalence of secondary amenorrhea in populations also sheds light on the potential demand for emmenagogues. What, then, do the data tell us about irregularity in populations, what factors could contribute to amenorrhea, and what is their impact on fertility for women who wish to conceive?

I examine possible causes of secondary amenorrhea and hypothesize about their role in suppressing fertility, using the Bongaarts and Potter (1983) model as a framework for a sensitivity analysis. Fertility models in demography account for postpartum and lactational amenorrhea but do not consider the impact of amenorrhea from other causes. Factors that have been associated with delayed menses include age, nutrition, psychological factors, strenuous physical exertion, disease, and environmental factors such as seasonality. I focus in particular on women in developing countries and in historical populations where the prevalence of amenorrhea is greatest. Finally, I discuss the ways in which oral contraceptives have altered the rules of the game by "correcting" irregular menses, yet creating new forms of amenorrhea.

Little information is available on the prevalence of secondary amenorrhea; data on menstrual irregularity generally focus on variation in cycle length and amount of blood loss rather than on the incidence of irregular or infrequent menses. This chapter thus represents an initial attempt at consolidating the literature and data on the prevalence of secondary amenorrhea. The link between amenorrhea and fertility is predicated upon the assumption that amenorrhea is indicative of anovulation. Although this is not always the case, the connection between menstruation, which is easily detectable, and ovulation, which is much more difficult to detect, forms the basis of the literature on amenorrhea and fertility.

THE DEMOGRAPHERS' DEBATE

The earliest demographic writings on secondary amenorrhea and fertility single out irregularity in the context of malnutrition as a proximate determinant of infertility. The connection between pathological amenorrhea and fertility was first made in 1946 in an article in the journal *Population*. The author, Jean Meuvret (1946), a historian of the Old Regime in France, noted that food crises resulted in a decline in the number of baptisms recorded in parish registers.

This notion was later explored by Le Roy Ladurie (1975) in a widely quoted discussion of "famine amenorrhea." He found that there had been considerable interest in "war amenorrhea" in urban Germany during World War I as a result of low-calorie diets, and similarly, in occupied France during World War II, where it was estimated that between 4 and 7 percent of women of childbearing ages were affected. Le Roy Ladurie notes the surprise of physicians at that time when confronted with what was considered an abnormal phenomenon. Statistics from the Dutch hunger winter of 1944–45 and from concentration camps indicate much higher percentages of temporary amenorrhea as a result of extreme malnutrition. A similar increase in temporary amenorrhea occurred during the siege of Leningrad. Jacobs (1972) notes that approximately 60 percent of women in a concentration camp in Hong Kong during World War II were amenorrheic.

The link between sporadic episodes of malnutrition and lack of menstruation was carried further by Rose Frisch, who associated amenorrhea with chronic malnutrition and suppressed fertility (Frisch and Revelle 1970; Frisch and McArthur 1974). Her thesis was adopted by anthropologists trying to explain the low fertility of hunters and gatherers, on the basis of Nancy Howell Lee's studies of the Dobe !Kung. However, although it is intuitively appealing to connect malnutrition-induced amenorrhea with low fertility, later studies failed to support the theory.

Over time, demographers largely debunked the theory of malnutrition as a means of explaining low fertility (Bongaarts 1980; Menken, Trussell, and Watkins 1981). The controversy played itself out in several prestigious journals, and most scholars agree that nutrition has little or no effect on fertility. Prevailing scholarly opinion holds that nutritional status has an effect on the age of menarche, but not necessarily through this route on fertility, as age at marriage, adolescent subfecundity, stress, and fetal wastage are also relevant factors in reducing fertility (Bongaarts 1980; Menken, Trussell, and Watkins 1981; Riley, Samuelson, and Huffman 1993). However, because these conclusions were drawn from aggregate data, it is not possible to entirely dismiss a connection between malnutrition and low fertility at the individual level.

THE MENSTRUAL CYCLE AND
SECONDARY AMENORRHEA

Anovulation (of which amenorrhea is a sign) affects fecundability, the probability of conceiving, which in turn affects fertility, or the actual bearing of children. No universally applied standard exists for the minimum duration of secondary amenorrhea, and it is not always clear from an individual study how many cycles a woman has missed before being considered amenorrheic. The absence of menstruation for at least 1 cycle is generally accepted as indicative of amenorrhea, although it is sometimes defined as the cessation of menses for 6 months or more. This divergence in definitions reflects the ambiguity in the literature, past and present, and acknowledges the concern that even 1 missed or delayed cycle may elicit in women.

The menstrual cycle, or ovarian cycle, is the result of a series of coordinated events that take place in different locations of the female body. If any hormonal event in the cycle occurs abnormally or fails to occur, amenorrhea may result. True menstrual retention, a rare event, occurs when an obstruction such as a congenital imperforate hymen, a blind double uterus, or an adhesion prevents the menstrual buildup from exiting. The menstrual cycle is an extremely complex system based on the precise interplay of a series of hormonal secretions; only a brief sketch will be provided here.

The cycle is traditionally divided into 2 phases based on changes that occur in the ovaries: the follicular phase, which is preovulatory, and the luteal, or postovulatory, phase. If a cycle lasts 28 days, each phase takes approximately 14 days to complete. Conventionally, the first day of menstrual bleeding is considered the first day of the menstrual cycle because it presents an obvious marker. At the start of the cycle, levels of estrogen and progesterone are low and the hormonally matured endometrial lining of the uterus begins to shed. In the ovaries, several follicles begin growing, one of which will produce the single mature oocyte (egg) for that cycle. Follicle growth is triggered by the aptly named follicle stimulating hormone (FSH), secreted by the pituitary gland, and gonadotropin-releasing hormone (GnRH), secreted from the hypothalamus. The hypothalamus plays a crucial role in regulating the ovarian cycle through the intermittent, or pulsing, secretion of GnRH.

As the follicle and its oocyte mature, the follicle produces increasing amounts of estrogen that stimulate the release of luteinizing hormone (LH) from the pituitary gland. Once estrogen production has reached a significant threshold, a sudden surge of LH occurs, about 36 hours before ovulation takes place. The spike in LH also stimulates the production of enzymes that rupture the follicle and expel the oocyte. The luteal phase of the ovarian cycle begins once the follicle has ruptured and takes on a new identity as a corpus luteum. The corpus luteum secretes estrogen and progesterone, a function that continues for a mean length of about 14 days. At this point, unless pregnancy occurs, estrogen and progesterone levels rapidly decline and the shedding of the uterine lining (menstruation) begins anew, signaling the start of a new cycle (Ferin, Jewelewicz, and Warren 1993; Hatcher et al. 1994).

If the hormonal events in the weeks leading up to menstruation do not occur normally, the shedding of the endometrium may not follow the regular pattern, or it may not take place at all, resulting in amenorrhea, the absence of menstrual function. An abnormal event in the follicular phase will have a deleterious effect on the luteal phase and on the development of the corpus luteum, which would impede menstruation. On occasion, an "especially exuberant" corpus luteum does not degenerate on schedule and develops into an ovarian cyst that continues to secrete estrogen and progesterone (Hatcher et al. 1994). This can inhibit the shedding of the endometrium for weeks or months. Another starting point for menstrual disruption is the hypothalamus, which, in response to factors such as stress and starvation, alters the pulsing of GnRH.

One particular kind of abnormal ovarian cycle is an anovulatory cycle, in which no oocyte is released. This may happen if the follicle fails to rupture or is empty, or the ovum remains entrapped in the follicle as a result of impaired follicular development or endocrine failure (Baird 1985; Healy, Trounson, and Andersen 1994). In some cases, a long cycle (which may be perceived as amenorrhea) is the result of extra time needed for follicular development. A long cycle may also be the product of 2 successive defective short cycles. This occurs when the oocyte is not fully matured and the follicular development is aborted. If one anovulatory cycle follows another in quick succession before withdrawal bleeding can occur, a series of anovulatory cycles may give the appearance of one very long cycle (Wood 1994).

Delayed menses may also be the result of unobserved early pregnancy loss. Various studies have attempted to estimate the probability of early fetal loss between fertilization and implantation and have produced probabilities varying from .08 (Whittaker, Taylor, and Lind 1983) to .43 (Miller et al. 1980) to .57 (Edmonds et al. 1982). These varying results reflect differences in procedures and criteria for defining pregnancy, and sampling errors. Wilcox et al. (1988) found a loss of 22 percent of clinically unrecognized pregnancies by highly sensitive immunoassay, excluding fertilized eggs that failed to implant.

Wilcox et al.'s (1988) study of the incidence of clinically unrecognized loss of pregnancy using hormonal criteria found that very early loss of pregnancy was associated with some delay in the onset of menses and with a slight increase in cycle length. The median length for cycles experiencing early loss was 32 days, in contrast with a median of 29 days for cycles in which no pregnancy occurred. Thus, pregnancy loss at this very early stage does not appear to have an effect on fertility. It is possible, however, that such small delays reflect an underlying problem that may ultimately lead to lower fertility. It is not clear whether very early loss of pregnancy occurs randomly throughout populations or if certain women are more likely to experience it than others.

SECONDARY AMENORRHEA AND FERTILITY

Far from being a consistent process, menstrual cycles vary for individual women, between women of the same population, and between women from different populations. And yet, when demographers model fertility levels, variation in the ovarian cycle is only implicitly taken into account through variations in fecundability. Fertility and fecundability models invariably use a period of 28 days as the length of the menstrual cycle for women of all ages; to incorporate variation in sophisticated deterministic models is extraordinarily complex, not the least because the distribution of various kinds of amenorrhea in a population is poorly documented and understood (see Leridon 1993 for a discussion of using data on amenorrhea to estimate fecundability and postpartum sterility). Moreover, medical researchers stress that "the clinical significance of . . . abnormal cycles as causes of infertility remains to be elucidated" (Healy, Trounson, and Andersen 1994: 1539).

   Although a cycle length of 28 days represents a mean found in many populations for which data exist, it masks considerable heterogeneity in menstrual cycles and ignores the possibility of sporadic pathological amenorrhea. Scholars suggest that the assumption of a regular, non-amenorrheic, 28-day cycle is likely to skew our understanding of fertility in historical populations and for women in developing countries today. Santow (1978:45) notes in her study of fertility models that fecundability estimates may be affected by menstrual abnormalities in a fraction of the population. Wood (1994:150) stresses that interpopulation variation in the fertile period "may exert a remarkably large influence on birth spacing via its effect on fecundability."

   Bongaarts and Potter (1983) proposed a demographic model distinguishing 5 reproductive states: single (e.g., not sexually active), post-partum infecundable, fecundable, pregnant, and permanently sterile. The single state and the sterile state flank both ends of the reproductive years. The 3 remaining stages form the reproductive cycle and are the main components of the birth interval in the absence of intrauterine mortality. The postpartum infecundable interval is largely determined by the duration and intensity of breast-feeding. The second component is the waiting time to conception, which is a function of fecundability, and the third component is full-term pregnancy.

In this model, amenorrhea could appear in 4 ways. First, an unrecognized early pregnancy may be perceived as secondary amenorrhea. Second, secondary amenorrhea could occur outside of a closed birth interval, typically affecting the first or last births of younger or older women respectively. In the case of young women, primary amenorrhea that occurs during the waiting time to conception before a first birth could increase the age at first birth. At the other end of the reproductive cycle, secondary amenorrhea setting in before menopause could reduce the proportion of years spent in the fecund period and hence could depress overall fertility by a birth or two. Third, pathological amenorrhea occurring during the postpartum infecundable interval would lengthen it beyond the normal effect of breast-feeding. Finally, it could appear as part of the fecundable period, if menstruation is interrupted or delayed after a first postpartum ovulation. In each interval of the reproductive period, with the exception of sterility, amenorrhea would prolong the time to conception. The cumulative effect of a lifetime of episodes of irregularity could conceivably affect a women's completed family size.

DATA: WHAT INFORMATION DO WE HAVE?

Relatively few empirical studies have been directed at gathering data on menstrual patterns, much less on the phenomenon of secondary amenorrhea. Empirical evidence of the incidence of infrequent menses in current populations is sparse and is impossible to gather from historical populations. A few studies of Western women indicate relatively low levels of secondary amenorrhea, although there is considerable variation. A 1934 study of women attending the Birth Control Clinical Research Bureau, directed by Margaret Sanger, found that 20 percent of women seeking birth control experienced irregular intervals between menses. These results cannot be generalized, however, given the obvious selection problem. An early attempt by Frances Drew to gather information on the prevalence of amenorrhea was limited to 3 bodies of nonrepresentative literature: medical studies of endocrinology, psychiatric literature, and concentration camp studies (Jacobs 1972). Results ranged from 1.6 percent amenorrhea among gynecological patients to 100 percent amenorrhea among female prisoners awaiting execution.

In a more recent study of 734 urban women, randomly chosen from a population in Warsaw, Poland, Skierska, Leszczynska-Bystrzanowska, and Gajewski (1996) found a frequency of secondary amenorrhea of 0.3 percent. However, in a study of 3,743 women, aged 15 to 44 years and selected at random from the county of Copenhagen, Denmark, prevalence of secondary amenorrhea of more than 3 months' duration was 4.6 percent (Munster, Helm, and Schmidt 1992). The duration of secondary amenorrhea was 6 months or less in 75 percent of women aged 15 to 34 years, but longer than 6 months in 55 percent of those aged 35 to 44 years. There is often some ambiguity in the collection of data on secondary amenorrhea. Even data on postpartum or lactational amenorrhea are not without problems. As Leridon (1993) notes, "[I]s the return of menses such a clear-cut event, especially for women who are undernourished or in poor health? Spotting and other bleeding episodes can be confused with the return of regular menses."

In the past, medical authors were often preoccupied with the abnormal phenomenon of pathological amenorrhea and devoted entire chapters to the topic (see, for example, Garrigues (1900) and Longshore-Potts (1896). Texts referring to "suppressed menses" appear early in antiquity, and the subject has been written about throughout human history. Not surprisingly, however, historical texts do not provide population-level estimates of various kinds of amenorrhea, so the full extent of the phenomenon can only be guessed at. Today, secondary amenorrhea continues to remain relatively undocumented, perhaps as a consequence of the discovery of the regulating properties of synthetic hormones that have reduced the need for greater understanding of menstrual irregularity.

Our understanding of variability in the menstrual cycle is largely drawn from 3 large-scale menstrual diary studies conducted in North America (Chiazze et al. 1968; Treloar et al. 1967; Vollman 1977).[3] Although these data sets provide a wealth of information about normal parameters of the menstrual cycle, they provide little information about menstrual abnormalities.[4] Because only healthy, noncontracepting, regularly menstruating women were accepted as subjects in the studies, the data are drawn from a nonrepresentative population and are restricted to normal patterns of menstruation.

A great weakness of the data in terms of secondary amenorrhea is that published reports generally present findings from cleaned data, from which all abnormal cycles or potentially abnormal cycles were eliminated. In the Treloar data, for example, if a woman experienced surgery, a major illness, or drug use, the data for that particular cycle were designated "anormal (sic) in the sense that there was reason to suspect it *might* be so. . . . Special study of anormal (sic) menstrual intervals is not appropriate to this paper" (Treloar et al. 1967: 81). Although the amount of data lost was not large (only about 1 percent), no effort was made to determine if, in fact, the cycles were abnormal or entirely missing. A recent study omitted 6 percent of women from its sample for similar reasons: "cases deemed to be anomalous were purposefully left out; these included cycles lasting for more than a hundred days, mono-phasic cycles, those coinciding with illnesses, and cycles with an incomplete record" (Monari and Montanari 1998).[5]

Given these shortcomings, what do these studies of menstruation tell us about the prevalence of secondary amenorrhea? Unfortunately, not a great deal. A major focus of studies of the menstrual cycle is variation in cycle length. That normal, healthy ovarian cycles vary in length is the rule, not the exception. Chiazze et al. (1968) found that 95 percent of the women in their sample had an average cycle length of 25 to 37 days, indicating considerable variation among women. Treloar et al. (1967) found that the average cycle length varied from 24 to 37 days at 20 years of age and declined to 23 to 32 days at 40 years of age. Collett, Wertenberger, and Fiske (1954) studied 302 complete cycles from 146 women and found substantial cycle variation, ranging from 16 to 41 days for women aged 20 to 39 years. Are longer cycles typical for the women who experience them, or do they reflect intermittent episodes of amenorrhea? Chiazze et al. (1968:380) note that longer cycles occur sporadically among women but that "reasons for reported long cycles are unclear. The extent to which factors such as missed periods, spontaneous abortion, and reporting errors are operative cannot be evaluated."

A longer ovarian cycle may mask a variety of biological processes, but available data on cycle length rarely distinguish between unusually long but physiologically successful cycles and defective cycles or early fetal wastage. Delayed menses due to an unrecognized early pregnancy are undoubtedly widespread. However, such data are impossible to recoup from the past and are rarely available for contemporary poor, high-fertility populations of the Third World. Reporting errors may also create the false impression of a longer cycle.

INTERPOPULATION AND ETHNIC DIFFERENCES

Menstrual cycles in non-Western women have received far less attention and are less well documented than those of Caucasians, "leaving unanswered the question of whether significant interpopulation differences exist in either cycle length or cycle quality. . . . Not surprisingly, we know nothing whatsoever about interpopulation variation in the fertile period" (Wood 1994:138).[6] The majority of menstruation studies undertaken in developing countries have focused on determining the mean age at menarche rather than assessing the prevalence of menstrual disorders and irregularity in a population. Moreover, studies in developing countries frequently use menstrual data from educated women, who are highly unlikely to be representative of all women in the nation (see, for example, Thomas, Okonofua, and Chiboka 1990 for a study of menstrual patterns among Nigerian university women).

The few studies that exist of the menstrual cycles of nonindustrial and nonurban women suggest cycles that are significantly different from those of Western women. A study of the menstrual diaries of 36 rural women in Papua New Guinea found that they experienced cycles that were about 40 percent longer than their North American counterparts (Johnson et al. 1987). A study of women in Zaire found a higher frequency of anovulatory cycles than in Western women and a significantly shorter length of menstrual bleeding than in U.S. women (Ellison, Peacock, and Lager 1989). The cycles of women of all reproductive ages in Bangladesh exhibit greater variability in length than cycles among women in developed nations, perhaps reflecting higher rates of fetal losses or lower proportions of ovulatory cycles (Menken 1975).

The extent to which various reproductive disorders, spontaneous abortions, chronic illness, malnutrition, and other stressors contribute to variations in the menstrual cycle among women in non-Western populations is unknown. Indeed, in past populations and in many developing countries today, menstruation is a fairly infrequent event, given frequent pregnancies and lactational and postpartum amenorrhea. In a study of Mayan Indian women in Mexico, one woman stated that she had not menstruated in 15 years because she had been either pregnant or breast-feeding (Beyene 1992). However, it is possible that, unbeknownst to her, other factors such as disease may have contributed to her amenorrhea. In sum, we know very little about the menstrual cycles of women in historical and developing countries, where the interaction between disease, nutrition, and physical exertion is most acute. The literature provides tantalizing suggestions of important interpopulation and ethnic differences in menstruation that warrant further exploration.

FACTORS ASSOCIATED WITH SECONDARY AMENORRHEA

We now turn to factors that may cause amenorrhea and anovulation in the absence of pregnancy. As researchers note, "[T]here are numerous conditions under which the menstrual cycle may become abnormal, that is, irregular, lengthened, shortened, anovulatory, or simply absent" (Ferin, Jewelewicz, and Warren 1993:114). What, then, could contribute to these delays? To what extent do these delays and missed menses suppress fertility?

Potential factors include age, nutritional status, disease, psychological influences, exercise, and environmental influences. However, only age and episodes of malnutrition have been considered by demographers as factors affecting fertility. Other factors that may have a salient impact on secondary amenorrhea, and hence anovulation, in historical populations and in developing countries today include infectious diseases, chronic malnutrition, strenuous manual labor, and sleep deprivation as a result of long hours of work.

Age

The most obvious factor associated with primary and secondary amenorrhea is age, a relationship that is recognized in demographic models of fertility. Patterns of menstruation are most clearly affected by gynecological age, defined as the time since menarche, rather than chronological age (Becker 1993; Wood 1994). It is possible that secondary amenorrhea is of particular concern to very young women (a fact that is confirmed in the literature of the past) and in women approaching the end of their fecund life.

The probability of a cycle being defective in any way is greatest during the years following menarche and rises again during the 5 years preceding menopause. Collett, Wertenberger, and Fiske's (1954) study of 146 women found greatest menstrual variations among women aged 17 to 19 years (including frequent anovulatory cycles) and 40 to 50 years. The development of the mature menstrual cycle is gradual and prone to irregularity in the years following menarche, when up to 50 percent of cycles may be anovulatory (Baird 1985; Petersen 1980). Munster, Helm, and Schmidt (1992) found the 1-year period prevalence of secondary amenorrhea of more than 3 months' duration among Danish women to be 7.6 percent, 3.0 percent, and 3.7 percent for women aged 15–24, 25–34, and 35–44 years respectively.

The effect of age on fertility through menstrual irregularity has been explicitly acknowledged in fertility models. The Bongaarts model excludes the years immediately following menarche and sets the upper limit of fecundability in the years just preceding menopause. Amenorrhea at both ends of the reproductive years is thus incorporated into the model, and its effects on fertility are considered rather small.

Nutrition

Researchers presently agree that only the most extreme cases of malnutrition will cause irregularity, and even severe malnutrition generally provokes only temporary amenorrhea. Famines leave a mark on the fertility curve, although the exact mechanism on lowering fertility is fairly complex. In the world today, the most malnourished populations also have the highest levels of fertility. Other factors, therefore, are clearly more important in suppressing fertility than the quality and quantity of caloric intake. To the effect of suddenly lowered calorie diets must be added loss of libido, separation from the spouse in times of famine, stress, and illness. One study of the Dutch famine of 1945 found that women who first experienced a cessation of menses during famine were likely to have been poorly nourished prior to the event (Stein and Susser 1975).

In a review of age at menarche, nutrition, and fertility, Riley, Samuelson, and Huffman (1993:61) conclude that "there is no strong evidence in the literature to support the hypothesis that nutritional status has a significant impact on fertility." Rahman and Menken (1993:67) reviewed studies from Bangladesh and New Guinea indicating that malnutrition may depress the age at menopause and conclude that "nutrition appears to play a role in determining age at menopause, but this relationship has not been clearly delineated."

Although malnutrition is an integral part of the history of humanity, the reproductive function is robust; we have been made efficient converters of energy through natural selection (Menken, Trussell, and Watkins 1981). The female body adjusts remarkably quickly to severe conditions, and menstruation, but perhaps not ovulation, generally resumes after a period of amenorrhea. Although some effects of malnutrition on fertility may persist, including subfecundity, spontaneous abortion, difficult birthing process, longer postpartum amenorrhea, and the shortening of the reproductive period at both ends, these effects are relatively minor. Thus the direct effect of malnutrition-induced amenorrhea on fertility is essentially minimal except in cases of famine, and even then the relationship is mitigated by other factors.

Disease

Interest in the relationship between nutrition and menstrual irregularity may have led demographers to neglect another cause of secondary amenorrhea. Physicians recognize that chronic disease and acute spells of illness result in irregularity. It is understandable that women in the past and in developing countries where mortality was high and the health status of the population was relatively poor, may have interpreted the cessation of menses as a cause rather than a consequence of illness.

Early textbooks on gynecology are replete with references to diseases or conditions that either lead to amenorrhea or are caused by it. One text from the turn of the century mentions amenorrhea as a "sequel of debilitating diseases, such as anemia, phthisis, malaria, typhoid fever, diabetes, or chronic mercurial poisoning" (Garrigues 1900:256). Discussion of these observations from the past barely exists in present-day biomedical literature; instead, exotic and rare conditions retain the interest of medical researchers.[7] Very little is known about the effect of common infectious diseases, such as malaria, tuberculosis, diarrhea, and fever, on the menstrual cycle.

McFalls and McFalls's (1984) review of disease and fertility is thorough and meticulous, yet it contains only a handful of references on the effect of disease on menstruation, reflecting a lack of knowledge and data on the subject. Instead, they focus on other pathways between disease and fertility, including coital frequency, fetal loss, and sexually transmitted diseases. Nonetheless, their extensive study brings together what is known about the impact of infectious diseases on menstruation and provides some indication of the magnitude of disease-related amenorrhea.

Tuberculosis has long been considered a cause of amenorrhea, and the connection has been cited in numerous gynecological studies. In 1943, Wharton notes that "amenorrhea is common in pulmonary tuberculosis and other acute and chronic illnesses" (107). As recently as

1975, Amiel notes that "pulmonary tuberculosis is one of the more important chronic illnesses associated with amenorrhea" (850). However, a recent text points specifically to genital tuberculosis as a cause of premature sterility in developing countries (Rahman and Menken 1993). Genital tuberculosis generally causes amenorrhea through damage or destruction of the endometrium, which leads to amenorrhea in 5 to 50 percent of all cases (Durgamba, Swany, and Rao 1972; Rozin 1968). Some researchers believe that genital tuberculosis was a significant cause of subfecundity in numerous historical populations (Gray 1977; McFalls and McFalls 1984).

Several other diseases common in developing countries have been linked to amenorrhea and are discussed by McFalls and McFalls. Filariasis, thought to affect more than 100 million people worldwide, may cause menstrual disorders and create an inhospitable endometrial environment, which may impede implantation and maintenance of a pregnancy. Schistosomiasis, affecting perhaps 200 million people, has also been implicated in menstrual disorders, including scanty menses, delayed menarche, and early menopause when the parasites lodge in the reproductive organs, which occurs in one-third to one-half of infected women (Charlewood 1956; Gilbert 1943). The Gambian sleeping sickness has been associated with menstrual dysfunction and amenorrhea, since it often attacks the endocrine system (WHO 1979).

Some studies of women suffering from schizophrenia and manic-depressive psychoses provide data on the prevalence of amenorrhea. These estimates range from 15 percent (Shader, Nahum, and DiMascio 1970), 33 percent (Israel 1967), and 30 to 40 percent (Siegler 1944). However, because relatively few women suffer from these mental illnesses (about 1 percent worldwide, according to McFalls 1979), it is unlikely that the prevalence of amenorrhea from psychiatric disorders has an important effect on fertility at the population level.

Documentation of the prevalence of disease-induced amenorrhea is scanty, due to underreporting and misreporting, unrepresentativeness, and the absence of normal values, particularly for women living in developing countries (McFalls and McFalls 1984). Perhaps also because it has ceased to be a significant problem in developed countries, it no longer attracts the attention of medical researchers. This may be due in part to easy treatment of menstrual irregularity with hormones but also to better treatment in the developed world of diseases that cause amenorrhea. A case in point is diabetes, which has historically been associated with amenorrhea, with 50 percent of diabetic women experiencing a total cessation of menses (Gold 1968). Today, insulin treatment not only brings on menstruation, but diabetic women also conceive and bear children.

The impact of disease on fertility through menstruation is undoubtedly underestimated if the aforementioned data provide any indication of the power of disease to disrupt the menstrual cycle. It is not surprising that women may have perceived a synergistic effect of disease and menstruation, believing that disease may cause amenorrhea and that amenorrhea contributed to disease. Given the absence of population data on disease and menstruation, it is impossible to determine the impact of disease on fertility through this means. Much better documented is the impact of disease on fertility through other means such as sexually transmitted diseases and fetal loss. It is, however, undoubtedly safe to say that disease may lengthen the waiting time to conception in susceptible populations if regular function of the hormones is jeopardized.

Psychological Influences

Relatively little research has been conducted on the psychological correlates of secondary amenorrhea. Nonetheless, there is accumulating evidence of the role of emotional and psychological factors in menstrual disorders, with amenorrhea representing one outcome of such disturbances. In a study of a random sample of amenorrheic and non-amenorrheic Swedish women, Fries, Nillius, and Petterson (1974) found that the amenorrheic women had experienced a higher incidence of stressful life events. Experiencing abnormal menstrual cycles or cessation of the menses can in itself result in psychological stress, which may in turn exacerbate irregularity, a situation perhaps not uncommon in the past and in many countries today.

Stress and fear are the primary psychological causes of amenorrhea (Coldsmith 1979). The menstrual cycle can be disrupted by an acute trauma such as rape, chronic stress, or relatively minor life events such as travel, courtship, exams, and other changes in the status quo (Amiel 1975; McFalls 1979; Saunders and Reinisch 1992). Periods of psychological stress have been linked to amenorrhea among college students in the United States (Osofsky and Fisher 1967; Siegel, Johnson, and Saranson 1979), a phenomenon that has also been observed among college students in Nigeria, particularly around the time of exams (Thomas, Okonofua, and Chiboka 1990). Many researchers now think that "war amenorrhea" is caused more by fear and anxiety than by malnutrition (Ihalainen 1975). It is not unusual for women to become amenorrheic when their husbands leave for war or when subjected to the stress of bombing raids (Rutherford 1965). The extent to which psychological factors affect menstruation in rural and non-Westernized women has not been studied.

Although there is less empirical support for the assessment of amenorrhea as a symbolic symptom of psychosexual conflict, the literature on psychoanalytic theory provides a rich source of explanations for irregular or missing menses. Some researchers view amenorrhea as a desire to avoid the adult female sexual role and pregnancy, while others view it as a rejection of femininity (Jacobs 1972; Saunders and Reinisch 1992). Others speculate that a fear of pregnancy or, conversely, intense longing for pregnancy can be an important determinant of amenorrhea (Israel 1967). This outlook is supported in historical medical texts, which frequently view secondary amenorrhea in psychosexual terms.

Exercise and Labor

Strenuous exercise can have a substantial effect on the ovarian cycle, causing delayed menarche, anovulatory cycles, and amenorrhea, all of which have been well documented in the literature (Cumming 1993; Davis 1997). Intensive athletic training may lead to changes in hypothalamic activity and to reduced pulsing frequency of GnRH, which can alter or eliminate menstruation. Sports amenorrhea may be related not only to the physical rigors of training but also to the emotional stress of competition, although the evidence is inconclusive (Cumming 1993). The impact of exercise on menstruation is exacerbated when weight loss is included.

It is, however, questionable to generalize subfecundity outcomes from extremely fit Western women with a low percentage of body fat to women in developing countries faced with strenuous daily exertion and poor diets. Studies of women having sports amenorrhea provide a weak proxy for malnourished, weakened women working long hours in the field or walking miles to collect firewood. Riley, Samuelson, and Huffman's (1993:51) comment about exercise and menarche is applicable to women of all reproductive ages: "Of particular interest is the daily activity of adolescent females in developing countries, such as carrying wood and water, harvesting, and pounding grain. These activities require considerable energy expenditure and strength, but do not place the same demands on the cardiovascular and muscular skeletal systems as do the athletic activities assessed in [Western] studies."

Unfortunately, very little is known about physical conditioning and menstruation in women in developing countries. A few studies provide some evidence that lifestyles of women in developing countries may be associated with infrequent menses. Researchers have theorized that the chronic, reversible, nonlactational ovulatory suppression experienced by the !Kung San women of southern Africa may be an adaptation to the needs of the hunter-gatherer; amenorrhea is necessary to space births so that a mother can walk 20 to 30 kilometers a day carrying a child. If, hypothetically, conception occurred every 24 months, the mother would be unable to meet the needs of her family, since carrying more than one child would limit the distance she could walk and her ability to bend and dig (Lee 1979; Prior 1996). Population data on the prevalence of such episodes of amenorrhea are unknown, however, so it is not clear whether hardworking women in other parts of the world experience similar kinds of amenorrhea.

The number of women affected by adaptive mechanisms to suppress the menstrual cycle under strenuous physical conditions is not known. However, studies of Western female athletes indicate that menstrual disruption is severe under conditions of rigorous training and weight loss, conditions not unfamiliar to past populations and to women living in rural areas in developing countries today.

Environmental Influences

A few intriguing studies have looked at the impact of seasonality and latitude on menstrual cycle variation. A study of menstrual cycles in an Alaskan village found significant seasonal variation in menstrual cycles and a widespread pattern of secondary seasonal amenorrhea (Graham, Stewart, and Ward 1992). The results of pregnancy tests given over a 2-year period to 273 women showed that 50 percent of the women were experiencing nonpregnancy amenorrhea. These cases were significantly associated with increasing hours of darkness and were the source of extreme anxiety for the women affected. In the absence of survey data, the full extent of seasonal amenorrhea of this sort is unknown.[8]

POST-1960: NEW ISSUES, NEW CONCERNS

Western populations have largely forgotten many of the menstrual problems associated with nutrition, disease, and long hours of arduous manual labor. Along with modernization, the synthetic production of various hormones has changed the rules of the game. As Ferin, Jewelewicz, and Warren (1993:166) note, "[M]edical induction of ovulation has been one of the most successful treatments in gynecologic endocrinology in the last 30 years, and is used extensively." Regulating hormones are sometimes prescribed for young women who suffer from menstrual irregularities. The increasingly popular hormonal treatment of perimenopause will, over time, obscure the observation of natural menopause.

Today, erratic or missing menses elicit much less concern than in the past. Modern medical textbooks often downplay the clinical significance of infrequent menses, particularly among adolescents. One textbook notes, "[W]hen there is merely infrequent spotting or staining, or late and delayed periods that are not very long or profuse, the physical significance is negligible" (Sturgis 1976:543). Because of the efficacy of hormones in regulating menstruation, research attention has focused on extreme cases of menstrual irregularity. Problems of the menstrual cycle that retain much attention concern anorexia nervosa, bulimia, and the amenorrhea of ballet dancers and athletes. These self-induced conditions, affecting relatively few women, receive more attention in the literature than that of poor women toiling in the Third World.

Somewhat ironically, in the changed world of synthetic hormones, new forms of "amenorrhea" have emerged. Injectable and oral contraceptives suppress not only ovulation but frequently withdrawal bleeding as well. Amenorrhea is very common during the 13-week interval of injectable protection and may continue for up to 8 months after the final injection (Davis 1997). Potter (in this volume) describes pill-induced "amenorrhea" that occurs if pills are taken continuously without a break between regimes. This is not truly a case of amenorrhea, since the ovarian cycle does not take place while a woman is on the pill. Nevertheless, this new kind of amenorrhea is now within the control of women and has no harmful side effects. The discontinuation of oral contraceptives may lead to a period of postpill amenorrhea of 6 to 10 weeks, although prolonged incidence of this type of amenorrhea is very low.

SECONDARY AMENORRHEA AND FERTILITY OUTCOMES

A review of the literature indicates that secondary amenorrhea is likely to affect most women at some point in their lives. Is any of the variation in ovarian cycles likely to have a discernible impact on fertility? This question has gained importance following the 1995 United Nations Population and Development meeting in Cairo, during which reproductive health was emphasized over fertility decline. In the case of secondary amenorrhea, improvements in women's reproductive health may contribute to increased fertility through shorter delays to conception. Following Bongaarts's decomposition of a woman's reproductive years into 5 successive phases, it is clear that secondary amenorrhea can manifest itself at any point in the reproductive cycle, lengthening any or all of the 5 segments. Under certain conditions, such as in populations with large numbers of chronically ill women facing daily physical demands, widespread secondary amenorrhea may help explain some variation in fertility. Let us first consider the impact of delayed menarche and early menopause on fertility.

The debate over whether delayed menarche, or primary amenorrhea, reduces overall fertility in natural fertility populations remains inconclusive but leans toward a negative finding. Riley, Samuelson, and Huffman (1993:60) conclude that "whether or not delays in menarche . . . translate into lower fertility in chronically under-nourished women is debatable." Since very few societies practice marriage before menarche, changes in age at menarche in these populations are not likely to have a generalizable impact on fertility and are therefore not likely to have an important demographic impact.

In some developing societies, marriage follows menarche after a period of approximately 3 years (Riley, Samuelson, and Huffman 1993). This raises the question of whether an upward shift in menarche would affect age at first birth, which could have some impact on total fertility. An interesting study by Foster et al. (1986) investigated age at menarche and age at first birth in Bangladesh and found *shorter* intervals for those experiencing late menarche. If these results can be extended to other populations, then a delay in menarche has no impact on fertility. Since the age at marriage in historical European populations was not tied to menarche, changes in the age at menarche in the past (which was generally quite high) would not have had an effect on fertility.

Our understanding of the effect of secondary amenorrhea on fertility at the end of a woman's reproductive life is similarly inconclusive. Rahman and Menken (1993) considered the impact of early menopause on fertility and conclude that "the extent to which disease and reproductive impairment contribute to [differentials in menopause] is not known" (82). They also note that countries having the highest levels of infecund women in their forties also have the highest levels of fertility, indicating that the link between early-onset sterility and fertility is not direct, but that many other factors contribute to the discrepancy. The relatively modest reduction in anovulatory cycles and corpus luteum failure in premenopausal women contrasts sharply with the major de-

Table 6.1   Standard Values of Proximate Determinants of Natural Fertility (in Years)

Age at marriage	22.5
Age at end of childbearing years	40.0
Duration of postpartum infecundability	1.0
Time added by intrauterine mortality	0.15
Standard gestation	0.75
Conception delay	0.60 (7.2 months)

SOURCE: Bongaarts and Potter 1983.

cline in fertility. Thus, ovarian cycle abnormalities reflect only a small proportion of the fertility decline, and increases in amenorrhea at the premenopausal stage are unlikely to affect fertility.

If primary amenorrhea and early menopause have a negligible impact on fertility, what of delays in the time to conception? Reductions in the probability of conception could lengthen the period of fecundability, postpartum amenorrhea, and lactational amenorrhea. These delays could be caused by any of the factors discussed earlier, including early fetal loss. Wood and Weinstein (1988) developed a model of age-specific fecundability, or the probability of conception, with a fixed reference period of 1 month, rather than 1 cycle, which permits modifications in cycle length. Assuming maximal coital exposure of at least 1 daily act of unprotected intercourse during the fertile period, the authors found that increasing cycle length at every age by 50 percent reduced fecundability by 20.9 percent; in addition, reducing ovulatory cycles by 50 percent reduced fecundability by 40.7 percent. Wood (1994:317) sums up the study by noting that "the sensitivity tests suggest that fetal loss, anovulatory cycles, the length of the fertile period, and the probability of conception within the fertile period are all potentially important sources of heterogeneous fecundability."

Applying a similar sensitivity test to the Bongaarts and Potter (1983) fertility model results in reductions in the total fertility rate. The proximate determinants of fertility and the standard values (in years) used in the Bongaarts and Potter model are presented in table 6.1. Using these values, which represent the average of a range of values from different natural fertility populations, the total fertility rate is 7 births per woman. This number is the quotient of the 17.5-year childbearing span divided by a mean birth interval of 2.5 years (the sum of a 1-year period of postpartum infecundability, 0.6 years of delay to conception during the fecundable period, 0.15 years of intrauterine mortality, and 0.75 of a year for pregnancy). The 0.6 years of conception delay concern us here, since amenorrhea is most likely to affect fertility by extending the delay to conception. Bongaarts and Potter (1983) present

Table 6.2 Changes in Delay to Conception during Each Birth Interval and the
Resulting Total Fertility Rate

Conception Delay (in months)	Total Fertility Rate
7.2 (standard)	7.00
8.0 (2-week delay)	6.82
8.2 (1-month delay)	6.78
9.2 (2-month delay)	6.57
10.2 (3-month delay)	6.41
11.2 (4-month delay)	6.18
12.2 (5-month delay)	5.99
13.2 (6-month delay)	5.83

a maximum delay to conception as .85 of a year, or 10.2 months. Their estimate is an average of the mean waiting time to conception for historical European communities and in 4 Latin American countries and Taiwan for women aged 20 to 24 years. These data are not representative of populations in contemporary developing countries or in the past, for which the delay to conception due to amenorrhea may be several weeks longer.

Table 6.2 presents the results of a sensitivity test applied to the Bongaarts and Potter model of proximate determinants of natural fertility, in which the time to conception during the fecundable period is altered beyond the boundaries in the original model to reflect different durations of amenorrhea, with the other values held constant. The total fertility rate is calculated as described above. In the absence of population level data on the prevalence of amenorrhea, the delay to conception is increased incrementally to reflect possible values of amenorrhea in a population. If women in a population suffer extensive periods of amenorrhea during each birth interval, the impact on fertility is not unimportant. For example, by increasing the time of conception delay from 7.2 months to 13.2 months, to account for a period of 6 months of amenorrhea added to each birth interval, the total fertility rate is reduced from 7 children to 5.83 children.

Perhaps more realistically, if a woman misses only one cycle due to amenorrhea during each birth interval, increasing the time to conception from 7.2 months to 8.2 months, the total fertility rate is 6.82 children, compared with 7. This sensitivity test indicates that even small episodes of amenorrhea in a natural fertility population have an impact on fertility. Bongaarts and Potter (1983) suggest that the largest variations in the total fertility rate are caused by variations in the age at first marriage and the duration of postpartum infecundability, but they may not necessarily be the principal causes of variation in natural fertility. They conclude by noting, "[T]he effect of variations in the conception delay, which cause the TFR to deviate 0.6 births from the standard value of 7 [using their maximum value], is quite respectable by itself, even though it is much smaller than the effects of age at marriage and postpartum infecundability" (Bongaarts and Potter 1983:46).

CONCLUSION

It is clear that studies of menstruation and fertility tend to neglect or downplay infrequent menses, focusing instead on the boundaries of normal experiences for healthy Western women. Although the literature indicates a strong connection between secondary amenorrhea and certain unfavorable conditions, the relationship is rarely quantified, and modern gynecological textbooks omit discussion of the prevalence of secondary amenorrhea altogether. At best, we are left with statements that assure us that "some" or "a few" women suffer from the condition without knowledge of whether "some" represents 1 percent or 10 percent of women. Simply increasing the waiting to conception by 1 month of amenorrhea for each birth interval, however, reveals that total fertility estimates are sensitive to episodes of infrequent menses.

The literature on menstruation reflects a dearth of information about secondary amenorrhea and women in the developing world. How many women experience secondary amenorrhea, and what is the distribution of causes for the cessation of menses? Are some women predisposed to infrequent menses, and, if so, do they experience regular episodes of amenorrhea, similar to the Dobe !Kung? We have much to learn about secondary amenorrhea in healthy women, and much more to learn about irregular menses in women from developing countries or in the past, where the interaction between disease, nutrition, and physical exertion is most acute and where infrequent menses seem to elicit a great deal of concern.

NOTES

1. *Primary amenorrhea* refers to the delay of menarche, or the first menstrual cycle, relative to one's peers. *Secondary amenorrhea* is the absence of menstruation in a woman having previously normal and regular menses

and is the most common type of amenorrhea. It may refer to postpartum or lactational amenorrhea or to pathological amenorrhea; in this chapter, however, it does not refer to lactational or postpartum amenorrhea, but only to pathological amenorrhea.

2. For example, Potts, Diggory, and Peel (1977:231) present a small graph claiming "estimated values" of nonpregnant menstrual delays; about 30 percent of women with menses delayed for 14 days were not pregnant. In a small pilot study by the World Health Organization to test "menstrual regulation" through a combination of mifepristone (RU486) and a prostaglandin sequential among young, healthy women whose menses were delayed by a few days, roughly one-fourth were not pregnant (WHO 1995).

3. One of the largest data sets on menstruation was collected by Chiazze et al. (1968). The data were collected from a populationwide survey given to 2,316 healthy American and Canadian women aged 15 to 45 years for a total of 30,655 cycles. The data set compiled by Treloar et al. (1967) began in 1934 and followed the menstrual cycles of 2,702 healthy, noncontracepting women for an average of 9.2 years.

4. There is some evidence that women altered data in order to avoid appearing abnormal. Both Treloar (1967) and Vollman (1977) found large discrepancies between objectively and subjectively reported menstrual data. For example, some women in the Treloar data set incorrectly reported cycles of 28 days in order to appear "normal."

5. A few studies focus on menstrual irregularity in adolescence but also exclude subjects who are experiencing other clinical symptoms. For example, in Venturoli et al.'s (1987:79) study of menstrual irregularity in adolescence, "subjects with additional clinical findings, such as severe acne, obesity, hirsutism . . . or physical or psychological disease were excluded from the study."

6. There is some evidence that ethnic differences also contribute to menstrual cycle differentials within the same Western population. Harlow et al.'s (1997) study of ethnic differences in the menstrual cycle during the postmenarcheal period found large ethnic differences between European-American and African-American adolescents. European Americans were more likely to experience an extremely long cycle and a larger between-woman cycle variance.

7. There are numerous pathological and congenital conditions associated with amenorrhea, although the majority are considered rare. Dysfunctional menstrual bleeding is most often associated with some form of hormonal imbalance and includes endometrial disease, prolactinomas, polycystic ovarian syndrome, thyroid disease, and other hematological defects (Amiel 1975; Davis 1997). Anomalies in the arterioles supplying the endometrium may also lead to menstrual abnormalities or amenorrhea. The prevalence of these and other conditions and the extent to which they cause amenorrhea remain undocumented, however.

8. A seasonal effect on menstruation is also evident, although much more subtly, in less extreme climactic conditions. Sundaraj et al. (1978) analyzed 10-year menstrual diaries kept by U.S. women (the Treloar data) and found a small but significant seasonal effect on menstrual cycle variation. They found longer cycles from October to January and a shift to shorter cycles for the rest of the year. In countries near the equator, the seasonal effect on menstruation is likely to be minimal, but women living farther from the equator or in high altitudes may be adversely affected. The extent to which women experience environmentally induced amenorrhea at high altitudes or in high temperatures is unknown.

REFERENCES

Amiel, G. J. 1975. "Disorders of Menstruation." *Update* 10:845–52.
Baird, David T. 1985. "Endocrine Basis of Menstruation and Its Disorders." In *Mechanism of Menstrual Bleeding,* ed. David T. Baird and Eileen A. Michie. New York: Raven Press.
Becker, Stan. 1993. "The Determinants of Adolescent Fertility." In *Biomedical and Demographic Determinants of Reproduction,* ed. Ronald Gray, Henri Leridon, and Alfred Spira, 21–49. Oxford: Clarendon Press.
Beyene, Yewoubdar. 1992. "Menopause as a Biocultural Event." In *Menstrual Health in Women's Lives,* ed. Alice J. Dan and Linda L. Lewis. Urbana: University of Illinois Press.
Bongaarts, John. 1980. "Does Malnutrition Affect Fecundity? A Summary of Evidence." *Science* 208:564–69.
Bongaarts, John, and Robert Potter. 1983. *Fertility, Biology, and Behavior: An Analysis of the Proximate Determinants.* New York: Academic Press.
Charlewood, G. P. 1956. *Bantu Gynecology.* Johannesburg: Witwatersrand University Press.
Chiazze, Leonard, Franklin T. Brayer, John J. Macisco, Margaret P. Parker, and Benedict J. Duffy. 1968. "The Length and Variability of the Human Menstrual Cycle." *Journal of the American Medical Association* 203: 377–80.
Coldsmith, D. 1979. "'Symbolic' Amenorrhea: Emotional Factors in Secondary Amenorrhea." *Medical Aspects of Human Sexuality* 9:95–112.
Collette, Mary E., Grace Wertenberger, and Virginia Fiske. 1954. "The Effect of Age upon the Pattern of the Menstrual Cycle." *Fertility and Sterility* 5:437–48.
Cumming, David C. 1993. "The Effects of Exercise and Nutrition on the Menstrual Cycle." In *Biomedical and Demographic Determinants of Reproduction,* ed. Ronald Gray, Henri Leridon, and Alfred Spira, 132–56. Oxford: Clarendon Press.

Davis, Ann. 1997. "A 21 Year-Old Woman with Menstrual Irregularity." *Journal of the American Medical Association* 277:1308–14.

Durgamba, K., S. Swany, and C. Rao. 1972. "Genital Tuberculosis." *Indian Journal of Chest Diseases* 14:32.

Edmonds, Keith, Kevin Lindsay, John Miller, Elsbeth Williamson, and Peter Wood. 1982. "Early Embryonic Mortality in Women." *Fertility and Sterility* 38:447–53.

Ellison, Peter T., Nadine R. Peacock, and Catherine Lager. 1989. "Ecology and Ovarian Function among Lese Women of the Ituri Forest, Zaire." *American Journal of Physical Anthropology* 78:519–26.

Ferin, Michel, Raphael Jewelewicz, and Michelle Warren. 1993. *The Menstrual Cycle*. New York: Oxford University Press.

Foster, Andrew, Jane Menken, Alauddin Chowdhury, and James Trussell. 1986. "Female Reproductive Development: A Hazards Model Analysis." *Social Biology* 33:183–99.

Fries, Hans, Sven Johan Nillius, and Folke Petterson. 1974. "Epidemiology of Secondary Amenorrhea." *American Journal of Obstretrics and Gynecology* 118:473.

Frisch, Rose E., and Roger Revelle. 1970. "Height and Weight at Menarche and a Hypothesis of Critical Body Weights and Adolescent Events." *Science* 169:397–99.

Frisch, Rose E., and J. W. McArthur. 1974. "Menstrual Cycles: Fatness as a Determinant of Minimum Weight for Height Necessary for Their Maintenance and Onset." *Science* 185:949–51.

Garrigues, Henry J. 1900. *A Textbook of the Diseases of Women*. Philadelphia: W. B. Saunders & Company.

Gilbert, Bruce. 1943. "Schistosomiasis (Bilharziasis) of the Female Genital Tract and Neighboring Tissues." *Journal of Obstetrics and Gynecology of the British Empire* 50:317–40.

Gold, Jay J. 1968. *Gynecologic Endocrinology*. New York: Harper and Row.

Graham, Effie, Martha Stewart, and Penelope Ward. 1992. " 'Seasonal Cyclicity' Effect of Daylight/Darkness on the Menstrual Cycle." In *Menstrual Health in Women's Lives*, ed. Alice J. Dan and Linda L. Lewis. Urbana: University of Illinois Press.

Gray, Ronald. 1977. "Biological Factors Other than Nutrition and Lactation Which May Influence Natural Fertility: A Review." Paper presented at the International Union for the Scientific Study of Population Seminar on Natural Fertility, Paris.

Harlow, Sioban D., Ben Campbell, Xihong Lin, and Jonathan Raz. 1997. "Ethnic Differences in the Length of the Menstrual Cycle during the Postmenarcheal Period." *American Journal of Epidemiology* 146:572–80.

Hatcher, Robert A., James Trussell, Felicia Stewart, Gary K. Stewart, Deborah Kowal, Felicia Guest, Willard Cates, and Micheal S. Policar. 1994. *Contraceptive Technology*. New York: Irvington Publishers.

Healy, David L., Alan O. Trounson, and Anders N. Andersen. 1994. "Female Infertility: Causes and Treatment." *The Lancet* 343 1994:1539–44.

Ihalainen, Olli. 1975. "Psychosomatic Aspects of Amenorrhea." *Acta Psychiatrica Scandinavica,* suppl. 262:1–139.

Israel, S. Leon. 1967. *Diagnosis and Treatment of Menstrual Disorders and Sterility.* New York: Harper and Row.

Jacobs, Theodore J. 1972. "Secondary Amenorrhea and Sexual Conflicts." *Medical Aspects of Human Sexuality* 6, no. 5:87–102.

Johnson, P. L., James W. Wood, K. L. Campbell, and I. A. Maslar. 1987. "Long Ovarian Cycles in Women of Highland New Guinea." *Human Biology* 59:837–45.

Lee, Richard B. 1979. *The !Kung San: Men, Women, and Work in a Foraging Society.* London: Cambridge University Press.

Le Roy Ladurie, Emmanuel. 1975. "Famine Amenorrhoea (Seventeenth–Twentieth Centuries)." In *Biology of Man in History,* ed. Robert Foster and Orest Ranum. Baltimore: The Johns Hopkins University Press. Originally published in *Annales: E.S.C.* (1969).

Leridon, Henri. 1993. "Fecundability and Post-Partum Sterility: An Insuperable Interaction?" In *Biomedical and Demographic Determinants of Reproduction,* ed. Ronald Gray, Henri Leridon, and Alfred Spira. Oxford: Clarendon Press.

Longshore-Potts, Anna M. 1896. *Discourses to Women on Medical Subjects.* San Diego: Self-published.

McFalls, Joseph A. 1979. *Psychopathology and Subfecundity.* New York: Academic Press.

McFalls, Joseph A., and Marguerite H. McFalls. 1984. *Disease and Fertility.* New York: Academic Press.

Menken, Jane. 1975. "Estimating Fecundability." Ph.D. diss., Princeton University.

Menken, Jane, James Trussell, and Susan Watkins. 1981. "The Nutrition Fertility Link: An Evaluation of the Evidence." *Journal of Interdisciplinary History* 11:425–41.

Meuvret, Jean. 1946. "Les crises de subsistance et la démographie de la France d'Ancien Régime." *Population* 4:643–50.

Miller, J. F., E. Williamson, J. Blue, Y. B. Gordon, J. G. Grudzinskas, and A. Sykes. 1980. "Fetal Loss after Implantation: A Prospective Study." *Lancet* 2:554–56.

Monari, Paola, and Angela Montanari. 1998. "Length of Menstrual Cycles and Their Variability." *Genus* 54:95–118.

Mphi, Mamoliephi. 1994. "Female Alcoholism Problems in Lesotho." *Addiction* 89:945–49.

Munster K., Helm, P., and Schmidt, L. 1992. "Secondary Amenorrhoea: Prevalence and Medical Contact—A Cross-Sectional Study from a Danish County." *British Journal of Obstetrics & Gynaecology* 99:430–33.

Osofsky, Howard, and Seymour Fisher. 1967. "Psychological Correlates of the Development of Amenorrhea in a Stress Situation." *Psychosomatic Medicine* 29:15–22.

Petersen, Anne C. 1980. "Puberty and Its Psychosocial Significance in Girls." In *The Menstrual Cycle: A Synthesis of Interdisciplinary Research,* vol. 1, ed. Alice J. Dan, Effie A. Graham, and Carol P. Beecher. New York: Springer Publishing Company.

Potts, Malcolm, Peter Diggory, and John Peel. 1977. *Abortion.* Cambridge: Cambridge University Press.

Prior, Jerilynn C. 1996. "Exercise-Associated Menstrual Disturbances." In *Reproductive Endocrinology, Surgery, and Technology,* ed. E. Y. Adashi, J. A. Rock, and Z. Rosenwaks. Philadelphia: Lippincott-Raven Publishers.

Rahman, Omar, and Jane Menken. 1993. "Age at Menopause and Fecundity Preceding Menopause." In *Biomedical and Demographic Determinants of Reproduction,* ed. Ronald Gray, Henri Leridon, and Alfred Spira, 65–84. Oxford: Clarendon Press.

Riley, Ann P., Julia L. Samuelson, and Sandra L. Huffman. 1993. "The Relationship of Age at Menarche and Fertility in Undernourished Adolescents." In *Biomedical and Demographic Determinants of Reproduction,* ed. Ronald Gray, Henri Leridon, and Alfred Spira, 50–64. Oxford: Clarendon Press.

Rozin, Samuel. 1968. "Genital Tuberculosis." In *Progress in Infertility,* ed. Samuel J. Berhman and Robert W. Kistner. Boston: Little, Brown.

Rutherford, Robert. 1965. "Emotional Aspects of Infertility." *Clinical Obstetrics and Gynecology* 8:100.

Santow, Gigi. 1978. *A Simulation Approach to the Study of Human Fertility.* Leiden: Netherlands Inter-University Demographic Institute.

Saunders, Stephanie A., and June M. Reinisch. 1992. "Psychological Correlates of Normal and Abnormal Menstrual Cycle Length." In *Menstrual Health in Women's Lives,* ed. Alice J. Dan and Linda L. Lewis. Urbana: University of Illinois Press.

Shader, Richard I., Jeremy P. Nahum, and Alberto DiMascio. 1970. "Amenorrhea." In *Psychotropic Drug Side Effects,* ed. Richard I. Shader and Alberto DiMascio. Baltimore: Williams and Wilkins.

Siegel, J. M., J. H. Johnson, and I. G. Saranson. 1979. "Life Changes and Menstrual Discomfort." *Journal of Human Stress* 5:41–46.

Siegler, Samuel L. 1944. *Fertility in Women: Causes, Diagnosis, and Treatment of Impaired Fertility.* Philadelphia: Lippincott.

Skierska, E., J. Leszczynska-Bystrzanowska, and A. K. Gajewski. 1996. "Risk analysis of menstrual disorders in young women from urban population" [in Polish]. *Przeglad Epidemiologiczny* 50:467–74.

Stein, Zena, and Susser, Mervyn. 1975. "Fertility, Fecundity, and Famine: Food Rations in the Dutch Famine 1944/5 Have a Causal Relationship to Fertility and Probably to Fecundity." *Human Biology* 47:131–54.

Sturgis, Somers H. 1976. "Menstrual Disorders." In *Medical Care of the Ad-*

olescent, ed. J. Roswell Gallagher, Felix P. Heald, and Dale C. Garell. 3d ed. New York: Appleton-Century-Crofts.

Sundaraj, N., M. Chern, L. Gatewood, L. Hickman, and R. McHugh. 1978. "Seasonal Behaviour of Human Menstrual Cycles: A Biometric Investigation." *Human Biology* 50:15–31.

Thomas, K. D., F. E. Okonofua, and O. Chiboka. 1990. "A Study of the Menstrual Patterns of Adolescents of Ile-Ife, Nigeria." *International Journal of Gynecological Obstetrics* 33:31–34.

Treloar, Alan E., Ruth Boynton, Borghild Behn, and Byron Brown. 1967. "Variation in the Human Menstrual Cycle through Reproductive Life." *International Journal of Fertility* 12:77–126.

Venturoli, S., E. Porcu, and R. Fabbri, et al. 1987. "Postmenarcheal Evolution of Endocrine Pattern and Ovarian Aspects in Adolescence with Menstrual Irregularities." *Fertility and Sterility* 48:78–85.

Vollman, R. F. 1977. "The Menstrual Cycle." *Major Problems in Obstetrics & Gynecology* 7:1–193.

Wharton, Lawrence R. 1943. *Gynecology with a Section on Female Urology.* Philadelphia: W. B. Saunders.

Whittaker, P., A. Taylor, and T. Lind. 1983. "Unsuspected Pregnancy Loss in Healthy Women." *Lancet* 1:1126–27.

Wilcox, J. Allen, Clarice R. Weinberg, John F. O'Connor, Donna D. Baird, John P. Schlatterer, Robert E. Canfield, E. Glenn Armstrong, and Bruce Nisula. 1988. "Incidence of Early Pregnancy Loss." *New England Journal of Medicine* 319:189–94.

Wood, James W. 1994. *Dynamics of Human Reproduction.* New York: Walter de Gruyter, Inc.

Wood, James W., and Maxine Weinstein. 1998. "A Model of Age-Specific Fecundability." *Population Studies* 42:85–113.

WHO (World Health Organization). 1979. *The African Trypanosomiases.* World Health Organization Technical Report Series, no. 635.

WHO (World Health Organization Task Force on Post-Ovulatory Methods of Fertility Regulation). 1995. "Menstrual Regulation by Mifepristone plus Prostaglandin: Results from a Multicentre Trial." *Human Reproduction* 10:308–14.

CHAPTER 7

Menstrual Regulation and the Pill

Linda S. Potter

Yet still I seek,
Month after month in vain,
Meaning and beauty in recurrent pain.
—Lesbia Harford, "Periodicity"

The birth control Pill is, in one sense, the ultimate menstrual regulator. Oral contraceptives are primarily meant for pregnancy prevention; they are 99.9 percent effective if taken consistently, although in typical use the pregnancy rate is at least 5 percent (Hatcher and Guillebaud 1998). Consistent use of oral contraceptive pills also regularizes menstrual cycles in frequency, timing, and amount of flow, so the Pill is sometimes prescribed specifically for that purpose. On the other hand, oral contraceptive pills taken inconsistently can instead deregularize the cycle. The third role of the Pill in the menstrual cycle is its post-coital use as an emergency "morning after" contraceptive.

Combined oral contraceptive pills contain synthetic estrogen and progestin, which augment the natural endogenous forms of those hormones. The pills are usually packaged in blister packs or dial packs, with 21 active hormonal pills followed by 7 placebo "reminder" pills. The increased and "smoothed out" hormonal levels caused by taking oral contraceptives mimic those of pregnancy, so the pituitary gland does not release the hormones that stimulate ovulation (FSH, the follicle-stimulating hormone, and LH, the luteinizing hormone that ruptures the follicle to release the ovum). Thus the active hormonal pill taken for 3 weeks, followed by a hormone-free week, artificially creates a 4-week lunar cycle but not a true menstrual cycle (Hatcher and Guillebaud 1998; Goldzieher 1994). (See the glossary following the introduction of this volume for a more detailed description of a normal menstrual cycle.)

As has been described throughout this volume, a regular cycle with fortnightly bleeding is taken in most cultures as a reassuring sign of reproductive health and fertility and even of general health and well-being. Consistent use of oral contraceptives virtually guarantees a regular cycle with a bleeding period that is almost absolutely predictable in timing, flow, and color. In addition, the increased hormonal levels reduce dysmenorrhea (menstrual pain) and other discomforts. The monthly bleeding period also confirms to a woman that she is "clean inside" and that there is no "obstruction" or "blockage" that could cause the blood to accumulate in her uterus or make later childbirth more difficult.

Ironically, this verification sometimes means that the lighter flow (reduced as much as 40 percent; see Hatcher and Guillebaud 1998) produced by the Pill can be disquieting in cultures where anemia is common, but the benefits of the lighter bleeding in controlling it is not known. In the United States and other countries where users, at least theoretically, better understand the dynamics of the Pill, the lighter bleeding is much preferred for its convenience. It may even be used specifically to reduce excessive bleeding during menses (menorrhagia) or in the case of anemia.

As long as sufficient levels of estrogen and progestin are in the bloodstream during the 3 weeks of taking hormonal pills, there will be no uterine bleeding. Cutting off the supply of these hormones during the last 7 days of each 28-day cycle imitates the sudden drop in hormonal levels that would occur with their natural endogenous equivalents at the end of a normal cycle. This in turn causes shedding of the endometrium (the lining of the uterus) which the Pill's hormones have built up during the previous 21 days. It is because the uterine lining is thinner than it would be in a true menstrual cycle that its shedding causes a lighter flow. What bleeding does occur tends to be deeper in color or, as some would describe it, "older" than during normal menses. These artificial menstrual periods are most accurately called "hormone withdrawal bleeds" or "letdown bleeds," to avoid confusion with true menses (Guillebaud 1991).

During the normal menstrual cycle, a woman is most likely to become pregnant at midcycle, immediately preceding ovulation; that is, about 15 days after the commencement of menstruation (Wilcox, Weinberg, and Baird 1995). Despite the fact that the lunar cycle created by using oral contraceptives is not a true ovulatory menstrual cycle, even in the most medically sophisticated societies the misconception persists that the "middle of the month [sic]" is the time one is most likely to become pregnant. In fact, clinical research strongly suggests the opposite. A Pill user would be more likely to ovulate and conceive immediately after the hormone-free fourth week of the cycle (Elomaa et al. 1998; Landgren and Czemiczky 1991). This can be especially problematic if pills have been taken erratically or the next pack is started late (Guillebaud 1987).

Another belief that surfaces from time to time is that the Pill's regularizing of the cycle can actually makes it easier to predict the timing of ovulation. However, its regularizing effect ceases as soon as the pill-taking ceases. More reassuring, however, is that the average time to return to fertility after pill-taking is stopped is only 1 month longer than it is for noncontraceptors, that is, an average of 4 months instead of 3 (Bracken, Hellenbrand, and Holford 1990).

Since the Pill was introduced in the early 1960s, the dosage of ethinyl estradiol—the estrogen contained in all oral contraceptives—has dropped by degrees from its original daily dosage of 80–150 milligrams, first down to 50 milligrams and now to just 20 or 30 milligrams. The nonmenstrual side effects of the early high-dose oral contraceptives, such as nausea and headaches, were very uncomfortable, but those original pills provided almost absolute cycle control, with virtually no intermenstrual bleeding, even when pills were missed. The dosage of the progestins, usually norethindrone or levonorgestrel, is now one-fifth of what it was 30 years ago, when the Pill was first introduced. These lower doses of the progestins have reduced the side effects but increased the chance of endometrial shedding, and hence the chance of unexpected "breakthrough" bleeding if the pills are taken inconsistently. Because of the greatly reduced hormonal doses, users must be especially careful not only to take the Pill every day but to take it about the same time each day to prevent this untimely bleeding.

USING THE PILL TO REGULARIZE MONTHLY CYCLES

The average cycle length among non-Pill users is 28 days, but anything between 25 and 31 days is considered normal. This range makes it harder to anticipate exactly when menses will occur. By creating a regularized 28-day cycle, the 21 days of hormonal pills followed by 7 days of placebo "reminder" pills, the cyclical rhythm is made familiar and reassuring. The precise 4-week cycle allows a woman to anticipate far ahead of time on which day of which week her bleeding period will begin, thereby also reassuring her that she is not pregnant when it does begin or providing a warning if it does not. In the United States at least, most clinicians recommend that an oral contraceptive user not be unduly concerned unless she has missed 2 menstrual periods in a row (Guillebaud 1991; Hatcher and Guillebaud 1998; Speroff and Darney 1992).

An early experiment in a Bangladeshi (at that time West Pakistan) village synchronized a lunar cycle of pill-taking for all 47 women using oral contraceptives. They were instructed to wait until the next new moon to begin the next cycle of pills. "All but two did so successfully and therefore generally experienced withdrawal bleeding during the dark of the moon" (Cobb et al. 1966). This very practical experiment was initiated because the women in this rural village were illiterate and did not know how to use a calendar. Levin (in this volume) has described a similar strategy used in Guinea, West Africa.

In the United States, virtually all women are told to start each pack of pills on a Sunday. This universal Sunday start was established in large part because it is easy to remember. It was also supposed to prevent menstrual bleeding on weekends. The theory was that if each week in a 4-week cycle begins on Sunday, the hormonal drop at the end of the third week would result in bleeding starting on Monday or Tuesday and ending by Thursday or Friday. However, a recent study found that 78 percent of Sunday starters do still have some bleeding on the weekend. Some do not start their period until Wednesday, and some continue for 4 or 5 days (Hertz and Dong 1994). One suggested alternative has been to start each Pill cycle a day or two earlier—on a Friday or Saturday. However, this may be a risky alternative. Those 2 weekend days are when schedules vary and women are most likely to forget to take their pills, thereby extending the hormone-free interval (Potter et al. 1996).

THE PILL AS A CYCLE DEREGULARIZER

Although the Pill generally reduces and regularizes bleeding, it also can cause breakthrough bleeding. In fact, surveys in both developing and developed countries have found that menstrual irregularities are the side effect most commonly named as the reason for stopping oral contraceptive use altogether. Providers interviewed in Egypt split evenly between those reporting that an advantage of the Pill is that it regularizes menses (15 percent) and those reporting that a disadvantage is that it causes irregular menses (also 15 percent) (Loza and Potter 1990). A focus group participant in that Egyptian study said, "Every week I get my period." Her husband was frequently away for a few days and she took the pills only when he was at home. One husband reported that he took his wife's pills with him when he migrated elsewhere to work for several months each year, "so she can't fool around," but then did not understand why she had so often become pregnant soon after he returned home each year. Neither realized that it can take up to 7 days for the pill to become fully effective, so it does not work if a couple resumes pill-taking on the same day as they resume sexual relations (Loza and Potter 1990).

When women start taking the Pill, about 30 percent experience some bleeding or spotting of blood between menstrual periods (metrorrhagia) (Hertz and Dong 1994). This midcycle breakthrough bleeding usually ends within 2 to 3 months after initiating use, unless doses are missed or, in the case of the very low-dose pills, are simply taken a few hours late (Rosenberg and Long 1992).

In developing countries especially, many women believe that any breakthrough bleeding is a menstrual period regardless of when or how often it occurs during the 28-day cycle. Several studies have shown that this confusion leads women to immediately stop pill-taking when they see any bleeding, wait for the bleeding to end, then start pill-taking again. One study by the author found that 7 percent of 500 Colombian women interviewed had interrupted pill-taking twice within a single 2-week interval because of unexpected bleeding (Potter et al. 1988).

As clearly demonstrated in previous chapters, women in some cultures have generally found that any kind of change in their monthly flow is disquieting. Any irregular bleeding while using oral contraceptives can be particularly distressing, as exemplified by Renne's description (in this volume) of Nigerian women directly attributing the irregularities *to* the Pill. A study in Mexico found that 10 percent of respondents complained about reduced menstrual flow, worrying that it signified a less robust uterus (Zúñiga et al. 1994).

Missing pills is the primary reason for breakthrough bleeding, but women have different definitions of "missed pills." Virtually all women know they should take the Pill every day. In fact, 98 percent of Pill users responded accordingly in the National Demographic and Health Surveys conducted in developing countries (Hubacher and Potter 1993). However, their understanding of what "every day" means varies dramatically, from "every day without fail" to "every day my husband is home" to "on the days we have sex" (Loza and Potter 1990; Zúñiga et al. 1994).

Another belief is that a woman needs to "rest" periodically from Pill-taking in order to "cleanse her system" and prevent side effects thought to result from a buildup of chemicals in the body or even an actual accumulation of pills in the uterus, believed by some to be the Pill's mode of action (Havanon, Kanchanansinith, and Potter 1992; Krieger 1982; Loza and Potter 1990; Potter et al. 1988). Despite the higher levels of understanding of the menstrual cycle in developed countries, misconceptions are still common.

For example, in the United States as late as 1989, a national survey of sex educators found that less than one-fourth of them knew that pill-taking did not have to be stopped periodically to give the body a rest (Forrest and Silverman 1989). When doses were 3 to 5 times higher than they are now, this may not have been an unreasonable idea with regard to safety. But, with the current low dosages, taking such a break has no real health benefits but is more likely to result in pregnancy.

A clinical survey of 161 Scottish women aged 16 to 35 years taking oral contraceptives found that 35 percent believed that the absence of bleeding is harmful to the body and 10 percent believed that this amenorrhea always indicates pregnancy (Finlay and Scott 1986). Furthermore, while there is a better understanding that missing pills can itself cause breakthrough bleeding, unexpected bleeding due to missed pills causes frustration. An African-American teenager in a Philadelphia focus group on teen pregnancy and contraception explained her concerns about her deregularized menstrual cycle this way: "Like the pill it change [sic] your menstrual cycle. That's very uncomfortable, walking around knowing that if I miss this pill for three days then I'm going to automatically come on my menstruation" (Crump et al. 1999).

WHY MENSTRUATE AT ALL?

"Recurrent menstruation . . . is a needless loss of blood," according to Elsimar Coutinho (Coutinho and Segal 1999:159). Several studies have found that active hormonal pills can safely be taken continuously, without the hormone-free intervals (de Voogd 1991; Hamerlynck et al. 1987; Kornaat, Geerdink, and Klitsie 1992), thereby preventing any monthly bleeding periods. The freedom from any discomfort and inconvenience of a monthly period would seem to be an attractive option. Yet the fascinating aspect of this apparent advantage of using oral contraceptives is how many women are not comfortable staying on active hormonal pills for an extended period. They cite concerns about not having the reassurance of a monthly period, the "unnaturalness" of not having one, of being "different" from other women (WHO 1981). Emily Martin, in her study of women in Baltimore, discusses this ambivalence in the U.S. context. The women she interviewed talked about the "disgusting mess," the "hassle," how "gross" and "dirty" their periods are, yet at the same time how their monthly bleeding period defines them as a woman (Martin 1987):

> Sometimes I wish I didn't have to have my period. I think everyone wishes that. But I've just gotten so attached to myself as a woman, it just seems so integral. I don't resent it anymore.
> When I have it, I think, I'm a woman, this is proof, that I get my period. (101)

One exception to this concern about uninterrupted pill-taking is that of taking 2 consecutive cycles (the "bi-cycle" or "honeymoon" regimen of 7 consecutive weeks of taking active hormonal pills), without a letdown bleed, for occasional special occasions—honeymoon, religious holidays, or sporting events. In a Netherlands study of a 7-week Pill cycle with 55 women, only 1 did not like the occasional bi-cycle regimen (Kornaat, Geerdink, and Klitsie 1992). A second Dutch study of a single continuous 11-week tri-cycle regimen found that about half of the 98 college students participating would favor extended amenorrhea of up to either 3 months or 6 months. The author notes that "for the other half this was unacceptable . . . for the emotional reason that this would be 'unnatural' despite the information that this prolonged bleeding interval would be without medical consequences" (Hamerlynck et al. 1987). Yet another study of 100 Dutch women (de Voogd 1991) who took the Pill for 11 consecutive weeks found that 91 percent said they would be willing to use the 3-month cycle again "if necessary." Thirty percent of those who had expected to be fully amenorrheic for those 11 weeks would not be willing to try it again because they eliminated their regular monthly bleeding period only to find they experienced unexpected breakthrough bleeds instead.

Similarly, researchers in Australia found that 54 percent of the 158 female patients and 45 percent of the 20 young female doctors in their study would choose to maintain a monthly bleed. The reasons given were "to allow the body to function normally, to copy what happens normally, to rid the body of waste and/or prevent the lining of the womb from building up" (Rutter et al. 1988). Nevertheless, 46 percent of the patients and 55 percent of the doctors participating said that they might choose to bleed at wider intervals if they could determine their own regimen.

There is very little quantitative data on continuous use of active hormonal pills in developing countries, but several researchers have reported that Muslim women likewise occasionally run 2 cycles of active pills together in order to avoid interruptions in prayers and fasting (especially during Ramadan). This exception is due to the strong prohibition against women participating in any religious activities while bleeding, since they are "unclean" at that time. (See Hull and Hull, this volume.)

EMERGENCY CONTRACEPTION

Oral contraceptive pills are being used increasingly for postcoital emergency contraception, whether or not they are the woman's regular method of contraception. The technique consists of taking a 100-milligram dose (2 pills containing 50 mg of estrogen or four 30-mg pills) within 72 hours of unprotected intercourse, followed by a second dose 12 hours later. This postcoital regimen is not a true emmenagogue, in that it does not bring on menstruation or even an immediate letdown bleed. Subsequent menses normally occur at the expected time but may be somewhat heavier than usual. For those returning to the regular Pill regimen, the timing of the first bleed may be somewhat less predictable.

Oral contraceptive pills can work as postcoital contraception in 3 ways: by interfering with the production or fertilization of the ovum, or by preventing the fertilized ovum from implanting in the uterus. The method is effective approximately 75 percent of the time (Glasier 1997; Trussell, Rodriguez and Ellertson 1999).

Any device or drug that acts *after* implantation is conventionally regarded as an abortifacient rather than a contraceptive (Glasier 1997). Therefore, it does fit into that hazy area between the use of emmenagogues and abortifacients, depending on beliefs about when life begins. Use of the Pill postcoitally is unacceptable to those who consider any intervention after the moment of conception to be an abortion.

Broader ambivalence about use of the Pill postcoitally is reflected in several ways. Clinicians have been using this high dose of oral contraceptives as an emergency contraceptive since the 1970s (Yuzpe and Lancee 1977), but only rarely have public or private providers of reproductive health care in the United States discussed this information with their patients until an actual emergency arose. Only since 1996 has information about using the Pill as an emergency backup method of contraception been provided to women when they are first counseled about using their chosen method of contraception effectively.

Another reflection of this ambivalence about using the Pill post-coitally is the fact than no U.S. manufacturer of oral contraceptives has been willing to petition the U.S. Food and Drug Administration to add this use of the Pill to the official product labeling. In fact, because no company would petition the FDA, the agency took the unusual step of independently issuing a statement of confidence in the safety and effectiveness of the Pill for emergency contraception (USFDA 1996). Thus far, just 1 percent of sexually active women in the United States have actually used oral contraceptives in this way, but openness in discussing and using the method have been increasing rapidly in the past 4 years.

CONCLUSIONS AND DISCUSSION

Oral contraceptives can be an extremely precise menstrual regulator, if taken as directed. They not only prevent pregnancy, but create cycles of exactly 4 weeks and reduce the length and amount of monthly bleeding. Yet, ironically, if they are taken inconsistently, they can disrupt the very rhythm they create, causing midcycle bleeding and even breakthrough ovulation.

Misconceptions about how oral contraceptives work and about their short- and long-term effects on fertility and general reproductive physiology, along with the mistaken belief that artificially induced monthly bleeding is a true menstrual period, reveal an important lack of education for all current and potential users. The importance of this point cannot be underestimated, because oral contraceptives, introduced just more than 35 years ago, are taken by more than 72 million women— 56 million of them in developing countries; worldwide, more than 650 million women have ever used the Pill (United Nations 1995). The United States alone has 10 million current users and 44 million former users (Abma et al. 1997).

Many women appreciate the ability to use oral contraceptives to regularize their monthly cycle. Many also appreciate the option to occasionally skip one or two bleeding periods for a specific event. Far fewer, however, are willing to eliminate or even appreciably reduce the frequency of what they themselves call the messy hassle of that monthly bleeding and the interruptions in sexual relations (Barnhart, Furman, and Devoto 1995).

The misconceptions and concerns so many women have about using the Pill to prevent menstrual bleeding raises fascinating questions. What characteristics distinguish women who strongly desire to maintain their monthly cycling from those who do not? Is this desire subject to change? How does this choice affect the rest of their lives? How might other changes in their lifestyles or environment influence their perspective? Might there eventually be greater acceptance of long cycles as women who are comfortable extending theirs share their stories? Could such change be brought about by direct education and counseling? What might be compelling reasons to encourage such change—political? economic? personal? Would encouraging such change be ethical? These questions reflect larger issues than the mechanical ability of oral contraceptives to regularize or extend cycles, but Pill users would make an excellent study population with whom to explore not only their own personal patterns and beliefs but also the role of menses in what it means to them to be female. They are the group most able to regulate menstruation and therefore to think through its ramifications.

Maybe the most telling aspect of the ambivalence about using oral contraceptives to prevent pregnancy and regularize the monthly cycle is that the cyclical letdown is not menstruation but is virtually always described as a "menstrual period," thereby denying that the cycle created by the Pill *is* artificial. What is most curious about this misrepresentation and misunderstanding of the letdown bleed as a menstrual bleed is that it can at least theoretically increase the risk of pregnancy at other times during the cycle when the Pill taker does not think she is vulnerable, especially immediately after her monthly bleeding period.

Therefore, use of the Pill as a menstrual regulator is not so *ambiguous* as the use of natural emmenagogues. Yet, although its mode of action and effectiveness have been precisely determined, users, prescribers, and the larger community have quite ambivalent feelings about the Pill. This is so in countries at all levels of development, even where the dynamics of the Pill are more or less understood. The desire for menses and its verification of fertility and femininity exceeds the desire for comfort, convenience, or even full protection against pregnancy, regardless of how safe and easy to administer—and discrete—the method is.

These observations about the use of the Pill as a menstrual regulator, in the most modern possible setting, are in line with what has been observed in virtually all societies, whether among the early Greeks or rural villagers in Africa, Latin America, and Indonesia, or through

the last three centuries in the United States and Europe. These findings confirm the kinship of women across time and culture, affluence,
education, and mores. The need of women—who could quite safely
never menstruate and never have an unintended pregnancy—to
menstruate regularly reveals the importance of *visibly* affirming their
femininity and fertility, thereby reassuring themselves and their
communities that they can continue their most essential role while
at the same time maintaining some sense of control over how and
when they do, however ambivalent or ambiguous their intentions may
seem.

REFERENCES

Abma, J., A. Chandra, W. Mosher, L. Peterson, and L. Piccinino. 1997.
*Fertility, Family Planning, and Women's Health: New Data from the 1995
National Survey of Family Growth.* Rockville, Md.: Centers for Disease
Control and Prevention, National Center for Health Statistics.
Barnhart, K., J. Furman, and L. Devoto. 1995. "Attitudes and Practice of
Couples Regarding Sexual Relations during the Menses and Spotting."
Contraception 51:93–98.
Bracken, M. B., K. G. Hellenbrand, and T. R. Holford. 1990. "Conception
Delay after Oral Contraceptive Use: The Effect of Estrogen Dose." *Fertil-
ity and Sterility* 53, no. 1:21–27.
Cobb, J. C., S. Farhat, N. A. Shah, S. I. Ameen, and P. Harper. 1966. "Oral
Contraceptive Program Synchronized with Moon Phase." *Fertility and
Sterility* 17, no. 4:559–67.
Coutinho, E. M., and S. J. Segal. *Is Menstruation Obsolete?* New York: Ox-
ford University Press, 1999.
Crump, A. D., D. L. Haynie, S. J. Aarons, E. Adair; K. Woodward, and B. G.
Simons-Morton. 1999. "Pregnancy among Urban African-American
Teens: Ambivalence about Prevention." *American Journal of Health Be-
havior* 23:32–42.
Elomaa, K., R. Rolland, and I. Bronsens et al. 1998. "Omitting the First
Oral Contraceptive Pills of the Cycle Does Not Automatically Lead to
Ovulation." *American Journal of Obstetrics and Gynecology* 179:41–46.
Finlay, I. G., and M. G. B. Scott. 1986. "Patterns of Contraceptive Pill Tak-
ing in an Inner City Practice." *British Medical Journal* 293:601–602.
Forrest, J. D., and J. Silverman. 1989. "What Public School Teachers
Teach about Preventing Pregnancy, AIDS and Sexually Transmitted
Diseases." *Family Planning Perspectives* 21, no. 2:65–72.
Glasier, A. 1997. "Emergency Postcoital Contraception." *The New England
Journal of Medicine* 337, no. 15:1058–79.

Goldzieher, J. W. 1994. *Hormonal Contraception*. Ontario: EMIS.

Greenslade, F. C., A. H. Leonard, J. Benson, J. Winkler, and V. L. Henderson. 1993. *Manual Vacuum Aspiration: A Summary of Clinical and Programmatic Experience Worldwide*. Carrboro, N.C.: IPAS.

Guillebaud, J. 1987. "The Forgotten Pill—And the Paramount Importance of the Pill-Free Week." *British Journal of Family Planning* 712: 35–43.

———. 1991. *The Pill and Other Hormones for Contraception*. Oxford: Oxford University Press.

Hamerlynck, J. V., J. A. Vollebregt, C. M. Doornebos, and P. Muttendam. 1987. "Postponement of Withdrawal Bleeding in Women Using Low-Dose Combined Oral Contraceptives." *Contraception* 35, no. 3: 199–205.

Hampton, Susan, and Kate Llewellyn, eds. 1986. *The Penguin Book of Australian Women Poets*. Ringwood, Victoria: Penguin.

Hatcher, R. A., and J. Guillebaud. 1998. "The Pill: Combined Oral Contraceptives." In *Contraceptive Technology*. 17th ed., 405–65. New York: Irvington Publishers.

Havanon, N., K. Kanchanasinith, and L. Potter. 1992. *Thailand: A Study of Pill Compliance among Drug Store Purchasers*. Unpublished report to the Ministry of Health, Thailand, and the U.S. Agency for International Development. Research Triangle Park, N.C.: Family Health International.

Hertz, R., and R Dong. 1994. "The Sunday Start for Oral Contraceptives: Its Effects on the Consistent Use and Timing of Bleeding." Unpublished report to Wyeth-Ayerst Laboratories. Arlington, VA: Rand Corporation.

Hubacher, D., and L. Potter. 1993. "Adherence to Oral Contraceptive Regimens in Four Countries." *International Family Planning Perspectives* 19, no. 2:49–53.

Kornaat H., M. H. Geerdink, and J. W. Klitsie. 1992. "The Acceptance of a 7-Week Cycle With a Modern Low-Dose Oral Contraceptive (Minulet)." *Contraception* 45, no. 2:119–27.

Krieger, L. E. 1982. *Body Notions, Gender Roles, and Fertility Regulating Method Use in Imbaba, Cairo*. Chapel Hill: University of North Carolina.

Landgren, B-M., and G. Csemiczky. 1991. "The Effect on Follicular Growth and Luteal Function of 'Missing the Pill': A Comparison between a Monophasic and a Triphasic Combined Oral Contraceptive." *Contraception* 43, no. 2:149–59.

Loudon, N. B., M. Foxwell, D. M. Potts, A. L. Guild, and R. V. Short. 1977. "Acceptability of an Oral Contraceptive That Reduces the Frequency of Menstruation: The Tri-Cycle Pill Regimen." *British Medical Journal* 2:487–90.

Loza, S. F., and L. S. Potter. 1990. *Qualitative Study of Oral Contraceptive*

Use in Egypt: Interviews with OC Users and Providers. Report to the Egyptian National Population Council and U.S. Agency for International Development. Research Triangle Park, N.C.: Family Health International.

Martin, E. 1987. "Menstruation, Work and Class." In *The Woman and the Body: A Cultural Analysis of Reproduction,* 92–112. Boston: Beacon Press.

Nabrink, M. L., Birgersson, A-S. Colling-Saltin, and T. Solum. 1990. "Modern Oral Contraceptives and Dysmenorrheoea." *Contraception* 42: 275–83.

Potter L., D. Oakley, and R. Cañamar. 1993. "MEMS Oral Contraceptive Study: Questionnaires 1, 2, 3, 4." Research Triangle Park, N.C.: Family Health International, and Ann Arbor: University of Michigan Center for Nursing Research.

Potter L., S. Wright, D. Berrio, P. Suarez, R. Piñedo, and S. Castañeda. 1988. "Oral Contraceptive Compliance in Rural Colombia: Knowledge of Users and Providers." *International Family Planning Perspectives* 14, no. 1:27–31.

Potter, L., D. Oakley, E. D. Wong, and R. Cañamar. 1996. "Measuring Compliance among Oral Contraceptive Users." *International Family Planning Perspectives* 28:154–58.

Rosenberg, M. J., and S. C. Long. 1992. "Oral Contraceptives and Cycle Control: A Critical Review of the Literature." *Advances in Contraception* 8, suppl. 1:35–46.

Rutter, W., C. Knight, J. Vizzard, M. Mira, and S. Abraham. 1988. "Women's Attitudes to Withdrawal Bleeding and Their Knowledge and Beliefs about the Oral Contraceptive Pill." *Medical Journal of Australia* 149:417–19.

Speroff, L., and R. D. Darney. 1992. "Oral Contraception." In *A Clinical Guide for Contraception.* Baltimore: Williams & Wilkins.

Trussell, J., G. Rodriguez, and C. Ellertson. 1999. "Updated Estimates of the Effectiveness of the Yuzpe Regimen of Emergency Contraception." *Contraception* 59, no. 3:147–51.

United Nations Population Division. 1995. *World Contraceptive Use 1994.* New York: United Nations.

USFDA (U.S. Food and Drug Administration). "Prescription Drug Products. Certain Combined Oral Contraceptives for Use as Emergency Postcoital Contraception." *Federal Register* 62, no 37:8610–12.

Voogd, W. S. de. 1991. "Postponement of Withdrawal Bleeding with a Monophasic Oral Contraceptive Containing Desogestrel and Ethinylestradiol." *Contraception* 44:107–12.

Wilcox, A. J., C. R. Weinberg, and D. D. Baird. 1995. "Timing of Sexual Intercourse in Relation to Ovulation." *New England Journal of Medicine* 333:1517–21.

WHO (World Health Organization Task Force). 1981. "Cross-Cultural

Study of Menstruation: Implications for Contraceptive Development and Use." *Studies in Family Planning* 12:3–16.

Yuzpe, A. A., and W. J. Lancee. 1977. "Ethinylestradiol and dl-norgestrel as a Postcoital Contraceptive." *Fertility and Sterility* 28, no. 9:932–36.

Zúñiga E., E. Ramón, C. Juarez, C. Cárdenas, and L. Potter. 1994. *Study of Oral Contraceptive Knowledge and Practices of IMSS Rural Midwives and their Recent OC Acceptors*. Mexico, D.F.: Academia Mexicana de Investigación en Demografía Medíca.

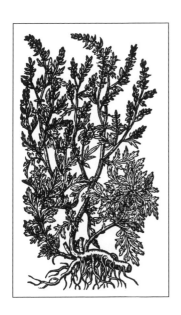

PART 2

ANTHROPOLOGICAL
PERSPECTIVES:
AFRICA, SOUTHEAST
ASIA, AND LATIN
AMERICA

The Meaning of Menstrual Management in a High-Fertility Society: Guinea, West Africa

Elise Levin

In Dabola, Guinea, menstrual management is a cultural practice used to maintain good reproductive health for the stated purpose of ensuring future childbearing. Women in rural Guinea use local pharmacopoeia to cure a variety of menstrual problems, including those associated with irregular timing of the monthly cycle. The plant-based medicines are ingested most frequently in the form of a tea or infusion, or added to the daily meal. In the Guinean women's view, this manner of inducing late menses provides them with an acceptable alternative to risking clandestine abortions. Abortion is illegal in Guinea, and it also violates deep-seated cultural norms. Most people find the very topic objectionable, although some women resort to abortion in the direst situations.

Distinct from abortion is the more socially acceptable practice that I call menstrual management, in which women pay close attention to the details of their menstrual cycle and respond to problems they observe. One common problem, menstrual lateness, is remedied with the help of an herbalist for the purpose of ensuring good reproductive health and future childbearing potential. Another effect of menstrual inducement is, in some instances, avoidance of an unwanted or poorly timed pregnancy; however, most explanations of menstrual management, from both healers and the women who use their cures, explicitly emphasize the positive health benefits of this practice. Because its stated purpose is to correct menstrual problems, not to end a pregnancy, this form of menstrual management is neither abortion nor contraception. Instead, it constitutes a separate category of reproductive action, one that is virtually unknown in contemporary Western societies.

The purpose of this chapter is to explain the practice of menstrual management in a contemporary town in Guinea, and the motivations of the women who use it. I conclude that trying to determine whether women induce their menses for the purpose of avoiding pregnancy or for maintaining their health misses the point. As a cultural practice, it is understood to accomplish both of these purposes. Providing a well-grounded understanding of the multiple meanings of this practice in its local context forms the content of this paper.

GLOBAL CONTEXT

Ethnographic evidence presented in several chapters of this volume, and in other papers from West Africa (Anarfi 1996; Renne 1996a, 1996b), Jamaica (Sobo 1993, 1996), India (Jeffrey, Jeffrey, and Lyon 1988), Colombia (Browner 1980), and China (Ngin 1985), indicates that the practice of menstrual management is quite widespread and not just a local Guinean phenomenon. The question of the origin of menstrual management is beyond the scope of this paper, although these studies help to place it in a wider context of practice. The fact that women in several locations in West Africa have now been found to practice some form of menstrual inducement makes it tempting to look for a direct cause, or a single source for what seems an arcane practice. Islam, or more specifically the importation of knowledge from the Islamic world, is sometimes identified as a source of cultural practices in West Africa. Although it is certain that historical linkages exist between West Africa and other parts of the Islamic world, it would be impossible to make such a claim for a specific practice. Distinctly Islamic forms of medicine, such as astrology and numerology, are practiced throughout much of West Africa, suggesting that health-related practices followed trade routes across the Sahara after the Muslim conquest of North Africa in the seventh century A.D. It is known that medical texts of ancient Greece were translated into Arabic during the eighth century A.D., and the works of Hippocrates, Galen, and others were consulted by physicians of the Islamic world in Egypt, Morocco, Spain, and elsewhere (Dols, in introduction to Ridwan [d. ca. 1068] 1984). This knowledge is likely to have been brought by travelers across the Sahara. The extensiveness of the area that was brought under Islamic control and the neighboring regions with which the Muslim scholars, traders, and others were in constant contact over seven centuries would have allowed for the medical practices of the ancient texts to find broad application. However, it is too great a leap to conclude that the specific concern with "suppression of menses" in the ancient texts gave rise to the problem of menstrual lateness described here.[1] Rather, problems of menstruation are culturally constituted in very specific ways within the Mande context of Dabola.

DATA SOURCES AND METHODOLOGY

The "discovery" of the practice of menstrual management revealed to me some of the shortcomings in standard social science research on reproduction in Africa. I came to learn about the practice of menstrual management by accident, having initially set out to complete a study of women's childbearing practices, focused on decisions about the timing and avoidance of pregnancy, in a part of West Africa known for high fertility.[2] Halfway through a household fertility survey conducted in Dabola, a community of 10,000 in Haute Guinée, several facts had become clear. Among them: women were quite willing to talk about their use of clinic-supplied contraceptives, to a greater degree than I had expected; and virtually none of the women had had an induced abortion, according to the survey responses. Yet I knew that some women in the town had indeed had an abortion, based on individual accounts in daily conversation apart from the survey. This discrepancy was not surprising, because the reluctance to talk openly about abortion was consistent with cultural norms and the national laws that forbid abortion. By contrast, the willingness to talk about contraception indicated a distinction between the meanings of these two practices.

At the same time, conversations with herbalists in Dabola revealed that the survey was missing something. As I followed an herbalist around in the woods at the edge of town one day, she pointed out different plants that she would harvest and prepare for women in order to cure various ailments. I had explained my interests in fairly narrow terms: plant medicines that could be used to prevent or delay a pregnancy, to help a woman become pregnant, or to cause an abortion. (All of the healers made it clear that they did not deal in this latter practice. None of them was willing to help a woman who wanted to abort a pregnancy, although one had provided this kind of medicine at a time in the distant past.) The herbalist explained that one of the main complaints from women was bellyache due to various causes. Among the causes are menstrual problems, including a range of symptoms, such as blood that was too dark or too light in color, too thick or too thin, too heavy or too light a flow, or too late in coming. At first,

I made the mistake of disregarding the concern with blood consistency, assuming that lateness was more important because it called for the inducement of menses, which I assumed to be a euphemism for early abortion. Over time, however, I learned that the practice of menstrual inducement was part of a wider practice of menstrual management, which constituted a completely separate cognitive category of reproductive action from either abortion or contraception.

In fact, by focusing on Western definitions of pregnancy, contraception, and abortion, many researchers have missed the menstrual management activity, and have concluded that in societies characterized by high fertility, respectable married women do nothing of consequence to control childbearing. One of my objectives in doing in-depth research on reproductive intentions and practices was to move beyond assumptions of this kind, learn about local women's management of their own fertility, and understand a system different from my own.

The conclusions I draw here are provisional, because this topic was not the initial or central focus of the research. No large-scale survey data exist on the prevalence of this practice in Guinea or West Africa. Rather, it is the consistency with which a variety of local sources pointed to the same conclusions that provides the main support for the argument. By piecing together information that emerged from open-ended survey questions in ethnographic research with young and old women, herbalists, doctors, and nurses over the course of a year of research, along with insights gained from my own observations and subsequently those of others about other West African locations, I have concluded that the practice that I have translated as "menstrual management" indeed plays an important part in women's reproductive lives (Levin 1996).

THE RESEARCH SETTING: DABOLA, GUINEA

Dabola, a community of about 10,000, lies along a geographical border separating the savanna of the Haute Guinée region from the Fouta Djalon highlands. Most of Dabola's inhabitants claim ancestral origins either in the Fouta Djalon or the Mande centers to the east and most speak primarily either Mandinka or Fula.

As in the past, this rural area is dominated by the cultivation of rice, groundnuts, and the local cereal, *fonio*. Now a part of the Haute Guinée region, the town of Dabola is an administrative seat for a *préfecture* (district) of 75,000 people where the average population density is 12 persons per square kilometer (low for Guinea, but typical for much of the savanna region in Guinea and Mali). Dabola has always been a market town, and many people are engaged in commerce. The road to Conakry was recently rebuilt, shifting commerce from Haute Guinée toward this capital city of Guinea.

All residents of Dabola are Muslims, except for approximately 20 civil servants and their families from the Forest region and several other foreigners, who are Christians. The local population has a number of options in seeking medical cures, and *fida toubabou* ("white man's medicine") is one of them. Dabola has both a hospital and a clinic for children and pregnant women, which since 1993 has provided contraceptives as part of a United Nations– and U.S. government–funded program. The presence of the hospital since the colonial time (Guinea was a colony of France until 1958) has likely diminished but not eliminated the appeal of a wide variety of other specialists, including healers who deal in magic; Koranic scholars, or *marabouts,* who also have healing powers; fetishists; herbalists; bone setters; traveling healers who sell medicinal powders; and other people known for their capacity to heal.

A Demographic and Health Survey conducted in 1992 in Guinea (Keita et al. 1994) reported high fertility (total fertility rate = 5.7), low contraceptive use (1.5 percent of all women using the so-called modern methods, 2.7 percent using all methods of contraception), long intervals between births (35 months), and relatively long periods of breast-feeding (23 months overall) and of postpartum abstinence (23 months). For the Haute Guinée region, the percentages of women using contraceptives were even lower: 0.6 for modern methods and 1.1 for all methods. In my 1995 community survey in Dabola, 14 percent of women used imported contraceptives, and the duration of both breast-feeding and postpartum sexual abstinence was 22 months on average for the previous 5 years.

MENSTRUAL MANAGEMENT IN DABOLA

Women in Dabola are keenly aware of their *fanka* (in Mandinka)— their physical robustness—which determines their capacity to recover from hardship, disease, pregnancy, and childbearing. All people are born with a certain level of *fanka* that is depleted over the course of one's life. More rapid depletion results from hardship, whether in the form of illness, a large number of pregnancies, particularly difficult pregnancies, labor, miscarriages, or other problems such as the death of family members or economic hardship. It is possible to restore one's *fanka* to some degree, and women who have suffered illness and difficult pregnancies must safeguard their health.

An important indication to a woman of her *fanka* and general health status is her menstrual health, which she measures by the regularity of the menstrual flow and the amount and quality of the blood. By being closely attuned to her menstrual cycle and acting quickly to treat problems, a woman can avoid serious problems common in this region, such as infertility, difficult pregnancy, miscarriage, hemorrhage, and death—her own or the child's. Consistent with the notion of *fanka* in the local system is the idea of a double spinal column in women, which gives them the additional strength they need to withstand pregnancy and labor. While this idea is mainly held by older women, many women express the exhaustion of repeated pregnancies in terms of the weariness of their bones. Similar expressions of depletion and fatigue are common in the Gambia (Bledsoe, Banja, and Hill 1998).

Menstrual problems are a sign of this depletion, and of fertility that may be compromised. Many menstrual problems are thought to be caused by a blockage, or *nyama* (in Mandinka),[3] which must be removed promptly. Blockages affect the color, quantity, and consistency of the menstrual blood but can cause more serious damage as well. For this reason, women who notice changes or problems in their cycle or in the menstrual blood seek help from one of several sources. They go to the hospital, where there is a reputable gynecologist, or to the clinic, where a well-known and trusted nurse can cure a variety of problems. Islamic specialists can also help women, as can others who use charms to heal. While the medically trained doctors and nurses are willing and able to help women who are pregnant, women who want to avoid pregnancy, and, to a lesser degree, women who are having difficulty becoming pregnant, they have fewer remedies for menstrual complaints. For this reason, many women seek the help of qualified herbalists who rely mainly on their knowledge of local botanical pharmacopoeia to treat both men and women for many illnesses. In my household survey, more than 20 percent of women reported having used plant medicines to either help them become pregnant, avoid pregnancy, or induce late menses. Most of these women had sought medicine from herbalists, although some medicines are available elsewhere, as described below.

Among the most common complaints for which women seek help from herbalists are painful menstrual periods; menstrual blood that is too dark, too light, too thin or thick, too abundant or too little; flow that is too heavy or too light; and menses that are expected but have not yet begun. As in many other societies, the Mandinka word for menstruation is the same word used for "month" or "moon": *karo*. Both the Mandinka and Islamic calendars use a 28-day month, which corresponds to the average length of a menstrual cycle. Women count months by cycles of the moon, and any cycle longer than 28 days represents a potential problem. (Another term used for menstruation is *mm'bolo ye gi ro* ["My hand is in the water"], referring to the large quantities of water needed to clean oneself and the menstrual cloth.) The ability to become pregnant when one wants to is extremely important; anything that would impair one's ability to do this indicates a possible *nyama*, or blockage, and must be corrected immediately. This concern is similarly expressed by some women when talking about contraceptive methods; the injectable contraceptive Depo Provera is known to stop menstrual flow during its use and to delay fecundity even after its use is suspended, which is an unfavorable property of a medicine otherwise seen as useful. Even the slightest hint that something is amiss in a woman's reproductive functioning is motivation to consult an herbalist and to take medicine.

Mariam is a pseudonym for a woman in Dabola who in 1995 was 30 years old, was married, and had one child, an 11-year-old daughter. Following several years of marital separation, Mariam was reunited with her husband, and although she thought her marriage was not secure, she wanted to have another child. In fact, she was under pressure from her own family, her husband's family, and other people to become pregnant. The following account of Mariam's situation suggests the importance of menstrual management and good menstrual health in curing infertility.

During 1995, Mariam was undergoing treatment for secondary infertility, having had one child and apparently unable to become pregnant again. Although several medical doctors had recommended surgery, she was reluctant to take such a drastic action. Instead, she sought advice from numerous practitioners and followed many different regimes in her effort to have another child. Among her doctors were a gynecologist at the local government hospital, and specialists in Conakry who had given her multiple courses of antibiotics and a type of water therapy. Upon returning to Dabola, she received help from two different healers, asked for advice from every herbalist and healer she met, and purchased medicine from the pharmacy when she could afford it. The plant medicines that she routinely took made her vomit frequently, but she would not be dissuaded from taking them. Mariam spoke openly about her remedies and her wish to become pregnant. She visited diviners to find out whether her efforts would be in vain. One day, she spoke enthusiastically about a plant medicine that she had recently found to be effective: "This medicine is extremely good. The blood is very good now, it isn't dark like it was before, it is very red, and healthy, and there is much more of it." I asked whether this would help her get pregnant. "I think so. I'm much healthier now, my period is much better, so I think I will be able to become pregnant" (Levin, 1995).

In this case, the herbalists are among several specialists consulted. Not only does Mariam seek a variety of medical and nonmedical healers for advice, but she also follows various treatments at the same time. She explains clearly the importance of good menstrual health in curing infertility. Crucial to this line of thinking is that the very goal of achieving good menstrual health is what allows women to seek help in inducing late menses; removing *nyama* that impede pregnancy is the first step in restoring good health. In addition, by establishing a relationship with herbalists and other healers, Mariam has given herself a basis for returning to them for other problems that may arise in the future. She has placed menstrual and reproductive health in the hands of healers, and her own responsibility for what happens is now partially, at least, reduced. No mother-in-law would think to impede a daughter-in-law's effort to have a child by questioning her reason for going to a specialist for care.

Late menstrual periods are one of the most frequent complaints for which herbalists treat women; another is a delay in becoming pregnant. The herbalists have a well-developed pharmacopoeia, including plants that can help women with menstrual complaints, and others that help in becoming pregnant (several plant medicines are used for both purposes). Women who seek treatment for "bellyaches" are questioned about their symptoms so that the herbalist can determine whether the bellyache is a menstrual complaint (including lateness), a pregnancy, or something different. The medicines used to treat menstrual lateness (emmenagogues) act by inducing menses. "Cleaning the belly" is one way of expressing menstrual inducement, although this term has other meanings as well. The herbalists also explain that their medicines can help to achieve a healthy, regular menstrual flow for a woman who has been unable to become pregnant.

Late menses, if one is not expecting to be pregnant, are often seen as a sign of a blockage. Many women do not expect or want to be pregnant during given times, for reasons that must be understood within the social context and local marriage and childbearing norms. The social requirement to maintain a 2-year interval between pregnancies provides an incentive to married women to carefully monitor their cycle. Sexual relations are forbidden during the postpartum period, but some women violate the rule by allowing their husbands to "visit" them (women generally have a room or a small house for themselves and their young children). In some cases, it is the fear that a husband will take a second (or third) wife that propels a woman to allow this transgression of rules. Similarly, women may find themselves in a relationship in which they do not want to have a child when their husbands are away for extended periods (men who work in the mines are typically away from home for months at a time), travel frequently for work, or are very old or sick, or when the women are visiting their own relatives for an extended time. The incentives for young women in school to avoid pregnancy are well known. And a woman who intends to leave her husband, or who expects her husband to leave, also tries to avoid having more children with him. All of these are reasons for married women not to be pregnant during specific times. For foreign observers, it is tempting to regard menstrual management simply as a form of early abortion when a woman has violated rules. Locally, however, the periods of pregnancy avoidance are highly charged with meaning; one must avoid pregnancy and tend to menstrual health so that, upon the end of the period of avoidance, pregnancy will be easily achieved and carried through to birth.

In Dabola, it is worth noting that menstruating women are not secluded, although they observe Islamic prohibitions against entering a mosque, praying, or observing the fast during Ramadan. Beyond the lack of obvious taboos, menstruation is a sign of good health, representing a woman's potential for future pregnancies and successful childbearing.

Women distinguish between menstrual management and abortion. Pregnancy is acknowledged only after the quickening (when the fetus can been felt moving), or when the pregnancy is obvious—approximately the fourth to fifth month. Although some women say that a pregnancy takes 10 months (in the lunar calendar), it is never really recognized until the time when it can no longer be denied. Most women refer to 9 months of pregnancy, counting from the time that an embryo is thought first to be formed. Reasons for reluctance to announce a pregnancy are the likelihood of miscarriage, or that an announcement will bring bad luck or invite jealousy and even witchcraft. Cases of abortion, while rare, always take place later in pregnancy. A study on maternal mortality in Guinea (Touré et al. 1992) found that most deaths due to abortion took place after the twelfth week of amenorrhea (due to pregnancy), pointing both to the higher risks attributed to clandestine abortion in later weeks, and to the secrecy around pregnancy as long as it can be concealed. Menstrual management, in contrast, appears to take place in the very first days, perhaps weeks, after a missed menses.

In Islamic writings, an early embryo is referred to as nothing more than a "clot of blood" that later forms into a human being (see also Hull and Hull in the present volume). The death of an embryo at this stage may not constitute the death of a person, leaving open the possibility that inducing menses during this time would not be considered an abortion, even in the case of conception.

LOCAL PHARMACOPOEIA USED FOR MENSTRUAL MANAGEMENT

Women who stated in interviews that they had used local plant medicines to clean the belly, either for the purpose of becoming pregnant or curing late menses, can obtain medicines from several sources, among them the local herbalists who work independently. Herbalists prescribe a variety of locally available plants and instruct women in the preparation of medicine for menstrual lateness, among a wide range of other problems. Two healers stated that menstrual problems were the most common complaint for which they were consulted. Their knowledge is highly specialized. It is not enough to know which plant to use; the plant must be picked at the right time of day and in the right season, and it must be handled in a manner known only to the herbalists. Sometimes the herbalist utters a phrase while picking and handling medicines. Among the local names of plants used are *kanin, sordon, popa,* and *sunsungbe.* Sometimes combinations of plants are made, to address certain combinations of symptoms or complaints. *Sunsungbe,* for example, can help a woman become pregnant, and, in combination with some other plants, is known to cure impotence in men. *Kanin* and *popa* are two medicines available at the market; they do not grow in the immediate vicinity of Dabola.

One of the advantages of herbalists is that one can consult them with far more privacy than is possible at the market. Both male and female herbalists treat women's problems; they diagnose an individual woman's problems carefully, focusing on not only the main complaint with which she initially arrives, but a range of symptoms that she might reveal over time. Most of these consultations, therefore, take place over a period of weeks or months. Healers generally want to have more than one session with a person seeking help.

I collected 18 plants that are used for reproductive purposes. Of them, 5 can be used to clean the belly, and, of these, 3 were reported by either doctors or herbalists to be effective in inducing an abortion. All 4 herbalists with whom I worked claimed knowledge of such plants. One herbalist also claimed to know of a plant that would prevent conception. Other plants are known to help women to become pregnant; those that help women who have previously had a child are distinguished from those that help women who have never given birth. All of the medicines used to clean the belly are also used to help ensure a good pregnancy. However, the herbalists insist that these medicines must not be used once a woman becomes pregnant, or they could cause a miscarriage. An important aspect of some of the medicines that help a woman become pregnant is that they induce menses as part of their cure. This procedure rids the body of problematic blood and blockages, and the medicines then correct the problem, the results of which are seen in the next menses.

By treating more than one problem at a time, the herbalist does not bring unnecessary attention to the fact that a woman's menses are late. Nor is there a reason to determine whether the lateness is due to an early pregnancy or some other problem. Instead, all aspects of the functioning of her reproductive system are treated simultaneously; the specific plant or plant mixture is chosen to remedy all of her complaints. Removing a potential blockage may be a part of the remedy, regardless of the source of the blockage.

AMBIGUITY AS A STRATEGY

I have argued that in Guinea, women are actively seeking help in treating menstrual problems in a deliberate effort to maintain their reproductive functioning and their ability to have a successful pregnancy. This activity includes the work of skillful and knowledgeable herbalists, whose involvement is important in legitimizing the activity as well as in providing essential medicinal plants and advice about their preparation and use. One element of menstrual treatment is the inducement of late menses, which women are eager to do, fearful that late menses may indicate blockages or other serious problems in their reproductive systems.

Menstrual inducement, I have argued, is seen as a measure taken in order to help maintain good health or to remove a blockage that is preventing pregnancy. It is a positive action undertaken with the intention of future childbearing. This is quite different, in local terms, from abortion, which is the removal of an unwanted fetus whose presence has announced itself to the woman by movement, a growing belly, or other signs. Abortions are the last resort in cases of premarital sex (particularly the seducing of young girls by older men), incest, extramarital sex that would be revealed by the pregnancy, a marriage about to dissolve, or in other situations in which the pregnancy is seen as misfortune. Abortions are done in secret; menstrual management may not be discussed publicly, but it is not subject to the same level of secrecy as abortion.

In herbalists' and women's own terms, the inducement of menses is a means of "cleaning the belly" to begin anew, to remove clots and blockages, to improve the quality of the blood, and to restore and maintain one's health and strength. Not knowing of the presence of a fetus, and not even wanting to know, is part of maintaining "cleaning the belly" as an activity that is wholly, conceptually different from abortion.

The local logic of menstrual management is internally consistent as a positive action that promotes reproductive health, and I believe that most women who practice it are concerned with their health, not with removing a pregnancy. Yet, there were indications that some women are using the same medicines once they suspect they are pregnant. One Guinean doctor told me, "The woman tells her friend, 'I have a bellyache.' The friend says, 'Here, take this,' and gives her a root. She aborts." While this statement represents a translation into medical terms, and points to a tension between biomedical views and local views about pregnancy, menstrual management, and abortion, it also provides a clue that intentions are not always stated directly. Other writers have pointed to the ambiguity that lies in this gray area between the use of emmenagogues and abortion (Sobo 1996; Carter 1995). In fact, ambiguity can provide women with the cultural space in this aggressively high-fertility context in which to control their fertility.

Ambiguity—the multiple meanings of menstrual management in the Guinean context—is in itself desirable precisely because it allows women to act on fertility intentions, and to control the timing of pregnancy without doing so in an obvious way that would be contrary to other norms. Within the field of reproductive action, menstrual management gives women a much greater degree of freedom, while being publicly consistent with the ideal of good reproduction. This does not mean that women who practice menstrual management are simply doing one thing (abortion) and stating that it is something else (fertility enhancement). There is instead a range of intentions and actions, all linked to specific situations and circumstances. And, without absolute knowledge of a pregnancy, it is impossible to say the degree to which actual pregnancies are avoided. A woman who simply cannot become pregnant in a given set of circumstances does not have to consider that possibility if she is regularly managing her menses.

The interconnections between intention, action, and explanation in individual situations are complex in the Dabola reproductive arena. Practices of reproductive enhancement and fertility control in this context are parts of the very same process. Giving birth to healthy children when it is considered appropriate and in good circumstances requires constant attention to one's reproductive health, and the avoidance of pregnancy during other times.

NOTES

I am grateful to Caroline Bledsoe for her contributions to this chapter, and to Mette Shayne, Patricia Ogendengbe, Mohamed Fofana, Robert Launay, Helen Schwartzman, Paola Scommegna, Fatou Banja, Alaka Basu, Peter Aaby, Gil Stein, and participants in a 1996 seminar, "Socio-Cultural and Political Aspects of Abortion from an Anthropological Perspective," sponsored by the International Union for the Scientific Study of Population. The research was conducted during 1994–95 with grants from the U.S. Fulbright Commission and the Program of African Studies of Northwestern University, under the auspices of the Sociology Department of the Université de Conakry.

1. The trade routes from the Islamic world into West Africa were indeed part of even larger networks that spanned Africa, the Mediterranean region, the Middle East, and much of Asia. Goods, technology, religious texts, and information traveled in all directions, and it is likely that ideas and practices followed circuitous routes. It would be most difficult to trace the route of specific remedies. Further, some of the remedies in the Greek texts, such as bloodletting, phlebotomy, and cupping (a practice involving the application of small hot bowls to the skin to create a suction) (Brain 1986), are not found in the ethnographic literature on West Africa. And women's health practices are less likely to have been disseminated in the medical texts of the Islamic scholars than other kinds of medicine (Launay 1998), even if health-related practices may travel in nontextual ways.

2. The total fertility rate in Guinea is 5.7; in the region of Haute Guinée it is 5.8 (Keita et al. 1994).

3. Extensive discussions of *nyama* in the literature on Mande link it to the life force and to blood (Paulme 1973; Conrad and Frank 1995; Dieterlen 1951). However, the present usage is probably best translated simply as "garbage" or "blockage" (Launay 1998).

REFERENCES

Anarfi, John. 1996. "The Role of Local Herbs in the Recent Fertility Decline in Ghana: Contraceptives or Abortifacients?" Paper presented to the seminar on Socio-Cultural and Political Aspects of Abortion from an Anthropological Perspective, International Union for the Scientific Study of Population, Trivandrum, Kerala, India.

Bledsoe, Caroline, Fatoumatta Banja, and Allan G. Hill. 1998. "Reproductive Mishaps and Western Contraception: An African Challenge to Fertility Theory." *Population and Development Review* 24, no. 1:15–57.

Brain, Peter. 1986. "Galen's Book on Treatment by Venesection." In *Galen on Bloodletting*. Cambridge: Cambridge University Press.

Browner, C. H. 1980. "The Management of Early Pregnancy: Colombian Folk Concepts of Fertility Control." *Social Science & Medicine* 14B:25–32.

Carter, Anthony. 1995. "Agency and Fertility: For an Ethnography of Practice." In *Situating Fertility: Anthropology and Demographic Inquiry*, ed. Susan Greenhalgh, 55–85. Cambridge: Cambridge University Press.

Conrad, David, and Barbara Frank, eds. 1995. *Status and Identity in West Africa*. Bloomington: Indiana University Press.

Dieterlen, Germaine. 1951. *Essai sur la religion Bambara*. Paris: Presses Universitaires de France.

Jeffrey, Patricia, Roger Jeffrey, and Andrew Lyon. 1988. *Labour Pains and Labour Power*. London: Zed Books.

Keita, Mohamed L., Mamadou C. Bah, Mamadou B. Diallo, and Bernard Barrère. 1994. *Enquête Démographique et de Santé: Guinée 1992*. Conakry, Guinea: Direction Nationale de la Statistique et de l'Informatisation.

Launay, Robert. 1998. Personal communication.

Levin, Elise. 1995. Field notes.

———. 1996. "Menstrual Management and Abortion in Guinea." Paper presented to the seminar on Socio-Cultural and Political Aspects of Abortion from an Anthropological Perspective, International Union for the Scientific Study of Population, Trivandrum, Kerala, India.

Ngin, Chor-Swant. 1985. "Indigenous Fertility Regulating Methods among Two Chinese Communities in Malaysia." In *Women's Medicine: A Cross-Cultural Study of Indigenous Fertility Regulation*, ed. Lucile Newman, 25–41. New Brunswick, N.J.: Rutgers University Press.

Paulme, Denise. 1973. "Blood Pacts, Age Classes and Castes in Black Africa." In *French Perspectives in African Studies,* ed. Pierre Alexandre, 73–95. London: Oxford University Press.

Renne, Elisha. 1996a. "The Pregnancy That Doesn't Stay: The Practice and Perception of Abortion by Ekiti Yoruba Women." *Social Science & Medicine* 42, no. 4:483–94.

———. 1996b. "Changing Assessments of Abortion in a Northern Nigerian Town." Paper presented to the seminar on Socio-Cultural and Political Aspects of Abortion from an Anthropological Perspective, International Union for the Scientific Study of Population, Trivandrum, Kerala, India.

Ridwan, Ali ibn. 1984 [d. ca. 1068]. *Medieval Islamic Medicine.* Ed. and trans. Michael W. Dols. Berkeley: University of California Press.

Sobo, Elisa. 1993. *One Blood: The Jamaican Body.* Albany: SUNY Press.

———. 1996. "Abortion Traditions in Rural Jamaica." *Social Science & Medicine* 42, no. 4:495–508.

Touré, B., P. Thonneau, P. Cantrelle, T. M. Barry, T. Ngo-Khac, and E. Papiernik. 1992. "Level and Causes of Maternal Mortality in Guinea (West Africa)." *Journal of Gynecological Obstetrics* 37:89–95.

CHAPTER 9

The Blood That Links: Menstrual Regulation among the Bamana of Mali

Sangeetha Madhavan and Aisse Diarra

The cow keeps the blood in herself in order to
give milk.

—Bamana proverb

Women in high-fertility populations are expected to bear numerous
children, yet they may also suffer from menstrual irregularity. Among
the Bamana of Mali, a regular menstrual cycle is seen as a sign of good
health, which, in turn, is a precondition for pregnancy and fertility.
Stated another way, menstrual blood links general good health to
healthy fertility. Irregular menstruation, on the other hand, is evidenced by numerous symptoms including a delay in menses, painful
menses, too little or too much bleeding, and dark or malodorous blood.
In a society where female status is earned through successful childbearing, it is not surprising that women endure substantial psychological
hardship when they attempt to reconcile desires for high fertility with
an irregular menstrual cycle. The failure to produce children can lead
to divorce or the acquisition of a co-wife, both of which can greatly
compromise a woman's position in her community. This is further
complicated by the fact that menstrual abnormalities along with many
illnesses are often seen as having nonphysiological causes such as jealousy between co-wives. We contend that menstrual irregularities evoke
particular anxiety not only because of their association with witchcraft,
but also because menstruation is so closely linked to childbearing.

In this chapter, we locate menstrual regulation within the context
of high fertility among the Bamana and argue that it is a necessity for
women whose ultimate fear is the inability to meet their childbearing
obligations. Specifically, we investigate (1) the perceptions of menstrual blood; (2) the perceived link between menstruation and fertility;
(3) the extent to which menstrual abnormalities are seen as a health

problem, and the most common treatments for them; and (4) the ambiguities surrounding abortion and menstrual regulation. We close with some observations on the psychological effects of menstrual irregularity. Our data come from a large-scale survey on social networks, a small survey on menstrual regulation, and qualitative interviews with elder women, traditional healers, clinic personnel, and herbalists.

RESEARCH SETTING

The research for this study was carried out in Mali, an impoverished West African country struggling to establish economic and political stability. While efforts are under way to provide adequate health care in all areas of the country, there remains a large unmet need for gynecological and obstetrical care, especially in the rural areas. The Bamana, a nominally Muslim[1] ethnic group, constitute 35 percent of the total population and inhabit the most arable area of the country. According to a recent fertility survey, rural Bamana women have a total fertility of 7.6 children per woman, a mean age of marriage of 16 years, a current contraceptive use rate of 1.5 percent, and a literacy rate of 10 percent (EDS 1996). Like the rest of the Malian population, they have not yet experienced a demographic transition. Bamana society is patrilineal and patrilocal, with a household organization system that places the most senior male member in charge of both production and reproduction of labor. Polygyny and extended family systems are common among the Bamana to meet the demand for agricultural labor. More than half of all married women are in polygynous unions. Household members are expected to work with one another for the greater good of the corporate structure. A strong pro-natalist ideology among the Bamana is strengthened by precisely such structural features (Brett-Smith 1994; Toulmin 1992).

The first indication that menstrual irregularities may be a widespread health problem in Mali came during data collection for a comparative study on women's social networks in Bamana and Fulbe communities (Adams and Castle 1995).[2] In contrast to the Bamana, the seminomadic Fulbe have a contempt for cultivation and instead idealize a life of herding cattle. A 9-part survey was administered to 500 rural Bamana and 500 Fulbe women of reproductive age. The women's anthropometry and health section included 2 self-reported health status questions. Among the many possible responses, the 2 that can be considered as potential indicators of menstrual irregularity are *maux de ventre* (belly-

ache) and *maux de seins* (painful or sore breasts). It should be noted
that *maux de ventre* and *maux de seins* are generic terms used to describe
symptoms associated with a whole range of illnesses, from heartburn
and indigestion to appendicitis. However, women tend to refer to these
two symptoms, in particular, when discussing ailments related to reproduction.

While *maux de seins* does not appear to be a significant problem,
maux de ventre is commonly reported. Sixteen percent of Bamana
women and 18 percent of Fulbe women who reported any health problems in the 2 weeks prior to survey complained of *maux de ventre*. In
addition, 23 percent of Bamana women and 20 percent of Fulbe
women who mentioned any problem at the time of survey specified
maux de ventre. The age distribution of the women suggests that *maux
de ventre* is a problem mentioned by women in all stages of the reproductive span, although it appears to be more common among older
women. Such a finding lends some support to the speculation that
maux de ventre is linked to menstrual irregularity, because menstrual
problems become more frequent as women near menopause.

In addition, during the course of qualitative interviews,[3] we noticed
that women often mentioned menstrual cramps and irregular cycles
as "illnesses" they had endured throughout their lives. In the case of
one 26-year-old Fulbe woman, her inability to have even one live birth
caused her to travel to the capital city to seek treatment. She had good
reason, given that her husband told us he would definitely get another
wife if the current one could not bear children for him. We found a
similar situation with a 19-year-old Fulbe woman who had lost both
her pregnancies and complained of severe bellyaches. Her husband
asked us for advice on treatments that would enable her to produce
children. These are but two examples of a recurrent concern we heard
from both Fulbe and Bamana women about reproductive mishaps and,
more important, irregular fertility.

Noting the preoccupation that women had with normal fertility and
the accompanying complaints about menstrual irregularities, we decided to collect data specifically on menstruation in 1 of the 2 ethnic
groups. We needed to learn how Bamana women perceive menstruation and what they consider to be abnormalities. Most important, we
wanted to see if and how they relate such problems to their fertility.
The discussion that follows is based on a semistructured questionnaire
administered to 20 women of reproductive age; in-depth interviews
with 5 postmenopausal women (older than age 50 years); and conversations with traditional healers and birth attendants. Given the sensitive nature of the subject matter, we conducted most of the interviews

in a village where we had made ourselves well known from previous work.

BAMANA PERCEPTIONS OF MENSTRUAL BLOOD

The anthropological literature on menstruation tends to focus on the negative aspects. We know that in many cultures there are taboos forbidding sexual intercourse during menses and prohibiting menstruating women from going near places of worship or food preparation (Buckley and Gottlieb 1988). Blood—the life force—in its menstrual form assumes the attributes of dirt and pollution. In accordance with such cultural notions and Islamic taboos regarding menstruation, we find Bamana women abstaining from prayer and visits to the mosque during their menses. They are also expected to abstain from sex by telling their husband that they "are sick." Among the Bamana, both men and women believe that sexual intercourse during menses could cause the man to fall sick. In some families, it is believed that menstruating women should not prepare food that will be eaten by others, a practice common to many cultures (Buckley and Gottlieb 1988). In addition, there is some evidence suggesting that Bamana men perceive each menses as a possible abortion, causing understandable apprehension among Bamana women (Brett-Smith 1998).

Many cultures see menstruation as a purification process through the expulsion of unclean blood from the body (Sobo 1993). In Bamana, *koli* (derived from the verb *ka kwo*, which means "to wash") is a common word for menstruation. However, its usage varies among women. In our survey, 7 out of 20 women explained *koli* as cleaning the menstrual blood itself, presumably of its "dirt," arguing that only after this impurity is purged from the body can pregnancy occur. A particularly graphic description came from a 62-year-old woman: "It [blood] is an impurity that must be detached from the body; if not, there will not be a pregnancy." The "dirt" in menstrual blood is also associated with illness, as explained by a 65-year-old woman who claimed that "[a] child conceived during menses will turn out to be a leper." The connection between menses and leprosy has been noted in Western cultures as well (Vosselman 1935). Other sources on Bamana beliefs suggest that a child conceived during a woman's menses will be sexually deformed (Brett-Smith 1994). Fear of either consequence reflects a general concern with inappropriate conceptions and unhealthy pregnancies.

The remaining 13 women defined *koli* as cleaning the cloth that is used to absorb the blood during menses. The preoccupation with keeping clothes and cloth clean, especially for young unmarried women, is fitting for a society in which women are expected to be discreet about sexuality and fertility. Bloodstains on one's dress or on the cloth amount to a public statement on one's fertility status. When we asked women what they were told about menstruation by their mothers and what they told their daughters, 9 out of 20 stressed the need to prevent staining. They explained that public appearance of menses not only would be shameful for the girl but also could be an invitation to young men to take advantage of her.

Bamana women are fiercely protective of their menstrual cloth because one's enemies can use it to perform acts of sorcery and cause sterility. A 63-year-old woman explained:

> Menses are considered to be impure; the cloth that is used is considered to be sacred; it should be well hidden because someone can use it against you and cause your menses to stop and subsequent sterility.

Traditionally, Bamana women have seen menstrual blood as a source of power because it is a part of one's womanhood and therefore can be used to thwart one's fertility. A 65-year-old respondent added, "Sterility comes not just from God but from people who do not like you." Nowhere is this better illustrated than in polygynous households, where we often find women competing for status through successful childbearing. Our interviews suggest that women do not see anything wrong with women having their menses together, just as they do not find anything particularly wrong about co-wives being pregnant at the same time. Yet, there is also some evidence that a woman is reluctant to divulge her menstrual status to a co-wife, either because of shame or because of the desire to keep such vital information from a potential competitor. In light of recent scientific evidence supporting the idea that there is synchronicity of menstrual cycles among cohabiting women (Angier 1998), co-wife competition becomes even more problematic. Moreover, an older study suggests that emotional more than physical closeness is needed for menstrual cycles to synchronize (Weller, Weller, and Avinir 1995).

MENSES AND FERTILITY

All but 2 of the 20 women in the survey stated that menstruation is a sign of a woman's fecundity. The 2 women who responded differently stated that it is a sign of physical maturity, which is another way of describing a woman's readiness for childbearing. Such consensus suggests that Bamana women, despite lack of any formal counseling on the reproductive process, recognize that the menstrual cycle is a precondition for fertility. This finding is consistent with other ethnographic research in West Africa (see Levin, this volume), which suggests that menstruation is not only a sign of good health but also a marker of a woman's reproductive capability. However, our discussions with both women and men about sexual intercourse suggest that most people do not have any deeper understanding about the menstrual cycle. We heard frequent complaints from newlyweds (both spouses) that it had been very difficult for the wife to become pregnant. Further probing about her last menses and their coital frequency revealed that neither partner knew that coitus needs to occur on certain days of the menstrual cycle.

The extent to which women connect menstruation and fertility is made clear in the comparison of menstrual blood with blood that is present at the time of delivery. A 55-year-old woman told us: "You should clean the sticky blood in order to be clean; it is like the blood that is there at the moment of delivery." The sticky blood is the menstrual blood, which needs to be purged in the same manner as blood during delivery. Most women note that there is greater volume of blood following delivery than during menses but that both are impurities. They classify the duration of bleeding of the former as "long" and the latter as "short." In short, the interviews give a strong indication that Bamana women see both menses and bleeding following delivery as cleaning mechanisms the body uses to prepare itself for the next birth.

While most women recognize that pregnancy stops menses, they also think of regular menses as having a positive effect on the probability of conception and having a healthy birth. Our study suggests that Bamana women attempt to correct menstrual irregularities through the use of emmenagogues in order to ensure regular and healthy childbearing. The use of menstrual regulation techniques offers an interesting twist to the notion of regular birth intervals in high-fertility populations with minimal contraceptive use (Bongaarts and Potter 1983). The mean duration to resumption of menses in our sample is 13 months. In the absence of any menstrual regulation (indicating that a woman is satisfied with the quality and regularity of her menses), birth intervals would be, on average, 2 years. If, however, women use emmenagogues with the intention of regulating their menstrual cycles to ensure healthy fertility, they may experience spontaneous abortions. This would lengthen the duration of the birth interval past 2 years. We present this hypothesis fully recognizing that data on spontaneous intrauterine mortality is very difficult to collect, let alone fetal mortality caused by emmenagogues. Moreover, it is highly unlikely that the use of emmenagogues is great enough in a given population to affect the proximate determinants of fertility. Nonetheless, it is precisely such ambiguity that should encourage us to scrutinize biomedical models of fertility that have assumed universal importance yet have not incorporated cultural variation. In Bamana society, where there is a high premium on healthy childbearing, women may attain more psychological security by using some form of menstrual regulation that they believe will guarantee a healthy birth, even if it means a longer birth interval.

PERCEPTIONS OF MENSTRUAL IRREGULARITIES

Regular menses are seen as a sign of good health. A delay in menses without a pregnancy was cited by 17 of the 20 women in our sample as a sign of "illness." While 18 of the 20 women surveyed said that once a month defines a normal cycle, their reported length of delays differed widely, ranging from a few days to several months, with a mean of about 3 weeks. Twelve women reported that they became concerned about any delay in their menses after a reasonable waiting period following the birth of their last child. Half of these 12 women worried about the possibility of illness, while the others feared that those who experience delays in their cycle would not fall pregnant quickly. These 2 responses evoke the linking blood metaphor wherein good health (good blood) is associated with a normal menstrual cycle, which in turn leads to healthy fertility. One 62-year-old woman summed this up nicely when she said, "The young women become worried because a missed month may mean that they will have to wait longer for a child." The remaining 6 women all gave answers related to pregnancy. They were concerned about an unnecessarily long wait until the next birth or the possibility of premature menopause. The 8 women who said that they were not particularly concerned with a delay in their menses simply stated that "it is normal for me."

Bamana women do not attribute menstrual abnormalities to hunger or hard work because the menstrual cycle is seen as a natural phenomenon that is part of being a "proper" woman. Our study also reveals that instead of seeing some physiological illness as a cause of delays, Bamana women see the delay itself as a physical malady caused by non-physiological forces. Quite often, these forces involve the efforts of a female rival who attempts to gain a "fertility advantage" by disturbing the menstrual cycle of another. While most women had difficulty articulating the precise cause of this "illness," there was consensus that it will cause delays in becoming pregnant and possibly sterility. The onset of menopause causes much apprehension in women because of their lack of knowledge as to its timing. Every Bamana woman is aware that she cannot bear children throughout her life but can only guess as to when the end of her reproductive life may be. As a result, a delay in her menses causes a woman to immediately contemplate her worst nightmare: premature menopause. The 4 women who reported not being concerned about a delay explained that they do not see the 28-day cycle as a norm for them and that it is, after all, God's decision. It is interesting to note that this rationale bears striking resemblance to the answer that women give when asked why they cannot specify a desired number of children. In Mali, any fertility-related phenomenon is in the hands of God (Madhavan 1997).

The older women, who tend to be the least inhibited and the most informed about traditional practices, explained their ideas about menstrual abnormalities. The most common cause is adultery, as explained by a 62-year-old woman: "One advice I give to women who have problems with their cycles is to be faithful to their husbands and avoid sex with a lover." This fits with the notion that menstrual blood is linked to the blood that carries a pregnancy to term. Blood that has been contaminated by a lover's semen causes physical discomfort and must be purged in order to ensure a successful pregnancy. Older women realize that imminent menopause could also explain some of these symptoms along with other reproductive ailments. Failure to conceive by women nearing menopause is generally accepted (though not always desired) as a normal occurrence. Whatever the cause, most women make great efforts to procure proper treatment that can come in many forms but has only one objective: to ensure healthy childbearing and thus secure status.

Two common Bamana terms are used to describe the menstrual cycle. The first is *kalo labo,* which refers to the periodicity of the lunar cycle. The idea of the menstrual cycle synchronizing with the lunar cycle appears to have universal resonance. Among the Bamana there are taboos about the new and full moons. One 18-year-old respondent explained, "When my cycle comes during the first two weeks of the month and it happens during the new moon, I become worried because I have heard that menses during the new moon indicates rapid

Table 9.1   Local Terms for Symptoms of Gynecological Ailments

Local Term	Description
Konnondimi	Lower bellyache
*Golocoroda**	Severe menstrual irregularity that can potentially cause sterility
Lodimi	Backache
Locodimi	Pain in the hips
Tonson nyimi	Pain of the placenta—can cause abortion if untreated
Bolodgioma	Discomfort during intercourse

* We understand this to be a general term to describe any fertility-related problem for both women and men.

fertility." The women in our sample also believe that menstruating during a full moon causes great difficulty in becoming pregnant. The second term, *m'bolo le ji la,* literally means "my hand is in the water" (referring to the quantity of water used to wash menstrual cloths repeatedly). Women use it as a polite way of letting their partners know they are menstruating and so cannot have sex. This same Mandinka expression is also used in Guinea (see Levin, this volume).

There appears to be no shortage of symptoms to describe what are potentially menstrual irregularities. Table 9.1 provides a list of the most common gynecological complaints, some of which encompass menstrual ailments.

For some women, *konnondimi* begins about 3 days before the menses and stops almost immediately, while for others it lingers until the end of the menses. Younger women experience especially painful menses along with nausea. *Lodimi* usually begins just before the onset of menses. Diakite (1993:31) defines *tonson nyimi* as a term that designates "all the illnesses responsible for stillbirths or repeated infant mortality." He observes that the term also classifies cases in which lesions on the placenta or on the body of the child are evident. A few women paid special attention to their menstrual blood itself in describing it as black or sticky or bad smelling. Three women reported that too much blood during menses is not normal and that it should be released as soon as possible.

COMMON TREATMENTS FOR MENSTRUAL IRREGULARITIES

Numerous studies in the developing world have found that women prefer to discuss sex and fertility with close friends or women of the same age group (March and Taqqu 1986). Bamana women consider problems related to the menstrual cycle as intimate or "female" issues that should be discussed only with close friends and family members, preferably women. In our sample, 15 out of 20 women said that they had sought advice from older women, and the remaining 5 consulted a traditional healer when they experienced such problems.

Menstrual abnormalities provide an ideal case for comparing use of traditional and modern health care because, from the Bamana woman's perspective, the etiology of the problems is not solely rooted in biomedical explanations. Bamana women attribute menstrual abnormalities to both physiological and supernatural factors, the latter referring to external efforts meant to thwart a woman's fertility. Therefore, most women seek treatment from traditional healers who are seen as better equipped than Western health practitioners to handle the wrath of spirits. A 63-year-old woman told us, "I advise a young girl to get advice from the elders on treatment. God can help and she falls pregnant." Not surprisingly, Western medicine is perceived as powerless in such cases, a common phenomenon that is well documented in anthropological and biomedical literature of the developing world (Kleinman 1980).

When women seek treatment for menstrual abnormalities, their goal is to regain synchronicity with the lunar cycle while avoiding the full moon. One simple method of avoiding this situation is bathing in water that has had hot coals in it. The most common emmenagogues, however, are infusions or powders made from plants. The prescriptions usually do not specify quantity measurements. One simply learns from trial and error the appropriate quantities much the way a good cook prepares a dish. Table 9.2 provides a partial list of some common emmenagogues and general treatments for gynecological ailments. The use of the talisman *(tafo)* is unclear, but it is consistent with a common belief in Mali that charms have the power to ward off evil spirits. Most treatments are often given by a traditional healer for free, although a payment of tea and kola nuts[4] is always appreciated. Women can also purchase some of these products in the local market or collect them in the forest and prepare the medicines themselves.

The last resort for the treatment of menstrual irregularities is modern medicine. Most midwives who work in clinics report seeing women of all ages seeking treatment for menstrual irregularities, sexually transmitted diseases, and menopause. Initial consultations cost CFA 700 (approximately US$1.50), which is not prohibitively expensive for most villagers. Being true to their training in Western medicine, midwives attribute menstrual abnormalities to hormonal irregularities and

Table 9.2 Common Traditional Treatments for Fertility-Related Ailments

Local Term	Scientific Name	Purpose	Method of Use
Manan	Generic name for a wild plant	Regularize menstrual cycles	Pound the bark and mix with water and drink.
Djiefelebe	N/A	Cures *bolodgioma* (discomfort during intercourse)	Pound the roots and mix with Karite* butter and apply to the genitals; can also mix with bathing water.
Belebele	*Maeru angolensis*	Cures *golocoroda* (menstrual irregularity)	Pound the roots into an ointment and apply to the stomach.
Dodotourou (leaves that are only found during the rainy season)	N/A	Regularize menstrual cycles	Boil the leaves and drink.
Nerecolokogniki	*Parkia biglobosa*	*Tonson nyimi* (pain of the placenta)	Fill an earthenware jug with cooked seed from the *nere* plant and then mix powder from the jug itself to make an infusion; drink with salt.
Tafo (talisman)	N/A	Prevent infection	Attach to a string and wear it around the kidneys.
Burned leaves found around a termite mound	N/A	*Tonson nyimi* (pain of the placenta)	Consume the powder daily with water.

* Karite is a tree commonly found in Mali. The "butter" made from the nuts is used in cooking and in ointments for a range of health problems.

illness, hard work, and hunger. They observe that young childless women express the greatest apprehension about delayed or missed periods because they feel the need to prove their fertility potential in their conjugal homes. One midwife explained, "Children are desired in Bamana society and menstrual irregularity is seen as an illness. The women first consult a traditional healer and then come see us." It should be clarified that *illness,* as used here, actually refers to symptoms of some illness that could have grave consequences for a woman's fertility schedule. Some patients are older women who do not want to have any more children and are worried that the delay is actually a pregnancy.

According to clinic midwives, modern treatments are categorized as either hormonal regulation (presumably in the modern family-planning usage of the term) or antibiotics. They explained that if the delay or quantity of blood is a result of hormonal imbalances, the woman is put on the birth control pill for 3 months, presumably to regularize the menses. One packet costs about CFA 100 (US$0.20). If the problem persists, she is given Dufaston, a generic antibiotic, or sent to a specialist in the capital city. These last two options are financially out of reach for many women. If the problem is diagnosed as being related to an infection, the treatment is usually some form of anti-biotic, anti-inflammatory, or antispasmodic such as Amoxcycline, Otrimoxazole, or Endometacyne. While women are beginning to have more faith in modern medicine's ability to handle "women's issues," they still prefer traditional treatments because they tend to be skeptical of the biomedical explanation of menstrual irregularity given by the clinic's midwife. Moreover, the formal health sector is increasingly us-ing a Westernized approach to fertility-related problems, which means that both menstrual abnormalities and menstrual regulation are mar-ginalized. Little attention is accorded to the Bamana notion of men-strual regularity that refers to the periodic cleansing of the body in preparation for the next birth. As a result, rural women for whom menstrual regulation is of primary importance feel alienated from "modern" health care.

MENSTRUAL REGULATION AND ABORTION

While we did not set out to investigate abortion practices in this study, the topic came up during conversations about treatments. Our data indicate that both women and traditional healers see a difference be-tween menstrual regulation and abortion and distinguish emmena-gogues from abortifacients, although they realize that the former can, in some cases, inadvertently cause an abortion. Part of the concern about keeping the two separate comes from the belief mentioned ear-lier that Bamana men suspect every menses to be a possible abortion. Notably, the women in our sample often described menses as a purg-ing, a depiction with a striking resemblance to the description of an abortion that expels the fetus. Describing emmenagogues, the 75-year-old woman who was the most trusted traditional birth attendant and healer in the village said,

> I know of a plant called *soro* which can regularize menstrual cycles when the sap is inserted into the vagina. However, it can also cause abortions, which is why I do not prescribe this treatment until the

woman has had a three-month delay in her menses, which would indicate that there is no pregnancy; in general, I do not talk about this with young women.

Her 3-month rule for ensuring that no pregnancy is aborted by accident is evidence of the distinction made between the use of emmenagogues for the purpose of restoring proper menses, which in turn enhances fertility, and abortifacients. Healers exercise much caution in prescribing emmenagogues to women who are in their prime reproductive years in order to prevent any accidental abortions. This lends support to a prevailing sentiment in strong pro-natalist cultures that abortion is only to be used in extreme circumstances (Caldwell and Caldwell 1994).

The situation is quite different for older women who have simply grown tired of childbearing and may, therefore, actively seek out abortifacients under the guise of menstrual regulation. Bamana women approaching menopause may be using emmenagogues as *post*-conception fertility management—a marked departure from the more familiar Western notions of *pre*-conception fertility control. In such cases, a traditional healer would understand that a client is actually looking for an abortifacient. Although abortion is illegal in Mali, women are aware that it can be done if needed, either through traditional emmenagogues or in clinics in the cities. In short, we advise caution in equating menstrual regulation with early-term abortion. Although it is often very difficult to distinguish the use of emmenagogues from abortifacients, we argue that in societies in which childbearing is still highly valued, women consider abortion only to avoid a potentially disastrous situation such as a birth from a forbidden union, or when they are close to the end of their reproductive life spans.

CONCLUSION

In closing, we would like to bring attention to one aspect of menstrual regulation that risks being marginalized: the psychological and emotional consequences of menstrual irregularity. These concerns, which came up consistently during our interviews, underscore the extent to which menstrual regularity is linked to successful childbearing. While menstrual abnormalities manifest themselves in pain and other physical symptoms, the actual source of worry for most women is the disruption to their fertility schedules. For newlyweds, who must establish their status in their husband's family, and for older women, who want to maintain their senior positions in their affined homes, the pressure to bear numerous healthy children is a constant source of anxiety. The fact that women on the extremes of the reproductive span are most likely to experience menstrual irregularities because of hormonal shifts (Treloar et al. 1967) makes these women particularly prone to psychological distress. While the physical aspects of menstrual irregularity are obvious, the psychological consequences require special attention. As a point of comparison, in Western countries with low fertility, we pay attention to the symptoms of premenstrual syndrome (PMS), which, for many women, include emotional and psychological hardship. Such a phenomenon is usually attributed to hormonal changes that occur prior to a menstrual period. For Bamana women who face enormous pressure to bear children, the psychological effects of irregular menstruation can be far more serious and last much longer than the periodic and short-term trauma that Western women experience from PMS. It is clear that in both Western and non-Western settings, menstrual aberrations have serious emotional and psychological implications.

It is not particularly surprising that women living in societies that place a high premium on fertility are judged to a large extent on their success in childbearing. Bamana women believe that healthy reproduction and regular menstruation are linked. It follows that menstrual irregularities cause much anxiety for women of reproductive age because they can lead to problems with conceptions. If, as Bamana women believe, a body purged of its impurities provides the ideal condition for a healthy pregnancy, there is little wonder that emmenagogues are frequently used. There is nothing paradoxical about Bamana women using emmenagogues to induce menses while expressing a strong desire to bear children. The former is an essential aspect of achieving the latter.

NOTES

The authors wish to thank Sarah Brett-Smith for her insightful comments and suggestions.

1. We describe the Bamana as nominally Muslim because historically they have always opposed Islam with Bamanaya, the traditional set of Bamana religious beliefs. People tend to identify themselves as Muslim because it is socially acceptable, but very few people are practicing Muslims.

2. This project was supported by the National Science Foundation and seeks to relate women's social network composition to maternal and child health outcomes. The authors took part in the fieldwork in Mali during the period April 1996 to April 1997.

3. These interviews were conducted by the authors during the fieldwork for the social networks project.

4. Tea and kola nuts, natural stimulants, are traditional gifting items in Mali. They are given as signs of respect and gratitude.

REFERENCES

Adams, Alayne, and Sarah Castle. 1995. "Women's Social Networks and Health: Linking Context, Process and Outcomes." Project funded by the National Science Foundation.

Angier, Natalie. 1998. "Study Finds Signs of Elusive Pheromones in Humans." *New York Times,* 12 March.

Bongaarts, John, and Robert G. Potter. 1983. *Fertility, Biology, and Behavior.* New York: Academic Press.

Brett-Smith, Sarah. 1994. *The Making of Bamana Sculpture: Creativity and Gender.* Cambridge: Cambridge University Press.

———. 1998. Personal communication.

Buckley, Thomas, and Alma Gottlieb. 1988. *Blood Magic: The Anthropology of Menstruation.* Berkeley: University of California Press.

Caldwell, John, and Pat Caldwell. 1994. "Marital Status and Abortion in Sub-Saharan Africa." In *Nuptiality in Sub-Saharan Africa,* ed. C. Bledsoe and G. Pison. Oxford: Clarendon Press.

Diakite, Djigui. 1993. "Quelques maladies chez les Bamana." In *Se soigner au Mali,* ed. Joseph Brunet-Jailly. Paris: Karthala and Orstom.

Enquête démographique et de santé: Mali 1995–1996. Bamako: Direction Générale de la Statistique et de l'Informatique and Calverton, Md.: Marco International Inc.

Kleinman, Arthur. 1980. *Patients and Healers in the Context of Culture.* Berkeley: University of California Press.

Madhavan, Sangeetha. 1997. Field notes from life history interviews. Kolondieba, Mali.

March, K., and R. Taqqu. 1986. *Women's Informal Associations in Developing Countries: Catalysts for Change?* Boulder: Westview Press.

Sobo, Elisa. 1993. *One Blood: The Jamaican Body.* Albany: SUNY Press.

Toulmin, Camilla. 1992. *Cattle, Women and Wells.* Oxford: Clarendon Press.

Treloar, A. E., R. E. Boynton, B. G. Behn, and B. W. Brown. 1967. "Variations in the Human Menstrual Cycle through Reproductive Life." *International Journal of Fertility* 12, no. 1, pt. 2:77–126.

Vosselman, Fritz. 1935. *La menstruation: Légendes, coutumes et superstitions.* Lyon: n.p.

Weller, L., A. Weller, and O. Avinir. 1995. "Menstrual Synchrony: Only in Roommates who Are Close Friends?" *Physiology and Behavior* 58, no. 5:883–89.

CHAPTER 10

"Cleaning the Inside" and the Regulation of Menstruation in Southwestern Nigeria

Elisha P. Renne

Medicines and procedures for "cleaning the inside" *(oogun fi f'onu),* the "inside" referring to a woman's womb or stomach, are used by Ekiti Yoruba women in Itapa-Ekiti, a small town in southwestern Nigeria, to clean "dirt" *(idoti)* from the body in order to promote regular, free-flowing, "pure" menstruation *(ase).* Unless thick and bright-red menses come regularly every month and last for 5 days, it is believed that a woman will have difficulty getting pregnant. Sometimes referred to as *nkan osu,* "sign of the moon" (Ojo 1966:174), the regularity of the menstrual period is calculated by some women in connection with cycles of the moon.[1] If menses do not appear according to calculation, if there is bleeding between menstrual periods, or if menstrual bleeding continues for more than 5 days, women may seek remedies, either from traditional healers or from chemist shops where they purchase patent medicines (Bleek and Asante-Darko 1986:345), described as emmenagogues in manufacturers' inserts. Some women may go for dilation of the cervix and curettage of the uterus (D&C), particularly if irregular menstruation is associated with a recent miscarriage (Renne 1996a). The treatment taken to remedy what is sometimes perceived as a physiological or a social imbalance depends, to some extent, on the perceived cause of the particular disorder.

These interpretations of menstruation and the means for regulating it have a temporal dimension as well. In the past, menstruation and virginity were the prerequisites of a system of arranged marriage; young women were expected to remain virgins until being brought to their husbands' houses as young brides, and only young women who had first begun menstruation could marry. Virginal brides who had menstruated were believed to become pregnant immediately after moving to their husbands' houses (Renne 1993, 1996b). Conversely, it was believed that those who had intercourse before beginning menstruation would subsequently become permanently infertile unless medicines were taken, and that those who were no longer virgins when marrying jeopardized their ability to become pregnant. Yet currently, when marital arrangements are often informally contracted and when a premium is no longer placed on virginity by many, some say that those who remain virgins past 15 to 20 years of age may delay the onset of menstruation. For them, first menstruation may be prompted by early intercourse, leading the way to subsequent pregnancy and marriage. Thus, while the idea persists that red, flowing menses directly contribute to a woman's fertility, the idea that women must not have intercourse before the onset of menstruation has changed. It is important to appreciate this reversal of the order of menstruation and intercourse in relation to beliefs about fertility, as it underscores the ways in which ideas about the regulation of menstruation may selectively change over time.

This observation relates to another aspect of the regulation of menstruation, namely the ambiguous uses of various herbal and chemical emmenagogues as well as D&C that may, on the one hand, "clean the womb" *(fo inu)* of retained menstrual blood or worms (Renne 1996a: 489) in order to enhance fertility, and, on the other, "clean the womb" of a pregnancy *(se ki oyun maa duro)* in order to abort (483). When the reasons for women's regulating their menstruation change—reflecting changes in marriage practices, education, and in the age of menarche—they have in turn affected the ways that substances for regulating menstruation are used. Nonetheless, as Richards (1935:25) astutely observed regarding social change more generally, such changes are part of "a process of differential adaption" in which appearances may be deceptive. While it may seem that everything has changed, as some elderly Ekiti Yoruba townspeople complain ("Women of today, they don't want pregnancies, they want pregnancies terminated." Interview #8-97, August 1997, Ilupeju-Ekiti), some older practices and ideas about "cleaning the womb" have been maintained. Presently, women may use traditional medicines that "clean the womb" to promote fertility, and, under different circumstances, they may use similar substances to "keep a pregnancy from staying" (i.e., abort). Thus, in this Ekiti Yoruba town, while new interpretations and techniques are being incorporated into local practices, many ideas about regulating menstruation continue, reflecting prior ideas about menstrual disorders and their cures.

SETTING

Itapa-Ekiti, the small rural town where this study was conducted, is located about 40 kilometers northeast of the capital of Ekiti State, Ado-

Ekiti, in southwestern Nigeria. While in the past, many Itapa towns-men were farmers and women were traders and weavers, many now have secondary school certificates or some higher education and are employed in schools and government offices in towns and cities. Others combine farming and trading with semiskilled occupations such as carpentry and hairdressing, practiced on a part-time basis. Although Itapa-Ekiti is a small town in terms of population (it had approximately 3,500 permanent residents in 1991, according to my town census), its educational facilities and location along a paved federal highway with easy transport to larger urban centers have exposed townspeople to outside trends and to the aspirations of those living elsewhere in Nigeria (Renne 1993; 1996a).

Initial research in this town was begun in June 1991 and continued through April 1992, although I have returned annually for shorter periods. In February 1992, 38 women were interviewed about virginity and how associated practices have changed (Renne 1993, 1996b). Quantitative data on the practice of D&C was obtained from 2 surveys of townswomen, the first in 1992 (Renne 1996a), with a follow-up survey in 1997. In July and August 1997, in-depth interviews focusing on the topic of menstrual disorders were conducted with 7 local traditional healers.

REASONS FOR MENSTRUAL DISORDERS

Physiological Explanations

Several physiological conditions are thought to affect the quality, regularity, and presence of menstrual blood. These are reflected in 3 particular menstrual disorders; one is characterized as black menstruation *(ase dudu)*, another as watery (or white) menstruation *(ase olomi, ase lilami;* Buckley 1985:73), and a third as an absence of menstruation altogether, amenorrhea (as when women fail to begin menstruation). If not treated with medicines that are said to "clean the womb," these conditions may lead to infertility.

The more common of these conditions, black menstruation, is said to be caused by the presence of dirt *(idoti)* in the womb, attributed to worms (Simpson 1980:100), incomplete menstruation or abortion, and sexually transmitted diseases (see Buckley 1985:87). One woman also mentioned incompatibility of blood, as when menstrual blood and semen do not mix well together (or if "what a woman discharges . . . and what a man discharges . . . combine" but are not compatible). This admixture, a form of dirt *(idoti)*, may block up the womb and prevent the free flow of menstrual blood, leading to black menses. Such obstruction of the free flow of pure, red menses may prevent pregnancy, as one Ekiti woman explained:

> When a menstruation is black, if a person is looking for a child, it will be difficult to get. Black menstruation is the one that is not pure, not clean. . . . Unless that impure or black menstruation is washed away, it may be difficult for such a woman to get pregnant. (Interview #2-97, July 1997, Itapa-Ekiti)

Alternately, the menstrual disorder known as watery or white menstruation *(ase olomi, ase lilami)* prevents pregnancy, not because the free flow of menstrual blood is blocked by dirt, but because such blood flows too freely. The term *watery menstruation* refers to the watery thinness and light color of this blood. It is said to be caused by sexual promiscuity that results in disease (possibly a sexually transmitted disease such as gonorrhea) that affects semen, so that when it is discharged, it will run out of the womb just like water. Although less common than black menstruation, this condition will also lead to infertility. In both cases, however, there are herbal cures that will restore a woman's fertility.

Another physiological condition that will result in infertility if not treated is a delay in the onset of menses, attributed to virginity. Some but not all women believe that the failure to begin menstruation may be caused by a virgin's thickened hymen, since "[i]t is said that as one grows older the *ibale* [hymen] will be getting harder" (woman, 25 years, married; Renne 1993:128). Thus, one woman said that "disvirgining can force the menses to come out," in other words, that menstrual blood will flow when the thickened hymen blocking it is penetrated. Another described a friend's painful menstruation as being remedied through the intentional loss of her virginity. This physiological explanation, the presence of a hymen causing menstrual disorders, has a social side as well as a physiological one, since a woman who is still a virgin (and perhaps not menstruating) by the time she is 20 years old would be referred to disparagingly as *suegbe,* antisocial (Renne 1996b:27).

Social Explanations

This social aspect of delay in the onset of menstruation—that antisocial young virgins are bringing this problem on themselves—may be seen in another menstrual disorder referred to as seized menstruation. This disorder is attributed to witches *(aje)*—disruptive social beings who, for reasons of malice or revenge, may attempt to stop or disrupt a woman's regular menses (Prince 1961:798; Simpson 1980:76). Seized menstruation, called *ase agba* (literally, "menses that one removes"),[2] was described by one woman diviner-healer:

> *Ase agba*, it is also called *ase dagba aje*. It is used to fight [harm] a woman as the pure menses will be seized. The witches use something to cover the womb, and the dirty things that should be coming out will stay in her. Then she will menstruate this dirty substance instead of pure menses. (Interview #1-97, July 1997, Ilupeju-Ekiti)

Again, there is reference to blockage causing impure, dirty menses, although the cause is not physiological but social, reflecting ideas about jealousy, social structural conflict, and extraordinary power—in particular, witchcraft (Beidelman 1986; Jackson 1989). In such cases, antisocial beings (witches) who invert the social order (e.g., they are thought to harm mainly immediate kin and to fly upside down at night) may invert normal fertility as well by blocking the womb and preventing menstruation (see Oyewumi 1989). As in the physiological disorders, if the absence of pure, red menstruation is not remedied, permanent infertility may result.

REMEDIES FOR IRREGULAR OR MISSING MENSTRUATION

Remedies for irregular menstruation associated with black menses, watery menses, failure to menstruate, or "seized" menses revolve around the idea of reestablishing order or balance, whether in social relations, sexuality, or in the constitution of blood amidst the disorder that contributes to this imbalance. Various things may be done or taken to alleviate the resulting dirt, water, blockage, or enmity that prevents the free flow of pure, red menses.

Traditional Remedies

In the case of complaints attributed to physiological problems such as dirt, menstrual blood itself may be used to ascertain what treatment should be used, as one older woman explained:

> In the past herbalists did make use of the blood itself. Just by testing the menstruation with cotton wool: you just have to take the rag used

[as a sanitary pad] to the *babalawo* [traditional healer-diviner] and he
in turn will use cotton wool to test this; or the woman could touch
it with the wool and take this specimen to her *babalawo* for a test;
and after the babalawo has studied this perfectly, he would be able
to prepare the matching medicine for the disease. (Interview #3-97,
July 1997, Itapa-Ekiti)

If black menstruation is diagnosed, a *babalawo* may prescribe various
sorts of *oogun fi f'onu* (medicines for cleaning the inside), usually consisting of a decoction made from ground roots and herbs, to alleviate
the problem. Similar sorts of medicines might also be prescribed to cure
white menstruation by thickening it.

In the case of "seized" menstruation, a diviner may be consulted to
ascertain the person or people believed to be responsible for the "sei-
zure" and what may be done to placate them:

> Any patient with this problem caused by wizards, witches, and herbal-
> ists should consult the *Ifa* oracle to know the cause. If the affected
> person can afford to provide whatever demand is made, then the di-
> viner will provide the medicine to cure it. The *Ifa* diviner will reveal
> everything—the source [of the problem] and how to get rid of it. [The
> woman] just has to take a little medicine and she will be cured. (Inter-
> view #1-97, July 1997, Ilupeju-Ekiti)

In cases when menstruation has not yet begun, traditional medicine
may also be taken to stimulate the onset of menstruation for young
women older than 15 years:

> Things can be done if a girl does not see her menses. Her parents will
> take her to a *babalawo,* and *iko odide* [red parrot feather; (Apter 1992:
> 113–114; Buckley 1985:228] with . . . *osun* [red camwood] will be
> mixed together with some other things and the girl will have to see
> her menses after she has used it. (Interview #4-92, 1992, Itapa-Ekiti)

This woman mentioned another means of activating the onset of menstruation, namely by sexual intercourse, although she did not believe
in this remedy herself. Nonetheless, several women did mention intercourse as a way to stimulate menarche, based on the idea that intercourse "forces" out menstrual blood, as one woman explained:

> Medicine can be done to bring it [menstruation] out. But losing one's
> virginity can make it begin. It depends on the body system of every
> body. Some people may have a strong body and they may not be able
> to see their menses on time. (Interview #5-92, 1992, Itapa-Ekiti)

Apart from this "mechanical" approach as well as the use of traditional herbal medicines and offerings made to malevolent beings, menstrual disorders may also be remedied by taking tablets known as patent
(or English) medicines, or the woman may go for dilation and curettage
(D&C) to "clean the womb" and reestablish regular menstruation.

Patent Medicines and D&C

Patent medicines are obtained without prescription in small patent-
medicine stores and pharmacies in villages and towns throughout
southwestern Nigeria. Those advertised and used as emmenagogues
include Dr. Bonjean's tablets, Menstrogen tablets, EP Forte tablets, Ergometrine tablets, Cumorit tablets, and Apiol and Steel pills.[3] Exactly
when these medicines were introduced to Nigeria is unclear. Tablets
manufactured in England consisting of various combinations of powdered aloes, ferrous sulfate, and ergot were probably introduced earlier
in the century,[4] with the British colonization of Nigeria. Menstrogen
and Cumorit were probably introduced during the 1950s, with the development of mass-produced steroid hormones.[5] More recently, oral
contraceptive tablets are also being prescribed to regularize menstruation.[6]

Imported emmenagogue tablets are sold singly or in packets, in
which case there is usually a manufacturer's insert with directions for
usage. While these directions describe their use for reestablishing delayed menstruation, these tablets were more often used as abortifacients by Ekiti Yoruba women, although it is unclear to what extent
they are effective for this purpose. It is possible, for example, that a
missed period is actually only delayed and that these drugs bring on
a "menstruation-like bleeding" that is interpreted as evidence of an
early-term abortion.[7]

Related to the use of these foreign patent medicines is the practice
introduced during the colonial period of using D&C,[8] particularly after
miscarriages, for clearing the uterus of endometrial materials that
could cause infection. Of the 71 women who mentioned going for
D&C in the 1992 survey, 24 (34 percent) went for "washing the
womb," usually after a miscarriage but sometimes when they are having difficulty getting pregnant.[9] They specifically referred to this sort
of D&C as *f'onu*, "washing the womb," using the same term as for traditional herbal medicines used to promote clean, thick, and red menstruation and, subsequently, fertility.

This association of D&C with menstrual regulation used to enhance
fertility is complicated by the fact that many women also go for D&Cs

to abort. There is a similar ambiguity surrounding the use of patent medicines by many young women, who said that they had taken these medicines with the intent to abort, even if they may have actually worked as emmenagogues. How these various forms of menstrual regulation are used by women—as womb-cleaning medicines to enhance fertility or as abortifacients to limit it—reflects the changing cultural and socioeconomic context in which these women live.

DISCUSSION

There have been many changes over the past 100 years[10] in the Ekiti Yoruba society, including shifts in social relations, reflected in the diminished authority of elders undermined through the introduction of court divorce, the demise of arranged marriage, and the increasing numbers of young people attending Western-style schools (see Renne 1993, 1996b). Furthermore, dietary changes have contributed to a lower age of first menstruation, and the introduction of various imported patent medicines and medical procedures such as D&C have expanded the means of securing an abortion.

These changes suggest that the ways of regulating menstruation as well as the reasons for doing so are closely linked to particular sociocultural contexts, and that these ways and reasons may change in time.

Social Change and Menstrual Regulation

For example, one older woman's description of menstruation, marriage, and fertility illustrates how these 3 factors were interpreted earlier in this century, when virginal unmarried women stayed in their family compounds and were given husbands through arranged marriage soon after menarche:

Q: When was it normal for young woman to begin menstruation in the past?

A: 20 years.

Q: When was your own?

A: 20 years.

Q: Had you been menstruating before you got married?

A: I had been menstruating. In the past if a woman has not been seeing her menstruation and she met a man, she will not be able to see the menses until medicine was done and she will have a delay in getting pregnant. (Interview #6-92, Itapa-Ekiti, 1992)

Such thinking—that one would cause menstrual disorder and a delay in pregnancy by premenstrual intercourse—discouraged young unmarried women from engaging in premarital sex that could mar their virgin status and marriage prospects. In other words, by following the socially approved sequence of virginity, menstruation, and marital intercourse, bodily disorder—amenorrhea and delayed fertility—could be avoided. This constellation of ideas—that a young woman's virginity must be guarded, that she should menstruate before marriage could occur, and that she would become pregnant immediately after marital intercourse took place—began to unravel with the introduction of procedures for divorce in the 1920s (Renne 1992), the subsequent demise of arranged marriage, and with attendance at primary school, away from the watchful eyes of female relatives.

Presently, in this Ekiti Yoruba town, most young girls attend primary school and many go on to secondary school. In the 1992 survey, it was found that 86.5 percent of women aged 15 to 19 years had some secondary schooling. Attendance at school not only gives these young women a certain freedom of movement but exposes them to new ideas as well. Unlike the past, when young men "would not attempt to have sex" with young women, as one older woman put it, such behavior is considered to be part of modern adolescent sociality by both young men and women (Renne 1993). Only the old-fashioned or antisocial would refrain from sexual forays.

The earlier age of first intercourse (15 years) reported by young women in the 1992 survey coincides with earlier ages for the onset of menstruation, related to dietary changes, as explained by one older woman:

Q: When is it normal for a young woman to begin menstruation now?
A: 15 years.
Q: Why has it changed?
A: It is the work of God and also the type of food we ate in the past is now different. In the past it was *agbo* [various types of herbal infusions] and *eko* [cornstarch gruel] throughout for a new baby but now it is [tinned] milk. All this has brought changes. (Interview #6-92, 1992, Itapa-Ekiti)

The combination of earlier menses, schooling, and premarital sex (as a prelude to subsequent marriage), referred to elsewhere as the "biosocial gap" (Gyepi-Garbrah 1985:30), has led to an increase in premarital pregnancies. This situation conflicts with young women's aspirations for salaried employment, which necessitates their completion of secondary and often postsecondary schooling, since pregnancy results in automatic suspension. Young women in such situations may decide, along with their boyfriends, to abort a pregnancy rather than end their education. Their options for doing so have increased through the availability of D&C as well an arsenal of patent medicine emmenagogues, the latter taken as overdoses or in combination with other substances in an attempt to abort (Renne 1996a).

Thus, for some young unmarried women in this Ekiti Yoruba town, the reasons and means for addressing an absence of menstruation have changed. Nonetheless, these changes do not mean that some older ways of thinking about menstruation have not been maintained. The use of traditional medicines and patent medicine emmenagogues to abort does not preclude young women's using the same medicines to cleanse their wombs of dirt and worms in order to promote fertility when they want to get pregnant. Nor does it mean that women never regulated menstruation in the past with the intention of aborting—in "the case of an emergency," as one herbalist put it. While knowledge both of medicine used to "clean the inside" *(oogun fi f'onu)* and of "medicine that keeps a pregnancy from staying" *(oogun ti won le fi se ki oyun maa duro)* existed in the past,[11] use of the latter was probably less common because there was little reason to do so.[12]

Comparing Past and Present Practices for Regulating Menstruation

When one woman diviner was asked who came to her more often, those seeking medicine to abort or those seeking medicine to regulate menstruation to get pregnant, she replied, "The two sides are frequent; to terminate pregnancies is common and people with irregular menstruation are many" (Interview with IM, July 1997, Ilupeju-Ekiti). The responses of townswomen who reported going for D&C (two-thirds for abortion, one-third for enhancing fertility), as indicated in the 1992 and 1997 surveys, lend support to her assessment.

It is more difficult to ascertain whether menstrual regulation was primarily meant to enhance or reduce fertility in the past. Several older people thought that previously menstruation was regulated mainly to "clean the womb" to facilitate a pregnancy, not to prevent one. It is likely that the use of menstrual regulation as fertility enhancement was more common, since the reasons for bringing on menstruation to induce an abortion would have been fewer. These would have included the need to conceal evidence of sexuality out of place: premarital sex,

sex during the 2-year postpartum abstinence period, and extramarital affairs. However, strong social sanctions, including the belief that premarital sex delayed fertility and that ignoring the postpartum abstinence "rule" resulted in infant mortality, discouraged these sorts of behaviors. Premarital and postpartum sex were not unheard of, but they were probably infrequent.

According to one older man, a traditional healer and diviner, "In the past, people did not terminate pregnancies as they do today. If there were a pregnancy that comes down itself [i.e., a spontaneous abortion], that is different" (Interview #7-97, July 1997, Itapa-Ekiti). Another traditional healer and diviner, a woman, compared the present-day regulation of menstruation with past practices:

> Some people have spoiled themselves, they have spoiled the inner selves, especially women of this day. They don't want pregnancies, they want pregnancies terminated. In the olden days, things weren't like this . . . men would sit around me and they would not attempt to have sex with me. Not only me, this was the general idea then. The past was better. Children of today can have sex at any available place and when pregnancy occurs they may terminate it and may throw the child into the bush; and this is why many women have irregular menstruation. (Interview #8-97, August 1997, Ilupeju-Ekiti)

One needs to be cautious about claims that nowadays many young women more often use medicines to abort, since nostalgia ("the past was better") and value judgments ("children of today can have sex [anyplace]") may color such statements. This judgmental thinking is also expressed by some (but not all) older women, who attribute earlier ages for the onset of menstruation to young girls' "corrupt" *(isekuse)*, promiscuous ways rather than to improved nutrition. While these older women disparage the new ways of the young, young women, on their part, view such thinking as old-fashioned and as associated with the backward practice of arranged marriage. For them, premarital intercourse and early menstruation are seen as signs not of social and bodily disorder but rather as signs of proper sociality and good health.

CONCLUSION

Presently in this southwestern Nigerian town, there are reasons both for "cleaning the inside" and for "keeping a pregnancy from staying." In some circumstances, menstruation may be regulated to enhance fertility—as when women take medicines to "clean the inside" of dirt or to remedy the conditions of black or watery menstruation, when they make offerings to placate beings who have "seized" their menses, or when intercourse is prescribed to induce menarche. In others, such regulation may represent an attempt to abort, contributing to a certain ambiguity in the ways that the absence of menstruation and other menstrual disorders are interpreted and treated. This ambiguity underscores the need to place women's regulation of their menses within a larger sociocultural and historical context (Gottlieb 1988:55). In this Ekiti example, the shift in the sequence from menstruation and virginity, marriage and fertility to premarital sexuality, menstruation, and fertility serves as a dramatic reminder that while bodily functions such as menstruation have a physiological basis, they also "must be regarded as a narrative of culture in anatomical disguise" (Laqueur 1990:236). The meanings attributed to menstruation and to the substances and practices used by women to regulate it—as emmenagogues or as abortifacients—cannot be understood outside of the changing sociocultural context in which sequences of bodily events are conceptualized.

NOTES

This study (1991–92) was initially conducted with funding from the Andrew W. Mellon Foundation in conjunction with a joint research project organized by Ondo State University, Ado-Ekiti, and the Health Transition Centre, The Australian National University, Canberra. The 1997 study was funded by the Wenner-Gren Foundation for Anthropological Research and the Mellon Foundation through my affiliation with Princeton University. I am grateful to all these institutions and foundations as well as to I. O. Orubuloye, Jack Caldwell, and Pat Caldwell for logistical support and to Kayode Owoeye, Comfort Ajayi, Adenike Oso, Iyabo Arunsoro, and Bose Ayeni for their research assistance.

    1. The way this calculation is made was described by one woman diviner-healer (Interview #8-97, August 1997, Ilupeju-Ekiti):

> The moon comes with twenty to twenty-one days, depending on the direction of the moon. So anyone who sees her menstruation in that moon period will expect it at the beginning of another moon; the first and second moon make a menstrual period. The moon counts its own days and women count days of menstruation, this is why the moon can be helpful in knowing the menstruation period.

The cycles of the moon are also used to calculate when a pregnant woman will deliver her child. Women with Western education are more likely to use a calendar to ascertain these dates.

2. Abraham (1962:231) gives an example of the use of the verb *gba* in relation to the blood of first intercourse: *o gba iba le omonge non,* "he deflowered that virgin" [he removed *(gba)* the hymen *(ibale)*].

3. For references to Menstrogen and EP Forte, see Greenhalgh 1986; Silverman, Lydecker, and Lee 1992; and Wolffers 1988; for references to all but Cumorit, see Bleek and Asante-Darko 1986.

4. For example, Hooper's Female Pills (which consisted of aloes and ferrous sulfate among other ingredients) were marketed in the United States as early as the mideighteenth century (Griffenhagen and Young 1959: 164). Apiol, "a crystalline substance obtained by distillation from parsley seeds" (*Webster's New Twentieth Century Dictionary of the English Language* 1983:85), has historically been a common ingredient of emmenagogues. The "steel" of Apiol and Steel Pills refers to ferrous sulfate, a purgative.

5. For example, the Dutch pharmaceutical company Organon that manufactures Menstrogen is said to have grown enormously:

> especially after the 1950s when it took a prominent role in the development and production of cortisone, steroid sex hormones, and other corticosteroids, pituitary hormones, and vitamins. (Silverman, Lydecker, and Lee 1992:114)

6. "One of the women interviewed today lost three children, all under five years of age. She was experiencing irregular menstruation and wanted to get pregnant so she went to a chemist to get something for regularizing it. He advised her to take family planning tablets which regularized her menses but she couldn't get pregnant. Her in-laws finally realized what the problem was" (Renne, field journal, 1997).

7. Women are specifically advised not to use Menstrogen or Menstrogen Forte if they are pregnant. The manufacturer's insert also warns women that using Menstrogen "for the diagnosis of early pregnancy [may risk] the possibility of virilization of female fetuses." The marketing of Menstrogen in India has been widely criticized because of its teratogenic effects (Wolffers 1988; Greenhalgh 1986; Silverman, Lydecker, and Lee 1992).

8. In the Ekiti area, induced abortions are performed by medical personnel using D&C rather than manual vacuum aspiration (MVA), available in university teaching hospitals elsewhere in Nigeria. People performing D&C in Ekiti have usually had some medical training but are rarely licensed physicians. They use D&C techniques because the necessary equipment is relatively inexpensive, replaceable, and easily available. The aspirators and associated equipment used for MVA are imported and hence expensive and not always obtainable.

9. These numbers were similar in a follow-up survey conducted in 1997. Of 305 women interviewed, 96 reported going to a clinic for a D&C; 32 (33 percent) went for "washing the womb" and 64 (67 percent) went to abort.

10. The Ekiti region was put under the authority of the British Travel-

ing Commissioner Major Reeve Tucker in 1899. He visited many parts of Ekiti in January 1900, and later that year convened a meeting of the rulers of the 16 Ekiti kingdoms, securing British rule in the area (Oguntuyi 1979:83).

11. There is some overlap in the ingredients used in herbal medicines to "clean the womb" and "bring a pregnancy down" (Renne 1996a:490).

12. Furthermore, since conception was associated with "quickening," which takes place around the fourth month of pregnancy, use of any medicine prior to this time would have been viewed as regulating menstruation to "clean the womb" *(f'onu)*. While women might notice that they had failed to menstruate, suggesting that they were pregnant, it was quickening that served as a confirmation of pregnancy. Since secondary amenorrhea is often caused by poor diet and weight loss (Franks 1987), it is possible that during periods of drought (or famine), such amenorrhea was common, and that failure to menstruate might not be assumed to mean pregnancy.

REFERENCES

Abraham, R. C. 1962. *Dictionary of Modern Yoruba.* London: Hodder and Stoughton.

Apter, Andrew. 1992. *Black Critics and Kings: The Hermeneutics of Power in Yoruba Society.* Chicago: University of Chicago Press.

Beidelman, T. O. B. 1986. *Moral Imagination in Kaguru Modes of Thought.* Bloomington: Indiana University Press.

Bleek, Wolf, and N. K. Asante-Darko. 1986. "Illegal Abortion in Southern Ghana: Methods, Motives and Consequences." *Human Organization* 45:333–44.

Buckley, Anthony. 1985. *Yoruba Medicine.* Oxford: Clarendon Press.

Franks, S. 1987. "Primary and Secondary Amenorrhoea." *British Medical Journal* 294:815–19.

Gottlieb, Alma. 1988. "Menstrual Cosmology among the Beng of Ivory Coast." In *Blood Magic: The Anthropology of Menstruation,* ed. Thomas Buckley and Alma Gottlieb, 55–74. Berkeley: University of California Press.

Greenhalgh, Trisha. 1986. "Drug Marketing in the Third World: Beneath the Cosmetic Reforms." *Lancet* (June 7):1318–20.

Griffenhagen, G., and J. H. Young. 1959. *Old English Patent Medicines in America.* Washington, D.C.: Smithsonian Institution.

Gyepi-Garbrah, Benjamin. 1985. *Adolescent Fertility in Nigeria.* Boston: Pathfinder Foundation.

Jackson, Michael. 1989. *Paths toward a Clearing.* Bloomington: Indiana University Press.

Laqueur, Thomas. 1990. *Making Sex: Body and Gender from the Greeks to Freud.* Cambridge, Mass.: Harvard University Press.

Oguntuyi, Anthony. 1979. *History of Ekiti.* Ibadan, Nigeria: Bisi Books.

Ojo, G. J. A. 1966. *Yoruba Culture.* London: University of London.

Oyewumi, Joseph. 1989. "Traditional Obstetrics and Gynaecology—A Case Study of Its Practice in Ife Community." Master's thesis, Institute of African Studies, University of Ibadan.

Prince, Raymond. 1961. "The Yoruba Image of the Witch." *Journal of Mental Science* 107:795–805.

Renne, Elisha. 1992. "Polyphony in the Courts: Child Custody Cases in Kabba District Court, 1925–1979." *Ethnology* 31, no. 3:219–32.

———. 1993. "Changes in Adolescent Sexuality and the Perception of Virginity in a Southwestern Nigerian Village." *Sexual Networking and HIV/AIDS in West Africa, Health Transition Review,* suppl. 3:121–33.

———.1996a. "The Pregnancy That Doesn't Stay: The Practice and Perception of Abortion by Ekiti Yoruba Women." *Social Science & Medicine* 42, no. 4:483–94.

———. 1996b. "Virginity Cloths and Vaginal Coverings in Ekiti, Nigeria." In *Clothing and Difference: Embodied Identities in Colonial and Post-Colonial Africa,* ed. Hildi Hendrickson, 19–33. Durham, N.C.: Duke University Press.

Richards, Audrey. 1935. "The Village Census in the Study of Culture Contact." *Africa* 8:20–33.

Silverman, Milton, Mia Lydecker, and Philip Lee. 1992. *Bad Medicine: The Prescription Drug Industry in the Third World.* Stanford, Calif.: Stanford University Press.

Simpson, George E. 1980. *Yoruba Religion and Medicine in Ibadan.* Ibadan, Nigeria: Ibadan University Press.

Wolffers, I. 1988. "De problemen rond hoge-dose oestrogeen/progestativum combinaties, zoals Menstrogen, in India." *Nederlands Tijdscrift voor Geneeskunde* 132, no. 8:364–65.

CHAPTER 11

Means, Motives, and Menses:
Use of Herbal Emmenagogues in Indonesia

Terence H. Hull and Valerie J. Hull

Indonesian women concerned about delayed menses access a wide variety of traditional and modern facilities to bring on the flow of blood. The focus of this paper is the widely accepted form of emmenagogues for early interventions to bring on menstruation, that are a subset of common herbal preparations called *jamu*. These preparations can be obtained from traveling *jamu* sellers and market vendors, or in the form of packets of dried herbal mixtures or powders that can be mixed at home. A stroll through the market and chats on the porch in community studies in Indonesia indicate wide knowledge of preparations to bring on menses. Particularly in the most populous island of Java, traditional and modern markets offer an abundance of herbal mixtures to regulate menses, with buyers coming from among women of all ages and marital statuses.[1] Inexpensive booklets on herbal remedies are widely sold, containing recipes to be followed for various ailments or conditions, including those relating to menstruation.[2] Case studies of these herbal concoctions collected in Java over recent years, combined with the limited literature available in English and Indonesian, indicate that *jamu* having emmenagogic or abortifacient properties covers an extraordinarily broad range of products directed to a variety of consumers. These, in turn, are a small subset of the wide variety of herbal medications available to most of Indonesia's 210 million population.

Westerners often think of *jamu* as being associated with bustling Indonesian markets, where colorful piles of aromatic powders and roots are wrapped in old newspaper and a price is set after a time of friendly haggling. The herbs are prescribed for a wide range of health- and fitness-related conditions, from colds and flu, through burns, strains, stomach aches, and diarrhea, to a deficit of stamina and sexual potency. Preparations can be drunk (sometimes mixed with eggs for "energy") or mixed into poultices that are placed on the temples, forehead, or painful limb. The traditional healers (*dukun*) do not have a monopoly on mixing and supplying the herbs. Rather, they are just one element in an elaborate system of growing, drying, and trading herbal preparations. Some villagers grow or gather their own supplies; others supply products for the large network of markets held in civic centers and crossroads across the countryside. Today, throughout the archipelago, supermarkets and modern shopping malls have large displays of hundreds of brightly colored boxes and packets of preparations, offered at fixed prices, and accompanied with detailed inserts describing indications and contraindications and giving a Department of Health registration number. The major regions for the manufacturing of *jamu* are Central Java (particularly around Solo and Semarang), East Java (Surabaya and Madura), West Java (Bandung), Aceh, and Kalimantan. Among the multiplicity of herbal mixtures—even restricting attention to the industrial versions, which have been processed and registered—there is a wide variety of preparations that can be used to regulate menses.

The herbal preparations having emmenagogic properties go by several euphemistic names, and are talked about in the context of good health as well as specifically in relation to possible pregnancy. Names are frequently indicative of the purpose to regularize menses:

- *Datang Bulan Terlambat:* Bring on the late "monthly"
- *Datang Bulan Tak Teratur:* Bring on the irregular "monthly"
- *Melancarkan haid:* Regularize menstruation
- *Terlambat Bulan:* Late "monthly"

One of the most common terms to appear in names is *peluntur* or *pluntur,* which is literally translated from Indonesian as "laxative." This is understood in common parlance as having a purgative effect on blood that is assumed to be late in flowing because it is "stuck" in the womb. Women in Java also take herbal mixtures (*jamu nifas*) in the postpartum period to cleanse the uterus of residual blood.

Despite the trappings of pharmaceutical modernity in the packaging, the contents range from hand-rolled pellets of dried herbs, to powders to be mixed in water or juice, to dissolvable capsules. Lists of ingredients are made to appear scientific through the use of Latinized names, but they range from the botanical to the comical, with relatively little overlap of ingredients among the many brands. The instructions also vary in terms of dosage, with the common "one pill three times a day before meals" having a very authoritative ring. Women are encouraged to continue the pills for 2 or 3 days. While most preparations are to be taken when the menstruation is delayed, some are promoted as appropriate preventive measures, to be taken in the week before menses are expected. *Sin lik* is aimed at the urban Chinese market, and promises to clear up white discharge as well as bring on late periods, but it can either be taken orally 3 times a day or administered vaginally a quarter of an hour before coitus. *Jamu Jago* brand is to be taken orally after sex. In a Jakarta study by Suharti and Wardhini (1982:9), some women took preparations only if their period was late, but others took the same type of *jamu* regularly at about the time they were due to menstruate.

The wide range of timing and methods of administration make it unlikely that women using these herbal products would assume they were invariably abortifacient. At the same time, some of these preparations are clearly labeled "Not to be taken by pregnant women" with the implication (and sometimes the explicit pronouncement) that it may provoke an abortion, hence attracting a market of customers seeking this result. Further, studies in abortion clinics have shown that a common reason for delay in seeking a surgical termination of pregnancy among unmarried women is repeated attempts to bring on menses through the consumption of large doses of herbal preparations (Hull et al. 1993).

From the above description it is obvious that the market for herbal emmenagogues is segmented: different women may take them for different reasons, and the same woman could seek these *jamu* for different reasons, depending on circumstances. In a small unpublished study conducted in 1983–84, Hull and Handayani attempted to systematically link the types of distributors with particular segments of the market, but this proved very difficult to establish. As mentioned, the preparations are sold widely, from door-to-door sellers to small corner kiosks to large traditional marketplaces and modern urban supermarkets. The study tended to focus on small shops, where sellers reported the "typical" consumer as being a housewife, but often commented specifically about "schoolgirls" or the "boyfriends of schoolgirls" as being notable purchasers of these herbs.

Interviews of users of these *jamu* in the same study show that despite written instructions, women follow their own prescriptions for use. They often take much larger quantities than the prescribed dosage; they combine a number of different purchased herbal products; or combine these preparations with the "traditional abortifacients" of unripe pineapple, mango or other green fruit, garlic, lime, pepper and chili. Medicinal wines are also taken as emmenagogues, either alone or in combination with other substances, and some women report relying on a combination of *jamu* and "prayer." The 1984 study also confirmed that timing of administration varies among women, from a matter of days after a missed period to weeks, and even up to 3 months. In the cases interviewed, it appeared that herbal preparations tend to be used in the first weeks after a missed period, with other interventions added if the herbal preparations alone do not produce the desired result.

In a community study in Ngaglik in central Java that followed women for 2 years after a birth, case studies yielded 7 fairly detailed stories told to field assistants by women faced with late periods. In all instances, women were not sure of their pregnancy status but had a sense of panic at the possibility of pregnancy, and undertook sometimes drastic measures to "bring on" their delayed menses. Of the 7, 3 cases ended in resumed menses, and 4 had confirmed pregnancies that were continued to live births. The methods to bring on menstruation were similar for all: they consumed capsules or pellets sold as "menstruation-regulating" preparations, followed or accompanied by a series of massages by a traditional midwife.[3] Amounts of the preparations taken varied: one woman took 3 bottles of the rather expensive variety of capsules, as well as eating *blimbing wuluh* (the fruit of *Averrhoa Bilimbi*, or cucumber tree), a sour fruit. Two of the women only took the capsules and, in one case, some medicinal wine as well (Hull 1984).

COMPOSITION AND EFFICACY OF EMMENAGOGUES

Seno Sastroamidjojo's (1948) compendium of Indonesian herbal preparations provides separate listings for *emmenagoga* (397–98) and *abortiva* (388), arranged according to the common Indonesian terms (see table 11.1). It is linked back to a medicinal guide and articles compiled by Dutch researchers in Indonesia from the turn of the century (particularly Kloppenburg-Versteegh 1909; reprinted in Indonesian in 1983) and includes analytical and bibliographic information on each plant. Drawing on a wide variety of scientific and medical sources, Sastroamidjojo's handbook is the basis for many recent publications on *jamu*. It did not, however, immediately spawn the sort of scientific testing of preparations and publication of results that Sastroamidjojo so admired in the European literature on herbal preparations because the stringencies of war and revolution encouraged readers to rely on the

Table 11.1 Indonesian Herbal Preparations

Number	Local Name	Latin Name	English Name
Preparations Listed as *Emmenagoga (Peluruh Haid)*			
8	*Akar teki, Mota, Kotehawaa*	*Cyperosus rotundus, C. tuberosus* L., *Cyperaceae*	Water chestnut
10	*Alim*	*Lepidium sativum*	(Seed)
14	*Aren*	*Arenga pinnata/saccharifera*	Sugar palm
24	*Besaran, Lampoong*	*Morus indica/alba, Moraceae*	White mulberry
41	*Dadap ajam*	*Erythrina variegata/indica*	Indian coral tree
60	*Daun Wungu*	*Graptophyllum pictum/hortense*	—
106	*Gandarusa*	*Justicia gendarussa*	—
147	**Kantil**	**Michelia champaca**	**Type of magnolia**
149	**Kapas**	**Gossypium abroreum/barbadense/Herbaceum**	—
154	*Kasumba*	*Carthamus tinctorius*	—
167	**Kelor**	**Moringa oleifera**	**Horseradish tree**
173	**Kembang merak**	**Caesalpinia pulcherrima**	—
175	**Kembang sepatu**	**Hibiscus rosa sinensia; Flos testalis**	**Variety of hibiscus**
189	*Ki bentili*	*Kickxia arborea*	(Tree)
193	*Kuma-kuma*	*Crocus sativus* L.	Saffron
204	*Legundi*	*Vitex trifolia*	—
225	**Meniran**	**Phyllanthus niruri/uninaria**	—
229	**Miana**	**Coleus atropurpureus/blumei/scutellarioides/ingrotus**	—
236	*Mungsi*	*Carum copticum*	—
238	**Nanas**	**Ananas comusus/sativus/sativa**	**Pineapple**
243	*Ojong, Gambas, Katjoor, Tjeme*	*Luffa acutangula* L., *Petota bengalensis*	Loofa, strainer vine
255	*Patjar djawa*	*Lausonia alba/inermis*	—
272	*Putjung (Peetjoong)*	*Pangium edule*	*Kluwak* nut used in *rawon* soup. All parts of the plant contain potentially deadly poisonous hydrocyanic acid.
278	*Sambangan*	*Spatholobus ferrugineus*	—

295	*Sere*	*Adropogon nardus/citratus/Schoenathus; Cymbopogon citratus*	Lemon grass
298	*Sawi, Sesawi*	*Brassica rugosa/juncea*	Swatow mustard, broad-leaved mustard
310	*Srigading*	*Nyctanthes arbortristis L.*	—
329	*Temu lawak, Koneng gede*	*Curcuma xanthorrhiza Roxb.*	Wild ginger
332	*Terate, Trate, Serodja*	*Nelumbium nelumbo Druce., N. speciosum Willd., N. nucifera Gaertn., Nymphea indica major Rumph.*	Lotus
337	*Tjendana, Tjandani, Tjandana, Tjandhana lakek*	*Santalu album L.*	Sandalwood

Preparations Listed as Abortiva (Obat Penggugur)

6	*Akar binasa, Tjeraka merah, Mehulatu*	*Plumbago indica L., P. rosea L.*	
16	*Asem djawa, Tangkal asam, Atjem, Tjelagi*	*Tamarindus indicus L.*	Tamarind
47	*Daun entjok, Ki entjok, Poksor, Bawa, Kareka*	*Plumbago zeylanica L.*	
79	*Djangkang, Kepuh, Kepok, Halumpang, Kolengka, Kalompang*	*Sterculia foetida L.*	
147	**Kantil**	**Michelia champaca**	**Type of magnolia**
149	**Kapas**	**Gossypium abroreum/barbadense/Herbaceum**	
167	**Kelor**	**Moringa oleifera**	**Horseradish tree**
173	**Kembang merak**	**Caesalpinia pulcherrima**	
175	**Kembang sepatu**	**Hibiscus rosa sinensia; Flos testalis**	**Variety of hibiscus**
197	*Kursani, Mursani, Pursane*	*Veronia antihelminthica Willd.*	
216	*Madja (Modjo), Bila, Gelepung, Madja lumut, Madja gedang, Madja pahit, Madja ghedang, Madja paek, Maos*	*Aegle marmelos Correa (fructus beloe)*	
225	**Meniran**	**Phyllanthus niruri/uninaria**	
229	**Miana**	**Coleus atropurpureus/blumei/Scutellarioides/ingrotus**	
233	*Modjar, Akar binasa, Auwarian, Tjeraka merah*	*Plumbago rosea L., P. indica L., Kadix vesicatoria Rumph.*	
238	**Nanas**	**Ananas comusus/sativus/sativa**	**Pineapple**
270	*Puring, Puding, Demung, Kotomas, Tomas, Karoton, Karotong*	*Codiacum varicyatum Bl.*	Croton plant
300	*Sidaguri, Guri, Sadagori, Otok-otok, Taghuri*	*Sida rhombifolia L., S. retusa L.*	
333	*Terong, Tjokrom, Entjung, Terong hutan, Tehung kanji*	*Solanum melongena L., S. rongum Poir., S. indicum L.*	Eggplant

SOURCE: Seno Sastroamidjojo 1948.

NOTE: Some entries corrected using information from Ochse et al. [1931] 1977. Entries in bold are listed both as emmenagogues and abortifacients.

handbook as a guide to medication rather than a source of hypotheses. As is true with so many folk medicine systems, the evident cases of real impact of herbal preparations are mixed with prescriptions and claims having seemingly little basis in either theory or verifiable practice (see, for example, Soeparto 1984 or Soemardjo-Sju 1980). This is particularly true with the wide variety of herbs associated with emmenagogic preparations.

The herbal mixtures sold in modern packaging include lists of ingredients that contain substances reported elsewhere as emmenagogues but many of which are common plants with important roles in cooking and aromatics. Some of these plants are regularly ingested by pregnant women as part of their normal diet or health regime. Turmeric and ginger, for instance, frequently appear on lists of ingredients as possible emmenagogues, but they are not identified as "food taboos" related to menarche, pregnancy, or lactation among women in rural Java (Hull 1986:257–58). A similar phenomenon is observed in the West, where Tierra's list of emmenagogues (1998) on the World Wide Web includes turmeric, wild ginger, saffron, and safflower. Hoffman's (1998) Web site also lists ginger, but does not include turmeric and saffron, substituting instead lavender, chamomile, peppermint, parsley, rosemary, raspberry, sage, red sage, thyme, fenugreek, and valerian.[4]

One Indonesian study notes that among the most commonly sold preparations, the components used to increase fertility have many similarities with the herbs used to suppress fertility. The difference lies in 1 or 2 additional herbal ingredients that are thought to have an abortifacient effect (e.g., *piper nigrum, Artemisia cina*) or an emmenagogue one (*Curcuma domestika, Corum copticum, Blumea balsamifera, Foeniculum vulgare, Baeckae frutescence,* and others) (Wardhini and Yasavati 1979:8). The study reported no antifertility effect in pregnant mice for a selection of 6 popular herbal preparations in pill and powder form, given in doses 10 times greater than the comparable recommended human dose.

Studies of possible teratogenic effects of one of the popular herbal preparations (P. T. Nyonya Meneer's *Jamu Peluntur*) showed no significant effect in terms of resorption or fetal mortality among pregnant mice given at proportionately 50 times the human dose (Rosmiati et al. 1984). A study in 13 birth clinics among nearly 5,000 women found that nearly 20 percent had tried to bring on menses during the first trimester of pregnancy through taking *Super Heporine* capsules (215 cases), medicinal wines, chili preparations, or saline injections (Muchtar et al. 1981).[5] Their investigation into possible birth defects linked to these efforts was reported to be inconclusive.

RESEARCHING THE EXTENT OF USE

Despite the qualitative research on emmenagogues in Indonesia and the large indigenous literature on traditional herbal medicine (Sastro-amidjojo 1948; Soepardi 1957), there is little quantitative evidence on the scale of use of herbs to regulate menses. Most of the cited evidence has tended to come from large-scale surveys set in the context of "family planning" questions, which would capture only *jamu* used for this purpose. In fact, such surveys give little indication of widespread use of *jamu* for contraception or abortion: percentages ever using emmenagogues range from 1 percent to a high of 6 percent (table 11.2). Suharti and Wardhini (1982) found in a study in Jakarta that only 48 out of 1,225 women were users of emmenagogues for abortive purposes; they cite a Department of Health study reporting an even lower usage rate of only 0.6 percent (Suharti and Wardhini 1982:11).

Some small-scale studies do provide indications that emmenagogues

Table 11.2   Reported Knowledge and Use of Herbal Preparations (*Jamu*) for "Family Planning" Purposes, Indonesia

Study Site	Data Source	Respondents	Year	Know of Method	Ever Used	Current Use
Jakarta	KAP Survey	Males and Females	1968	14.0	X*	0.7‡
W. Java Urban	FM Survey	Ever married	1973	39.5	X	X
W. Java Rural	FM Survey	Ever married	1973	27.6	X	X
C. Java Urban	FM Survey	Ever married	1973	22.7	X	X
C. Java Rural	FM Survey	Ever married	1973	16.5	X	X
E. Java Urban	FM Survey	Ever married	1973	17.9	X	X
E. Java Rural	FM Survey	Ever married	1973	12.8	X	X
National† 23+	SUPAS II	Ever married	1976	6.2	X	X
Java-Bali	SUPAS III	Ever married	1976	20.1	3.4	0.7
Java-Bali	SUPAS III	Exposed	1976	22.1	4.2	1.1
Java-Bali	SUSENAS	Currently married	1979	X	X	6.3
National-20	CPS	Currently married	1987	12.4	2.8	X
National-27	DHS	Currently married	1991	5.2	1.8	0.6
National-13	IFLS	Currently married	1993–94	28.6	5.8	0.4
National-27	DHS	Currently married	1994	7.1	2.2	0.8

SOURCES: Various survey reports.

* X Indicates that the question was either not asked, or the answers were not published.

† "National" figures have sometimes been based on samples excluding particularly difficult provinces or parts of provinces. These are indicated by a reference to the number of provinces covered in the survey. The 1976 sample marked 23+ indicates 23 full province samples, plus one regency each in Nusatenggara Timur, Maluku, and Irian Jaya.

‡ 1968 Question was asked of both males and females and referred to use in the last month.

are more widely used than family planning surveys suggest. A study investigating delayed menstruation in the capital city of Jakarta and nearby West Javanese city of Bogor (Toha et al. 1992) found that more than half of married and unmarried women reported they had experienced delayed menses. Of those taking action, nearly two-thirds consumed herbs as their first response to the perceived delay. Community-based studies undertaken by teams from Gadjah Mada University in Sriharjo, Maguwoharjo, and Ngaglik in the Special Region of Yogyakarta in the Javanese heartland have always found far greater familiarity and use of *jamu* for bringing on menses than is indicated in family planning surveys.[6] And in Palembang, on the east coast of Sumatra, Agoes and colleagues (1976a; 1976b; 1978) have found high levels of *jamu* use among women of all ethnic groups. They detail the use of reproductive health remedies including *jamu* to augment lactation, tighten the vagina, and increase libido, as well as to bring on menstruation. Their survey findings indicated that about half of the women used some form of *jamu* regularly and 6 percent of all women reported using emmenagogues (Agoes, Syamsuir, and Tamzil 1976b:243–44). In a study of 227 women giving birth in a local maternity hospital between October 1975 and January 1976, one-third had taken some form of *jamu*. One in 10 of the mothers took *jamu peluntur* early in their pregnancy in order to prevent the birth, but they had "failed" to bring on menses (Agoes, Chaidi, and Suryadi 1976:249, 250). While such studies are plagued by questions about representativeness and reliability, they are suggestive of more common use of emmenagogues than might be assumed on the basis of national surveys. Can the discontinuity between family planning surveys and other evidence be explained solely by the fact that women are using *jamu peluntur* for reasons other than "family planning," or is the reality more complex?

TRANSLATING THE CONCEPTS

There are problems in translating words and concepts concerning the means and the motives of menses control. While the preparations are well known in Indonesia, and there is no strict taboo associated with talking about them, it is difficult to phrase questions that can determine whether the use of particular herbs is intended to prevent or terminate pregnancy or to promote fertility.

Furthermore, since the 1970s, government population control campaigns have appropriated words associated with contraception and family planning and cut them off from association with traditional behavior related to the control of elements of the reproductive system. The term *keluarga berencana* ("family planning") has become the universal term covering birth control and contraception (though not abortion), and it is all but totally connected to the government's official program, comprised largely of modern technical measures. The pervasiveness of this program has resulted in a strong bias among both survey interviewers and respondents to restrict any notions of family planning methods to those officially promoted by the national program. This may help to explain why the reported knowledge and use of herbs for "family planning" in surveys since 1968 has been low, even though impressions from contacts in markets indicate that the availability of preparations has, if anything, been high and even increasing.

Confusion surrounding the link of means and motives is compounded by the fact that delayed menses, even for some weeks, are not necessarily regarded as a specific sign of pregnancy, perhaps related to some Islamic beliefs in this predominantly Muslim country. One school of thought, for example, defines ensoulment as occurring 120 days after conception. Prior to that, stages of development each last 40 days as follows (Musallam 1983):

- *Nutfa:* seminal
- *'alaqa:* bloodlike clot
- *mudgha 1 and 2 (80 days):* unformed

It is only after these stages that the fetus is "quickened" and acquires a human state (in the second 40 days of the *mudgha* phase, which also involves the formation of organs). Consequently, it is only after 120 days that the "crime" of abortion is defined in at least one school of Islamic thought (Hull 1995). On this basis, some Hanafi jurists permit women to terminate pregnancies up to the fourth month of gestation, even without their husbands' permission (Musallam 1983:54–55, 57). One notable aspect of this interpretation is the idea that in the second month following conception, the development is denoted as a "bloodlike clot," which would be the commonsense observation of women experiencing a miscarriage or heavy flow following delayed menses. From this language it is a small step for women to refer to termination of pregnancy as simply "bringing on menses" and to distinguish this from any notion of "abortion" that is defined in the popular mind as removal of a fetus. The fact that some women[7] do not consider the bringing on of menses in the early months of pregnancy as being an abortion means that, even if women were willing to be frank about pregnancy termination on a survey, specific questions about herbs as abortifacients can result in underreporting.

Public figures in Indonesia routinely condemn "abortion" and declare that attempts to procure abortion are immoral. In recent years the precise legality of abortion has become confused, as successive legislation has codified criminal and civil offenses related to pregnancy termination, but with sometimes contradictory language (Hull et al. 1993). One result is that newspaper articles and political speeches frequently declare that induced abortion is totally illegal when in fact it is legally restricted but widely practiced by specialist practitioners and some general practitioners. The English term *menstrual regulation* for vacuum-aspiration abortions is translated into Indonesian as *induksi haid* ("menstrual induction"). Popularized in Indonesian cities in the 1970s with the importation of electric pumps and Karman cannulas by the U.S. Agency for International Development, the procedure is available in all major cities, and in many regency capitals. In Manado, North Sulawesi, some elite women have menstrual regulation done quarterly in preference to using modern forms of contraception.

The anti-abortion rhetoric does not define when precisely an abortion might be said to occur, and seldom is mention made, in the course of public debate, of the range of traditional practices including consumption of herbs that might cause abortion in the medical sense of the term. Instead, attention is directed to doctors in cities or midwives in private practices who carry out medical terminations of pregnancy. In surveys, respondents and interviewers alike tend to avoid discussion of herbs if the context was deemed to be related to unwanted pregnancy rather than "delayed" menstruation. Confusion of intention surrounds the various medical procedures and modern medications termed menstrual regulation, but technically intended to induce menstruation following the implantation of an embryo. Such uncertainty, we will argue below, can be an adaptive response for women and medical practitioners who regard abortion with moral ambiguity and use the technical ambiguity to assuage their consciences.

A more accurate picture of the scale of use of herbal preparations might be obtained if researchers asked women about the use of specific preparations and sidestepped the issue of the purpose of their use. Thus, for example, women could be asked if they have used any form of herbal emmenagogue (*jamu peluntur*) in the weeks or months prior to a survey, or they could be asked to report on use of a list of specific brands or types of preparation. No national surveys have ever attempted this in Indonesia. Such an approach would have a good chance of obtaining fairly accurate quantitative data on the use of emmenagogues. Trying to discern women's motives for their use would require more qualitative approaches and would demand careful attention to potential biases.[8]

MOTIVES FOR RESORTING TO MENSTRUAL CONTROL

For most Indonesian women over much of recorded history, menstruation was regularly suppressed by pregnancy or disrupted by the lengthy
period of breast-feeding post partum. Very long periods of postpartum amenorrhea have been reported for Java, and even recent Demographic and Health Surveys indicate mean durations of postpartum
amenorrhea of more than 8 months. This is especially true among
older, less educated rural women. It is also true that the time before
the resumption of normal menses post partum is declining. Urban
women in particular are likely to have an average duration of postpartum amenorrhea of less than 4 months, but overall Indonesian women
have long been accustomed to substantial periods of their fertile life
being "menses-free," as they were either pregnant or breast-feeding.

A study conducted by the World Health Organization in the late
1970s found that nearly half the respondents in Java reported that they
were not worried about a form of contraception that might cause
amenorrhea. This was in contrast with many of the other cultures represented in the multicountry study (WHO 1981:12). This has been confirmed over the past decade and a half as Indonesian women have
adopted injectable contraceptives in great numbers. Though users of
injectables and implants report disruption to their menstrual patterns,
they seem to be more concerned about excessive or irregular bleeding
than the absence of bleeding.

Older women (over age 40) we have interviewed over the years have
often been accepting, even welcoming, of irregular menses as a sign
that they are approaching the end of their fertile period. *"Haid sudah
tidak teratur"* ("irregular menses") is their matter-of-fact response to the
question of why they are not currently using contraception.

Of course the birth control pill, widely used in Indonesia, can be seen
as a main method of "menstrual control" in terms of producing regular
periods. But more than that, some Islamic women report taking hormonal pills continuously during the fasting month, to ensure they do
not menstruate and hence can avoid this perceived time of impurity
during a holy time of the year. In the 1980s the government family
planning program in West Sumatra promoted oral contraceptives as
the *"pil Ramadhan"* for just this purpose, and some women going on
the pilgrimage to Mecca also start taking the pill in advance of their
journey to avoid menstruating at an inopportune time. In a less benign
variation, some employers encourage, or even force, their female em-
ployees to take the contraceptive pill continuously so they will not
claim the "menstrual rest leave" guaranteed under some of the nation's
labor regulations.

Some may pose the question "why the emmenagogues?" if lack of menses or irregular menses are acceptable or even desirable under many situations. Although women, or some women at certain times in their lives, undoubtedly use these preparations simply to regulate menses as a sign of health, for many others emmenagogues probably have more to do with preventing pregnancy than is revealed in surveys and even in more-intensive research approaches. Herbal mixtures are seen as the first and most private and self-controlled option to bring on delayed menses in the case of an unwanted pregnancy.

In such cases, the more-intrusive methods such as saline solution injection (usually by nurses/trained midwives) and very vigorous massage (usually by traditional midwives) might be reserved for use after emmenagogues did not bring the desired result. Herbs, then, are an important step in the management of delayed menses, but women do not regard them as foolproof means of terminating pregnancy, nor does research to date confirm their efficacy. Of course, in many cases of late menses, menstruation resumes either naturally or as a result of early spontaneous abortion. Women who have turned to herbal preparations or other interventions in the intervening period would be likely to attribute success to their chosen method, allowing the perpetuation of methods through what is a reasonable if rough "cost-benefit" analysis of their use. What is lacking in Indonesia is research on the frequency of these use patterns for different motives and among different populations. What is difficult about this research is the fact that the motives are not easy to define. The many dimensions of meaning attached to perceptions of delayed menses convert into motives of such ambiguity that both researcher and respondent may be unsure of what is in question, and what interpretations might be attached to the answers.

MENSTRUAL CONTROL AS A REPRODUCTIVE HEALTH ISSUE: POLICY IMPLICATIONS

The practice of regular resort to medications purporting to bring on late menstrual periods raises a number of important questions in the context of reproductive health. First, little is known of the actual impact of herbal preparations, massage, or the improper dosage of "modern" drugs (such as the popular capsules sold under the brand name Super Heporine) on the volume of menstrual flow. Where the majority of adult Indonesian women are anemic, frequent attempts to induce menstruation may be of clinical significance quite apart from the issue of pregnancy. Such literature as exists in Indonesia does not specifically address this issue, nor does public policy consider the promotion of modern commercial *jamu* to be an area of significant health interest. At this stage, the cautionary principle would seem to call for further pharmacological study on the potential health impact of regular or excessive use of the major forms of *jamu*. Such studies should consider both the impact on the general health of women and that on the health of developing fetuses in women who attempted to "bring on menses" at an early stage of the pregnancy.

Second, while we know much about the variety of menstrual regulation technologies in Indonesia, we have little data on the frequency or intensity of their use. For well over a century, medical researchers have catalogued herbs, but there has been little priority given to research on how commonly they are used by women of different classes, ages, occupations, or ethnic groups across the nation.

The questions on *"jamu* for family planning" in demographic, health, and other major surveys have been unhelpful, since they underestimate past or current use of herbal preparations. It should be possible to design questions to gain reliable data on consumption of specific types of *jamu* purchased by women, focusing on the group of preparations related to menstruation. The major forms of *jamu terlambat bulan* or *peluntur* are well known, and women would be willing and able to say if they had ever or if they had recently purchased such preparations. Rather than assuming motives, the question of the purpose of specific *jamu* should be determined in a different way, with efforts to determine the links to pregnancy prevention or termination.

While the link between menses and pregnancy may not always be clear and direct, there is no doubt that control of menstruation is important for Indonesian women. It is time that the research and policy agendas recognize this as a central issue of reproductive health.

NOTES

Our interest in the topic was stimulated while living and conducting research in a Javanese village in 1972. The herbalists in the market were bemused that we would buy herbs for infertility on one visit, and on our next visit purchase herbs to induce menses.

1. Although the use of *jamu* is most prevalent on the island of Java, studies cited by Suharti and Wardhini (1982) claim that 70 percent of Indonesians use traditional herbal medications of some type. Even beyond

Java, packets of instant *jamu* from Java or Madura (an island off East Java) are available in relatively isolated markets, and it is common to see a Javanese or Madurese *jamu* seller going house to house in towns and cities.

2. A sample recipe for "irregular menses" given in one booklet mentions coriander root, turmeric, nutmeg, cardamom, cumin, cloves, and the leaves of Srigading (*nyctanthes arbortristis*), showing many similarities to the ingredients of a South Asian culinary dish. Many of the cooking herbs and spices used in the subcontinent are not used in central Indonesian cuisine, but rather as *jamu*, and Javanese served Indian food can be heard to remark that it "tastes like medicine."

3. Abdominal massage, sometimes in a painful and robust manner, is performed by a traditional healer. In general, this procedure is done after more considerable time of delay of the menses, with the specific intention of aborting a fetus. When performed soon after a missed period, there is still some uncertainty as to whether the women regard themselves as being pregnant at the time of the massage (and thus are intentionally procuring abortion) or if they see the delayed menses as a precursor of the state of pregnancy (and thus think of the procedure as a preventive measure). In a study of traditional midwives in Ngaglik, most said that women requested abortion services from them, several admitted to performing the massage technique, and two reported that they "often" did them (Yitno and Handayani 1980).

For hundreds of years, traditional midwives in Java have also practiced a particular massage (*pijat walik*) said to retroflex the uterus to prevent pregnancy. In the folklore this procedure is said to be very effective, and has the benefit of being reversible, though reportedly only if performed by the same *dukun*. While this type of massage is well known across Java, it is rare to find a woman who admits to having had one performed, and rarer still to have any reports about the effect of the procedure on the regularity or volume of menses.

4. Both Terra and Hoffman include a variety of less common herbal preparations, providing Latin names for ease of comparison.

5. In the Ngaglik study, one woman's case study reported that she took Super Heporine capsules in large doses in an effort to bring on her menses, without success. She rationalized that if it was fated that she would not be pregnant, the medicine would bring on menses, but that if it were her fate to be pregnant, Super Heporine would help make the baby healthier.

6. The late Professor Masri Singarimbun, as head of the Population Institute at Gadjah Mada, always encouraged his researchers to treat traditional behavior seriously, and thus was able to collect much more detailed information on herbal preparations than was done in community studies of population dynamics elsewhere in Indonesia in the 1960s and 1970s. At the time it was believed that the difference was a contrast of Ja-

vanese behavior with that of other ethnic groups, but now there are indications that virtually all groups in Indonesia have long established traditional pharmacopoeia, including emmenagogues. The challenge is to record them.

7. Although some 80 to 90 percent of Indonesians report themselves as Muslim, a much smaller proportion actually follow Islamic tenets and practices strictly. While it is unlikely that large numbers of Indonesians would be aware of the formal classification of fetal development presented, it may be that many are influenced by a more generalized idea that termination of a pregnancy in the early months is not a fetal death.

8. In the Ngaglik study (Hull, unpublished material), for example, the question about emmenagogues was prefaced by the following introduction: "Sometimes a woman who thinks her period is late may drink some herbal mixture/medicine or do something else to bring on the menstrual flow. She may do this because she feels a delayed period may upset her health; or that she may be pregnant when she doesn't want to be or, alternatively, some women regard menses as a sign of fecundity, and want to bring it on because they are trying to become pregnant." Even with such a lengthy introduction, the limits of a survey approach were apparent. Assessment of the researchers was that use of these preparations was underreported for a variety of reasons, including the fact that field assistants tended to be young women. Respondents on the survey were asked about perceptions of the situation in their community as well as their own experience, and this tended to yield higher levels of usage. In other words, herbs are used "by other women, but not by me."

REFERENCES

Agoes, A., Jusup Chaidi, and Suryadi. 1976a. "Penggunaan jamu pada wanita-wanita di Palembang" (The use of traditional herbal preparations by women in Palembang). Paper presented to the Third Congress of Obstetrics and Gynaecology, Medan.
Agoes, A., Syamsuir, and Sutomo Tamzil. 1976b. "Pengaruh obat-obat tradisional pada keluarga berencana" (The influence of traditional medicines in family planning). Paper presented to the Third Congress of Obstetrics and Gynaecology, Medan.
Agoes, A., Sjamsuir Munaf, Lailani, Ali Ghanie, and Sjahril Aziz. 1978. "Kebiasaan minum jamu dan hubungannya dengan berat lahir" (The practice of taking traditional herbs, and its relation to birth weight). Paper presented to the Fourth National Congress of Pediatrics, Yogyakarta.
Hoffman, David L. 1998. "Emmenagogues: Are They or Are They Not?"

Found at ⟨*http://www.healthy.net/library/books/hoffman/reproductive/ emmenagog.htm*⟩ on 3 July 1998.

Hull, Terence H. 1995. "Competing Rights: The Mother, the Foetus and the State." *Development Bulletin* (Australian Development Studies Network) 34:33–35.

Hull, Terence H., Sarsanto Sarwono, and Ninuk Widyantoro. 1993. "Induced Abortion in Indonesia." *Studies in Family Planning* 24, no. 4: 241–51.

Hull, Valerie J. 1984. *Breastfeeding and Fertility in Yogyakarta.* Monograph no. 5, Population Studies Center, Gadjah Mada University, Yogyakarta.

———. 1986. "Dietary Taboos in Java: Myths, Mysteries and Methodology." In *Shared Wealth and Symbol: Food, Culture, and Society in Oceania and Southeast Asia,* ed. Lenore Manderson, 237–58. Cambridge: Cambridge University Press.

Kloppenburg-Versteegh, J. [1909] 1983. *Indische Planten en haar Geneeskracht.* 3d ed., reprinted in 1983 as *Petunjuk Lengkap Tanam-Tanaman di Indonesia dan Khasiatnya Sebagai Obat-Obatan Tradisionil* (A complete guide to Indonesian plants and their use as traditional medicines), vols. 1 and 2. Yogyakarta: Yayasan Dana Sejahtera and Rumah Sakit Bethesda.

Muchtar, A., I. Darmansyah, K. S. Suharti, Hedi Rosmiati, and F. D. Suyatna. 1981. "Survai efek teratogenik jamu super heporine capsules di Jakarta" (A survey of the teratogenic effect of Super Heporine capsules in Jakarta). *Medika* 7, no. 4:245–50.

Musallam, B. F. 1983. *Sex and Society in Islam: Birth Control before the Nineteenth Century.* Cambridge: Cambridge University Press.

Ochse, J. J. and R. C. Bakhuizen van den Brink. [1931] 1977. *Vegetables of the Dutch East Indies (Edible Tubers, Bulbs, Rhizomes and Spices Included).* Canberra: Australian National University Press.

Rosmiati, Hedi, Azalia Sinto, Siti Siswoyo, Moehammad Martoprawiro, and Suharti Suherman. 1984. "Uji teratogenisitas jamu peluntur pada mencit" (A test of teratogenicity of menstrual regulation herbs in mice). *Majalah Kesehatan Indonesia* 34, no. 9:509–18.

Sastroamidjojo, Seno. [1948] 1967. *Obat Asli Indonesia* (Traditional Indonesian Medicine). Reprint, Djakarta: Penerbit Dian Rakjat.

Soepardi, Raden. 1957. *Obat-Obatan dari hasil Hutan* (Medicines from the forest). Djakarta: Dinas Penerbitan Balai Pustaka.

Soeparto, Soedarmilah. 1984. *Jamu Jawa Asli* (Traditional Javanese herbal medicine). Jakarta: Penerbit Sinar Harapan.

Soemardjo-Sju. 1980. *Resep Obat-Obat Tradisionil Jamu Jawa* (Recipes for Traditional Javanese Herbal Medicines). Surabaya: Karya Anda.

Suherman, Suharti and S. Wardhini. 1982. "Survai penggunaan jamu sebagai kontrasepsi" (Survey on the use of herbal preparations as contraceptives). *Warta Kontrasepsi* 5, no. 1.

Tierra, Michael. 1998. "The Emmenagogues: Herbs that Move Blood and Relieve Pain." Found at ⟨*http://www.plantherbs.com/articles/BloodHerb.html*⟩ on 3 April 1998.

Toha, Muhaimin, Asri Adisasmita, Luknis Sabri, Tris Eryando, and Yovsyah. 1992. "Study to Identify Knowledge, Attitude and Behavior about Delayed Menstruation, as Well as Variables Affecting Attitude toward Access to Comprehensive Reproductive Health Services for Low/No Income Women in Jakarta and Bogor." Study Group on Reproductive Health, School of Public Health, University of Indonesia, Jakarta.

Wardhini, S., and Yasavati Kurnia. 1979. "Skrining antifertilitas beberapa jamu peluntur pada mencit" (Antifertility screening of menstrual regulation herbs in mice). *Majalah Farmakologi Indonesia* 1, no. 2:3–9.

WHO (World Health Organization). 1981. "A Cross-Cultural Study of Menstruation: Implications for Contraceptive Development and Use." *Studies in Family Planning* 12, no. 1:3–16.

Yitno, Amin, and Tri Handayani. 1980. *Sang Penolong: Studi Tentang Peranan Dukun Bayi Dalam Persalinan di Ngaglik, Yogyakarta* (The honored helper: A study of traditional birth attendants in Ngaglik, Yogyakarta). Yogyakarta: Pusat Penelitian dan Studi Kependudukan, Universitas Gadjah Mada.

CHAPTER 12

Regulating Menstruation in Matlab, Bangladesh: Women's Practices and Perspectives

Heidi Bart Johnston

Regular menstruation is good for women's health.
If menstruation is regular, then women will not
attract disease. Women with regular menstruation
do not feel weak.

—Older Muslim woman, Matlab

Menstruation is seen as both a purifying and a polluting event in many cultures, including those in Bangladesh. While seemingly contradictory, this way of thinking is actually two manifestations of the same concept. Menstruation is valued as a means of regularly flushing "bad blood" from a woman's body, cleaning the woman, and signifying that she is fertile. Once out of the body, however, menstrual fluids are believed to pollute anything they contact. To limit menstrual pollution, the general movements and religious and household activities of menstruating women have been severely restricted by social proscription (Blanchet 1984; George 1994; Maloney, Aziz, and Sarkar 1981; WHO 1981a, 1981b).

Few studies have been conducted on women's perceptions and practices regarding menstruation. Bangladesh is a particularly attractive setting to conduct such a study because rapid increases in availability and use of hormonal contraceptive methods, which affect menstrual regularity, may be influencing these attitudes and behaviors. An even more significant factor may be the existence of a government program that countenances the use of menstrual regulation as postconception birth control in a country where abortion is illegal. Because Bangladesh's menstrual regulation program is unusual, a brief description of its development and issues regarding its acceptance follow.

By assuming its name, the Bangladesh National Menstrual Regulation Program took advantage of the positive association in women's minds between health and the regularity of menses. Officially, menstrual regulation (MR) is "an interim method of establishing nonpregnancy" for women with delayed menses who are "at risk of being pregnant" (Ali, Zahir, and Hossein 1978; Dixon-Mueller 1988). The program provides uterine vacuum aspiration to women up to 10 weeks after the expected date of the missed menstruation. Since the program's establishment, MR provision has spread to urban and rural hospitals, health complexes, and clinics throughout the country.

In its evolution, the MR program never directly challenged Bangladeshi national or Islamic law. National abortion law, based on the British penal code of 1860, states that abortion is illegal except to save the life of the pregnant woman (Akhter 1988). This legislation was liberalized briefly in the early history of Bangladesh to allow abortions for women raped during the 1971 Independence War. After the law was reinstated, the Menstrual Regulation Program was gradually introduced, partly in response to high numbers of complications resulting from unsafe abortions.

Dixon-Mueller (1988) and Amin (1996) attribute—to varying degrees—the acceptance of the Menstrual Regulation Program to the use of the culturally acceptable concept of MR as opposed to "inducing abortion." Even more important to the early success of the program, according to Amin, was the government's legitimization. In a widely distributed government memorandum, aborting a known pregnancy (illegal) was distinguished from inducing menstruation when pregnancy status is unknown (legal) (Amin 1996; Government of Bangladesh 1980).

Islamic doctrine, Amin points out, allows "a range of interpretations with a considerable degree of tolerance for early term abortion in some cases" (Amin 1996). The Hanifi School of Jurisprudence, dominant in Bangladesh and elsewhere in South Asia, permits abortion before ensoulment, but forbids it afterward. The *Hadith*—guidelines of the prophet Mohammed—clearly states that ensoulment occurs 120 days after conception (Amin 1996; see also Hull and Hull, this volume, for Indonesia). The limit of MR to 10 weeks after a missed period falls within the allowance provided by the Hanifi School. Anthropological evidence from Bangladesh indicates that respondents who view MR favorably believe the fetus has no life at the early gestational stage at which MR is performed (Aziz and Maloney 1985). From this perspective, there is little if any difference between removing a fetus prior to ensoulment and inducing menstruation.

Rural Bangladeshi women place a positive value on regular menstruation. Perceptions of menstruation and amenorrhea among these women are strongly influenced by the current confluence of persisting traditional thought, rapidly decreasing family size desires, and exposure to modern medicines and medical techniques. Through an analysis of qualitative and quantitative data, this chapter explores the perceived causes of stopped menstruation and responses to this event among reproductive-age women in rural Bangladesh. The particularities, ambiguities, and ironies surrounding menstruation, amenorrhea, and the use of emmenagogues in this region are commented on.

RESEARCH SETTING AND METHODS

The research upon which this analysis is based is the product of a study measuring the prevalence of induced abortion in Matlab, located in the deltaic plain of southern Bangladesh. The Matlab area is characterized by a subsistence agriculture economy, poor infrastructure and communication, and high landlessness and illiteracy rates. Its population is predominately (88 percent) Sunni Muslim, subscribing to the Hanifi School described earlier (Aziz 1994), with the remaining population almost entirely Hindu. As elsewhere in rural Bangladesh, a system of purdah restricts women's physical mobility, rendering them unlikely to leave the vicinity of their village or *bari* (family compound) without a male family member, even to procure basic health services (Koenig et al. 1994; Simmons, Mita, and Koenig 1992).

Matlab's population is unique in rural Bangladesh because of the intensive family planning activities that have been supported since the mid-1970s by the International Centre for Diarrhoeal Disease Research, Bangladesh (ICDDR,B) research program. Monthly since 1966, the roughly 200,000 residents of the Matlab study area have reported births, deaths, marriages, divorces, in- and out-migrations, and internal movements to the Demographic Surveillance System (DSS) (Aziz and Mosley 1994).[1]

While the provision of maternal care services continues to improve in the Matlab maternal and child health and family planing (MCH-FP) area, services beyond basic care remain difficult to access, as elsewhere in rural Bangladesh. Both the MCH-FP and comparison areas are served by static clinics handling a population of about 20,000 to 25,000 each. These clinics offer curative maternal and child health care services, clinical contraception, and treatment for contraceptive complications (Koenig et al. 1994). Some clinics and the *thana* (rural administrative unit) health complex offer MR services. More complicated procedures, such as cesarean sections and blood transfusions, are available at government district hospitals and some private clinics in Nara-yanganj, to the north of Matlab, and Chandpur, to the south. By boat and/or bus, the trip to a district town would be between 2 to 4 hours for the residents of Matlab *thana* who can arrange access to transport (Ronsmans et al. 1997).

The data presented in the following section are drawn from quali-tative and quantitative studies on the practices and perceptions of women regarding induced abortion. Because of the strong associations between pregnancy termination and menstruation in Bangladesh, multiple aspects of menstruation were explored in the qualitative re-search that preceded and informed the survey research. To distinguish between spontaneous and induced abortion, and between inducing menstruation and inducing abortion, the retrospective survey also in-vestigated aspects of amenorrhea such as durations of amenorrheic events, perceived causes and symptoms, and strategies for treating amenorrhea.

Fieldwork took place from January to September 1997. The qualita-tive data come from 51 in-depth interviews with 19 married women of reproductive age and 7 local health care providers. Interviews were conducted in the MCH-FP and comparison areas of the ICDDR,B study area in Matlab. Informants were selected to broadly represent women in the community in terms of age, Muslim or Hindu religious affilia-tion, the family planning services provided to their community, and the distance of their residence from a modern health facility. In the first interview, women were asked general questions about their re-productive health, and the interviewer probed for details on relevant topics. In subsequent interviews, women were asked direct questions about their experiences, or the experiences of other women in the com-munity with abortion, amenorrhea, MR, and fertility promotion.

In addition, 9 interviews were conducted with 7 health care provid-ers from Matlab, 5 of whom assist women in the Matlab area to induce abortion and menstruation. Two interviews were conducted with a healer, or *kobiraj,* who provides traditional health care. Two family wel-fare visitors (government-sponsored paramedics) who provide manual vacuum aspiration at the hospital in Matlab were interviewed once each. One interview apiece was conducted with a village "doctor" who distributes allopathic medicines from a village market stall, and a ho-meopath[2] who treats women who want to induce menstruation or abortion when their cycle is delayed. Two interviews were conducted with an ICDDR,B community health worker from the MCH-FP area, and 1 interview was conducted with a community health worker from the comparison area.

The second data source is the semistructured, retrospective Abortion

Frequency Survey (AFS), conducted between July and September 1997. A total of 909 married women of reproductive age responded to a survey for estimating the Matlab abortion rate. In an attempt to eliminate misreporting of unwanted pregnancies as irregular menstruation and induced abortions as spontaneous ones, interviewers explored respondents' reports of irregular menstruation. They asked for the dates that menstruation stopped and resumed, symptoms of stopped menstruation, respondents' perceptions of why menstruation stopped, and how menstruation started again. In the section that follows, data presented in italics are quotations from the in-depth interviews, and data presented in standard text are paraphrased reports from the semistructured AFS.

RESULTS: "THERE ARE NO BAD SIDES TO MENSTRUATION"

Amenorrhea—broadly defined as absence of menstrual bleeding in reproductive-age women and women making the transition from reproductive age that does not result in birth—is a common occurrence among the women interviewed. In the year prior to the survey, 58 percent (n = 524) of AFS respondents reported having experienced the event; 1,538 cases were reported by the 909 respondents.

While the reporting of amenorrheic events is known to be highly subject to recall bias (WHO 1981a, 1981b), these results are illuminating, as they show the variety of perceived causes of stopped menstruation and give some indication of the relative occurrence of each cause. Injectable contraception (DMPA) and postpartum amenorrhea each were reported to have caused about 40 percent of reported incidences of amenorrhea. Anemia and weakness, pregnancies not carried to term, menopause, and supernatural spirits were named as causes of most of the remaining cases (see table 12.1).

The aim of this analysis is to describe, in rural Bangladeshi women's terms, the perceived principal causes of stopped menstruation and women's responses to it. The 3 principal named causes of the absence of menstruation are injectable contraceptive use; poor health, including anemia and weakness, spirits, and other elements; and pregnancy.

Contraceptive Use: "I am an injection user, so my menstruation has stopped. I am swollen"

According to AFS data, 42 percent of perceived episodes of amenorrhea were caused by use of injectable contraceptives, making this practice

Table 12.1 Causes of Irregular Menstruation in Matlab, 1991–97

Cause	Frequency	Percentage
Injectable (DMPA)	644	41.9
Postpartum amenorrhea	591	38.4
Anemia/weakness	103	6.7
Pregnancy resulting in induced abortion	64	4.2
Pregnancy resulting in spontaneous abortion or stillbirth	32	2.1
Menopause	20	1.3
Evil eye	10	0.6
Other (don't know, etc.)	74	4.8
Total cases	1,538	100.0

SOURCE: Responses from 909 women interviewed in the Abortion Field Survey.

the chief cause of stopped menstruation. The Matlab MCH-FP area has a high rate of injectable use compared with other areas of Bangladesh. With 35 percent of all married women of reproductive age using the injectable, it is the most popular method of contraception in the MCH-FP area (van Ginneken et al. 1998). Although its rate of use is low in the rest of the country, it is increasing more rapidly than that of any other method: in 1989, 0.6 percent of modern-method users used the injectable (Huq and Cleland 1990); in 1996–97, 6.2 percent used it (NIPORT et al. 1997).

Results of the qualitative research demonstrate that informants generally associate irregular menstruation caused by use of family planning methods with perceived rheumatic pain, swelling of the body, and storage of bad blood. Regular menstruation is also upheld as a religious ideal:

> *If women use FP they will suffer rheumatism. Women stop menstruating when they use FP. If a woman has regular menstruation, then the* kharap racto *(bad blood) comes out. It's the rule of Allah. So when women use the pill or injection, they become swollen and have tingling.* (Middle-aged,[3] Muslim, MCH-FP area)

Other informants accepted the amenorrhea associated with injectable use:

> *My menstruation has stopped for one year. I don't feel any problems, so I don't go to the doctor. If I feel a problem, I will go to the doctor.* (Middle-aged, Muslim, MCH-FP area)

Some women experiencing amenorrhea from the injectable feel a need to menstruate. Strategies for menstruating in this circumstance include method switching from the injectable to oral contraceptives back to the injectable; dilatation and curettage (D&C); and more traditional herbal methods. The Pill is the principal method of inducing menstruation from amenorrhea related to injectable use. The following two reports recorded by AFS interviewers are typical:

> After being amenorrheic from taking the injectable since before 1991, the respondent wanted her menstruation to start so she dropped the injectable and took the pill for two months. After two months of regular menstruation she took the injection again. (Age 42, MCH-FP area)

> The respondent takes the injectable for six months and then takes the pill for one month to menstruate. Then she starts the injectable again. (Age 36, MCH-FP area)

One respondent took oral contraceptives to induce menstruation while continuing to take the injectable:

> After the respondent had been taking the injectable regularly for about four years she took a packet of pills, while still on the injectable, over a month period to start her menstruation. Despite taking the packet of pills her menstruation did not start. (Age 44, MCH-FP area)

One respondent had a D&C to start menstruation after amenorrhea associated with injectable use:

> The respondent had not menstruated for five years because she used the injectable. She felt abdominal pains and backache so she dropped the injectable to allow her menstruation to start. Five months after dropping the injectable she still had not menstruated. The respondent discussed her situation with the family welfare assistant, who told her to go to Chandpur. The respondent's husband took the respondent to a doctor at Gouripur Hospital. After checking, the doctor told them that inside the uterus there was some infected blood that was preventing menstruation. The problem was caused by use of the injectable. The doctor performed a D&C to clear out the infected blood. (Age 30, comparison area)

Traditional methods are used on their own and in combination with modern techniques to induce menstruation, as demonstrated by the following two examples:

> The respondent had nine months of amenorrhea after dropping the injectable. At that time she had abdominal pains and felt something round inside her belly. Her body became swollen. She went to the *kobiraj* for treatment. She took the *kobiraj* treatment for two months

and began to menstruate. She had five days of bleeding black fluids. (Age 35, comparison area)

After four months of amenorrhea while on the injectable the respondent took the sap from a tree, iron syrup, and seven iron tablets to start her menstruation. She menstruated then experienced amenorrhea again. (Age 30, MCH-FP area)

These data reveal that traditional and modern practices are being used by rural women to remedy amenorrhea—the negative connotations of which are rooted in traditional beliefs. The modern medical technology implemented includes inappropriate use of hormones, contraceptive method switching, and D&C.

The finding has widespread and important implications for family planning counseling in Bangladesh. While injectable use is still uncommon there, the injectable-pill-injectable method switching pattern is not limited to Matlab. Rahman et al. and Haque et al. report similar findings from the rural areas of Abhoynagar in southwest Bangladesh and Sirajganj in the northwest. Irregular menstruation is reported by 21 percent of long-term users of the injectable (Rahman et al. 1997). Many women who dropped the injectable did so after a long period of use, suggesting that irregular menstruation is tolerable for some time, but not indefinitely. The data also show a pattern of method switching from the injectable to the pill back to the injectable. Such switching is associated with periods of no contraceptive protection, unwanted pregnancy, and induced abortion (Ahmed et al. 1996; Haque et al. 1997; Rahman et al. 1997).

These findings emphasize the importance of offering appropriate counseling with the injectable contraceptive and other family planning methods that disrupt regular menstruation. Such counseling is incomplete if it does not inform women of the possible side effect of amenorrhea; address the stigma associated with long durations of amenorrhea; and address the hazards of method switching and more-invasive techniques of starting menstruation.

Poor Health: "If menstruation is regular, there are fewer chances that disease will be attracted"

Regular menstruation is associated with good health where such indicators are few, and maternal health is generally poor. Bangladesh is a case in point: 70 percent of its women suffer from nutritional deficiency anemia (World Bank 1995). While the literature suggests that only in the most extreme cases would malnutrition cause amenorrhea (Bongaarts 1980; Warriner, this volume), there is also the opinion that insufficient knowledge is available, particularly regarding the effect of chronic malnutrition on menstrual patterns of women from developing countries (Cumming 1993; Warriner, this volume). It is generally agreed that malnutrition delays menarche (Bongaarts and Potter 1983), and studies have linked malnutrition with extended periods of postpartum amenorrhea (Becker, Chowdhury, and Leridon 1985; Huffman et al. 1978; Huffman et al. 1987). Furthermore, amenorrhea is linked with dieting, weight loss, low body weight, and reduced body fat (Cumming 1993).

Regardless of the scholarly literature, women interviewed perceive amenorrhea as linked with poor nutrition, general weakness, and poor health. Irregular menstruation associated with physiological or spiritual poor health is the third most common cause of amenorrhea after injectable use and postpartum amenorrhea. Over a 6-year period, respondents to the AFS reported experiencing 187 amenorrheic events not associated with a recognized pregnancy, contraceptive use, or menopause. Fifty-five percent of this reported amenorrhea was caused by general weakness and 5 percent by a supernatural spirit, whereas 25 percent was from an unknown cause and 14 percent was due to another cause. Some informants indicated that irregular menstruation can occur for no reason. The qualitative data indicate a coexistence of traditional and modern medical beliefs and practices regarding anemic amenorrhea.

The coexistence of traditional and modern beliefs is marked by the following two respondents. The first recognizes only *kalir suut* (evil god's eye) as a cause of stopped menstruation not related to pregnancy. The second recognizes both traditional and allopathic explanations.

> *Menstruation is stopped by* kalir suut. *When women have* kalir suut *they will catch diseases.* (Older, Muslim, comparison area)

> Q: What kind of disease caused the large gap between your pregnancies?
> A: *The* kobiraj *said it was caused by* alga *[supernatural spirit]. The doctor said the gap was caused by insufficient blood and vitamins.* (Middle-aged, Hindu, MCH-FP area)

Anemia and conditions associated with physical weakness are perceived by women as common causes of irregular menstruation. Regular menstruation is associated with good health, showing that a woman has enough blood and adequate nutrition:

If women suffer anemia—if a woman has no blood—she has no menstrua-tion. (Younger, Muslim, MCH-FP area)

Regular menstruation is good for women's health. If menstruation is regu-lar, then women will not attract diseases. Women with regular menstrua-tion do not feel weak. (Older, Muslim, comparison area)

Strategies of regulating menstruation range from use of amulets and herbal medicine from the *kobiraj* to D&C from a modern hospital. While women do still go to the *kobiraj* and the homeopath for treat-ment to regulate menstruation, the following informant demonstrates a pull away from traditional medicine:

Q: What can women do to encourage regular bleeding again?
A: *The woman can go to the hospital. The doctor will advise her to eat vege-tables and foods with vitamins. Sometimes the village women go to the kobiraj. The kobiraj will give her herbal medicine. I don't believe in herbal medicine.* (Older, Hindu, MCH-FP area)

Oral contraceptives are the most common method of starting men-struation. Informants could name the brand of pills used to regulate menstruation:

When menstruation is irregular women use the pill to make menstrua-tion regular. For example, my sister-in-law had irregular menstruation. Her husband lived in another country. She suffered abdominal pain. Then she used FP pill to regulate her menstruation. (Younger, Muslim, MCH-FP area)

I heard that when women have stopped menstruation for two to three months then they take the pills called "ovasted" and other names. Then their menstruation will start. One woman in this area told me about this process.

The same informant continues:

Now there are different kinds of FP pill methods in the market. When a woman goes to the doctor for this problem [amenorrhea] then the doctor tells the patient the FP pills the woman can take to make her menstruation start. (Middle-aged, Hindu, MCH-FP area)

Iron pills and vitamins are also recommended as treatments for amenorrhea associated with anemia. The family welfare visitor pro-vides modern medicine to start menstruation, and the village doctor has a host of modern treatments for "insufficient" menstruation:

If malnourished, the woman will menstruate but an insufficient amount of blood will come out. In that situation we give iron tablets and vitamins, and give FP pill for regular menstruation. If they do not have regular menstruation, then we refer them to Dhaka for D&C. (Village doctor, comparison area)

Several informants associated what they perceived as potentially fatal tumors with stopped menstruation. One informant had a uterine tumor removed several years prior to the interview. Her unusual bleeding pattern indicated to her that she needed health care from a professional provider:

One time my menstruation stopped for three months. Afterwards I started heavy bleeding. I went to Chandpur for a gynecological exam. The doctor diagnosed a tumor in my uterus. The doctor operated to remove the tumor. (Older, Hindu, MCH-FP area)

Six months after the operation the informant conceived and successfully carried the unwanted pregnancy to term.

For these informants, regular menstruation is a positively valued physiological event. When menses are irregular, it is a sign or a symptom of anemia, weakness, or a physiological spiritual problem. Women's methods of bringing on menstruation include traditional techniques from the *kobiraj* and homeopath, but as is the case with amenorrhea associated with injectable contraceptive use, women are also using family planning pills and other modern medical technology to reinstate regular menstruation.

Unwanted Pregnancy: "When menstruation starts, the woman thinks she is fine, otherwise she feels tense, and thinks she has conceived a child"

The most important aspect of menstrual regularity is its relationship with fertility. In rural Bangladesh, menstruation is regarded as a sign of good reproductive health, as it marks a woman's ability to bear children (Blanchet 1984; Maloney, Aziz, and Sarkar 1981). Furthermore, stopped menstruation, with nausea and tiredness, are the principal signals of early pregnancy. Among women who want to delay or have completed childbearing, stopped menstruation can signify unwanted pregnancy, forcing them to make difficult decisions about continuing it.

In Bangladesh, the ideal family size is 2.5 children, almost 1 child lower than the total fertility rate (TFR) of 3.4 (Mitra et al. 1994). In

Matlab, the TFR is 3.0 (2.7 in the treatment area and 3.5 in the comparison area) (Mostafa et al. 1998), and 32 percent of Matlab AFS respondents reported having experienced 1 or more unwanted pregnancies. For women who have achieved their ideal family size or who are not ready for a pregnancy, regular menstruation is an important sign that they are not pregnant. Late menstruation can represent having to face the decision of adding a financial burden to the household or terminating a pregnancy. The importance of regular menstruation with regard to pregnancy status is explained by this informant:

> *Sometimes women feel physically uncomfortable and have abdominal pain. When menstruation starts they feel easy, more comfortable. When menstruation starts the woman thinks she is fine, otherwise she feels tense, and thinks she has conceived a child.* (Middle-aged, Hindu, MCH-FP area)

Despite legal, religious, physiological, and terminological ambiguities regarding induced abortion in Bangladesh, evidence suggests that women perceive themselves as able to distinguish between pregnancy- and nonpregnancy-related amenorrhea (Johnston 1998; Maloney, Aziz and Sarkar 1981). The 51 in-depth interviews and 909 completed surveys yielded no evidence suggesting MR is sought for reasons other than to terminate a pregnancy. Interestingly, D&C, a procedure similar to MR, is sought to stimulate fertility.

The expressions used in Bangla by informants are indicative of how the menstrual regulation procedure is perceived. In Matlab, and probably in most rural areas of Bangladesh, the term *menstrual regulation* and its abbreviation MR are unknown to the majority of potential clients. However, the service, provider, and, for some women, even the technique is known. Informants used terms such as *boccho fallai* ("drop the child") and *boccho nosto* ("waste the child"), referring not to starting menstruation, but to terminating a pregnancy. The vacuum aspiration procedure officially called menstrual regulation is perceived as a means of terminating a pregnancy. The ambiguity lies in the official and even household-level terminology. However, from potential clients' perspectives, the purpose of the procedure is not ambiguous.

Terminological ambiguity at the household level is demonstrated by informants who clarified that they were speaking of pregnancy only by mentioning the presence of a fetus. To informants, stopped menstruation can mean either pregnancy- or nonpregnancy-related amenorrhea. Some differentiated between the two without probing on the part of the interviewer, but often when discussing stopped menstruation with an informant, researchers were unaware that she was discussing pregnancy until she mentioned the fetus. The ambiguity in terminology is demonstrated by the following two examples:

A: *If a person wants to have regular menstruation she will go to the village doctor.*

Q: Then what treatment does the doctor give?

A: *The doctor will give an injection and medicine.*

Q: Does the medicine and injection work?

A: *No. I hear sometimes after using the medicine and injection, the fetus does not come out.*

Q: Then what does the woman do?

A: *She does not get treatment again. The fetus stays inside, and after nine months of waiting it comes out.* (Middle-aged, Muslim, MCH-FP area)

A: *Regular menstruation is good for health.*

Q: What are some bad things about irregular menstruation?

A: *If menstruation is irregular, then sometimes there will be a swelling of the body. And rheumatism attacks the body.*

Q: When women suffer irregular menstruation, what will they do?

A: *They will take medicine from the* kobiraj. *Some women will have a wash. Some women will keep the fetus.* (Young, Hindu, comparison area)

Modern and traditional techniques are being used to terminate unwanted pregnancy. The family welfare visitor uses manual vacuum aspiration to perform MR, ostensibly free of cost. However, for multiple reasons, including corruption in the system of obtaining MR supplies and a substantial demand for MR services, these providers charge clients. In Matlab, the unofficial fees associated with the MR procedure and the lack of confidentiality provided by the family welfare visitor drive women to less safe, less expensive, but perhaps more confidential providers for pregnancy termination. The village doctor provides allopathic medicines to induce abortion, the homeopath provides homeopathic tablets and syrups, the *kobiraj* uses herbal tonics and invasive techniques. Many women attempt to self-induce abortion using the contraceptive pill, well known in Matlab as a method of regulating menstruation (Johnston and Akter 1997). Caldwell et al. (1997) identifies the same general types of abortion providers in Abhoynagar Thana in western Bangladesh.

Menstrual regulation from a trained provider is the safest method of pregnancy termination available in rural Bangladesh. Most respondents to the AFS reported no problems after having had an MR, but several reported postprocedure vaginal bleeding and abdominal pain. The following demonstrates the secrecy women use when seeking to terminate a pregnancy, even when using the government-provided service:

> When the respondent understood that she was pregnant she asked her husband for permission to go to her parents' house. Without her husband knowing she and her brother's wife went to the Jurainpur Hospital for the respondent to have an MR. The family welfare visitor performed the MR for 150 taka. The respondent experienced no bleeding and no discomfort. (Age 22, comparison area)

Village doctors provide tablets and intramuscular injections (Menstrogen and Gynocib were named) to induce abortion. Women who attempt to abort using this option have a high failure rate: of 21 attempts, only 6 pregnancies were terminated. An AFS interviewer documented the following unsuccessful abortion attempt by a village doctor:

> The respondent wanted to space her births but she became pregnant four months after giving birth when she was a nonuser. When she was one month pregnant she bought seven tablets from the village doctor, but the medicine did not work. The village doctor told her that if the medicine does not work she should return. But her husband disagreed, so she kept the fetus. (Age 30, MCH-FP area)

Homeopathic medicine in rural Bangladesh is said to combine local traditional treatments with allopathic ones. The homeopath admits that his techniques often fail to induce abortion in women. AFS results show that of 29 attempts to induce abortion using homeopathic techniques, only 4 attempts were successful. Despite the widely acknowledged poor success rate, many women turn to the homeopath for a first attempt to induce abortion when they have an unwanted pregnancy:

> The respondent became pregnant while using the pill. When she realized she was pregnant she stopped taking the pill. When she was three months pregnant she took two bottles of homeopathic medicine to induce abortion. The medicine cost 50 taka. After taking the medicine she experienced five days of heavy bleeding with belly pains. The first day of bleeding she saw a clot of blood come out. For 15 days more she had normal bleeding. (Age 23, comparison area)

Women with unwanted pregnancies also use traditional medicine, even though it is known by many to be unsafe. *Kobiraj* abortions are less expensive and more confidential than abortions from other providers—if there are no post-abortion complications (Johnston and Akter 1997).

Informants described several techniques *kobiraj* use to induce abortion, which include giving herbal tablets or blessed water to the pregnant woman. The *kobiraj* we spoke with only described one method of inducing abortion. She explained that she uses herbal medicine and a creeper (a stiff jungle vine), which is inserted into the uterus (Johnston and Akter 1997). Of the 15 attempts to induce abortion using *kobiraj* techniques that were reported to the AFS, 6 attempts actually terminated the pregnancy. The respondent referred to below reported her traumatic experience to the AFS interviewer:

> In 1991, when the respondent was one and a half months pregnant her husband bought two tablets from Chandpur which were supposed to induce abortion. She took the tablets, but nothing happened. When she was two and a half months pregnant she went to the *kobiraj* to induce abortion. The *kobiraj* gave her a creeper. After the respondent inserted the creeper a clot of blood came out. Then the woman withdrew the creeper but she did not bleed anymore. After 10 or 12 days the woman felt something round inside of her belly. She again bought a creeper from the *kobiraj*. Her husband forbade her to use the creeper. When the respondent was three months pregnant she suffered severe fever and severe belly pains one night. The next day at noon the fetus came out. Then a lot of blood and clots came out. In the evening the doctor came and gave her medicine to stop the bleeding. After taking the medicine she experienced 17 or 18 days of normal bleeding. (Age 23, comparison area)

Self-aborting unwanted pregnancies using family planning pills is a common, if fairly ineffective, strategy among Matlab women, and is replacing homeopathic medicine:

> *There is no need for homeo medicine to treat stopped menstruation. At that time take* Maya Bori *[brand name of oral contraception], and menstruation starts. . . . After two to three months, then family planning methods don't work. After one or one and a half months, then medicine works. When menstruation has stopped for three months, then the* boccho *[child/fetus] grows. Then the woman needs the treatment from the doctor.* (Middle-aged, Muslim, comparison area)

Of the of 34 attempts reported to the AFS to abort using oral contraceptives and iron tablets (used as the placebo pills in oral-contraceptive cycle packets distributed in Bangladesh), only 8 succeeded. The following is an example of a reported success:

The respondent's fourth pregnancy was unwanted. After one and a half months of pregnancy the respondent took several hormone pills at a time to induce abortion, but nothing happened. She took seven iron tablets at once. One day afterwards she started bleeding. She experienced three days of heavy bleeding and another five days of light bleeding. (Age 39, comparison area)

Of the 108 pregnancies that women attempted to abort which they reported to the AFS, 64 were terminated and 44 were not. When the first attempt failed, more than half of the women made a second attempt. Almost half of the women experiencing a second failure made a third attempt. Thirty-two percent of the 90 failed attempts overall used medicine from the homeopath. Twenty-nine percent were attempts to self-induce abortion—mostly by using hormone pills and the accompanying iron tablets in the contraceptive pill cycle packet. Twenty-three percent used medicine from the village doctor; 11 percent used medicine from the *kobiraj*. Women are rarely if ever informed of potential side effects of methods used. As the following example demonstrates, failed attempts to abort represent potential morbidity to the woman and possibly to the fetus:

The respondent took 3 hormone pills after she realized she had conceived, but her menstruation did not start. She went to the village doctor's house for treatment. The village doctor gave her 8 small tablets. She took all the tablets but did not abort the pregnancy. After 4 days passed, she took 8 more tablets. Then she felt dizzy and became weak. She bought a bottle of syrup from a doctor in Nandalalpur Bazaar. She recovered, but did not abort the pregnancy. In the end she kept the pregnancy. (Age 29, comparison area)

CONCLUSION

Research results show that for women not wanting a pregnancy, regular menstruation is an indication that they are in good physical and spiritual health. Menstruation is a sign that a woman is fertile, nonpregnant, and has sufficient blood to menstruate. In addition, menstruation is perceived as a regular purge of bad blood stored in the body. Regular menstruation is in harmony with God's design. The principal causes of stopped menstruation other than postpartum amenorrhea range from the traditional—unexplained amenorrhea related to poor health and unwanted pregnancy—to those associated with modern contraceptive technology. When menstruation is irregular, many women choose to treat it. Both traditional and allopathic medicines are applied to induce menses. Data suggest that traditional techniques of inducing menstruation, using *kobiraj* or homeopathic remedies, are decreasing in popularity as women turn to the Pill or other allopathic techniques available from the village doctor and elsewhere.

In rural Bangladesh, the most important application of allopathic medicines to induce menstruation—in terms of potential numbers of women influenced by the use of the technique—is discontinuing the injectable contraceptive and switching to the contraceptive pill to induce menstruation. Such contraceptive method switching has been found to result in unwanted pregnancies and induced abortions. This finding emphasizes the need for appropriate counseling associated with injectable acceptance, particularly as injectable contraception use is increasing more rapidly than that of any other family planning method in Bangladesh.

Other results from this research suggest that the allopathic technique referred to as menstrual regulation or MR at the government level is unmistakably thought of and used as a technique to terminate pregnancies. While the use of menstrual regulation using manual vacuum aspiration equipment is not considered a technique to induce menstruation (other than that resulting from unwanted pregnancy), other more-invasive techniques, such as dilation and curettage, are.

Any family planning campaigns offering injectable contraceptive services should apply lessons learned from Bangladesh's MR program. Since its inception, the MR program has capitalized on the culturally relevant concept of the importance of regular menstruation while providing pregnancy terminations—a culturally stigmatized activity. Accordingly, at these early stages of a large-scale injectable contraception introduction in Bangladesh, there is a need to latch on to a culturally valued aspect of women's reproductive health to compensate for the common association between injectable contraception use and culturally unacceptable amenorrhea.

Modern contraception and medical techniques have influenced the way rural Bangladeshi women perceive, experience, and respond to irregular menstruation and unwanted pregnancy. Strategies of inducing or regulating menstruation and inducing abortion are being adapted as allopathic medicines and practices become increasingly available. The medicines and practices used to start menstruation from a state of nonpregnancy are probably less dangerous than traditional techniques of menstrual regulation. At the same time, however, they are probably often unnecessary. Techniques of terminating unwanted pregnancies other than MR from a trained provider are not reliable, can prolong the gestational age of the fetus before proper care is sought, and can cause morbidity and even death to the pregnant woman.

While women perceive regular menstruation as an indication of good health, many methods of MR available to rural women can actually be physically damaging. The increasing availability of modern medical techniques and providers, accompanied by appropriate information, has and will continue to reduce morbidity related to inducing menstruation among women, whether pregnant or nonpregnant.

NOTES

Research was funded by a grant from the Andrew W. Mellon Foundation through the Johns Hopkins University Population Center with the institutional support of the International Centre for Diarrhoeal Disease Research, Bangladesh. The assistance of Shefali Akter in data collection, translation, and analysis is gratefully acknowledged, as are the helpful comments by Sajeda Amin.

1. In 1978, the Matlab study area was divided into a maternal and child health and family planning (MCH-FP) area and a comparison area. A community-based contraceptive distribution system was established in the MCH-FP area to document replicable means of decreasing fertility and mortality.

2. The self-proclaimed homeopath had no formal training, but apprenticed with homeopaths in nearby villages. When treating a client, he claims he attempts to understand the patient's symptoms, then gives medicine that mimics those symptoms. Thus his philosophy is akin to traditional homeopathic thought. He imports his medicines from Dhaka and sometimes distributes allopathic medicines to clients.

3. Younger women are between 18 and 24 years of age; middle-aged includes women aged 25 to 39 years; older women are age 40 years or older.

REFERENCES

Ahmed, Shameem, Indrani Haque, Barkat-e-Khuda, Bazle Hossain, and Shahidul Alam. 1996. "Abortion in Rural Bangladesh: Evidence from the MCH-FP Extension Project (Rural)." Paper presented at the Annual Meeting of the Population Association of America, New Orleans.

Akhter, Halida H. 1988. "Abortion: Bangladesh." In *International Handbook on Abortion*, ed. P. Sachev. New York: Greenwood Press.

Ali, M. S., M. Zahir, and K. M. Hossein. 1978. "Report on Legal Aspects of Population Planning, Bangladesh." Dhaka: The Bangladesh Institute of Law and International Affairs.

Amin, Sajeda. 1996. "Menstrual Regulation in Bangladesh." Paper presented at the International Union for the Scientific Study of Population Seminar on Socio-cultural and Political Aspects of Abortion from an Anthropological Perspective, Trivandrum, Kerala, India.

Aziz, K. M. A. 1994. "Matlab: Physical Setting and Cultural Background." In *Matlab: Women Children and Health*, ed. V. Fauveau, 13–27. Dhaka: International Centre for Diarrhoeal Disease Research, Bangladesh.

Aziz, K. M. A., and C. Maloney. 1985. *Life Stages, Gender and Fertility in Bangladesh*. Dhaka: International Centre for Diarrhoeal Disease Research, Bangladesh.

Aziz, K. M. A., and W. Henry Mosley. 1994. "Historical Perspective and Methodology of the Matlab Project." In *Matlab: Women Children and Health*, ed. V. Fauveau, 29–50. Dhaka: International Centre for Diarrhoeal Disease Research, Bangladesh.

Becker, Stan, Alanddin Chowdhury, and Henri Leridon. 1985. *Seasonal Patterns of Reproduction in Matlab, Bangladesh*. Unpublished manuscript.

Blanchet, Therese. 1984. *Women, Pollution and Marginality: Meanings and Rituals of Birth in Rural Bangladesh*. Dhaka: The University Press Limited.

Bongaarts, John. 1980. "Does Malnutrition Affect Fecundability? A Summary of Evidence." *Science* 208 (9 May):564–69.

Bongaarts, John, and Robert G. Potter. 1983. *Fertility, Biology, and Behavior: An Analysis of the Proximate Determinants*. New York: Academic Press.

Caldwell, Bruce, Barkat-e-Khuda, Shameem Ahmed, Fazilatun Nessa, and Indrani Haque. 1997. "The Determinants and Consequences of Pregnancy Termination in Rural Bangladesh: A Client Perspective." Paper presented at the Annual Meeting of the Population Association of America, Washington, D.C.

Cumming, David C. 1993. "The Effects of Exercise and Nutrition on the Menstrual Cycle." In *Biomedical and Demographic Determinants of Reproduction*, ed. Ronald Gray, Henri Leridon, and Alfred Spira, 132–56. New York: Oxford University Press.

Dixon-Mueller, Ruth. 1988. "Innovations in Reproductive Health Care: Menstrual Regulation Policies and Programs in Bangladesh." *Studies in Family Planning* 19, no. 3: 129–40.

George, A. 1994. "It Happens to Us: Menstruation as Perceived by Poor Women in Bombay." In *Listening to Women Talk about their Health*, ed. Margaret E. Bentley, Joel Gittelsohn, Pertti J. Pelto, Moni Nag, Saroj

Pachauri, Abigail D. Harrison, and Laura T. Landman, 168–82. Delhi: Har-Anand Publications.

Ginneken, J. van, R. Bairagi, A. de Francisco, A. M. Sardar, and P. Vaughan. 1998. *Health and Demographic Surveillance in Matlab: Past, Present, and Future.* Dhaka: International Center for Diarrhoeal Disease Research, Bangladesh.

Government of Bangladesh. 1980. Memorandum No. 5-14/MCH-FP/ Trg./80/358/1(96).

Haque, Indrani, Thomas T. Kane, Nikhil Ch. Roy, Khorshed A. Mazumder, and Barkat-e-Khuda. 1997. "Contraceptive Switching Patterns in Rural Bangladesh." In *Reproductive Health in Rural Bangladesh: Policy and Programmatic Implications,* vol. 1, ed. T. T. Kane, Barkat-e-Khuda, and James F. Phillips, 217–44. Dhaka: International Centre for Diarrhoeal Disease Research, Bangladesh.

Huffman, Sandra A., A. K. M. A. Chowdhury, J. Chakraborty, and W. H. Mosley. 1978. "Nutrition and Postpartum Amenorrhea in Rural Bangladesh." *Population Studies* 32:251–60.

Huffman, Sandra L., Kathleen Ford, Hubert A. Allen, and Peter Streble. 1987. "Nutrition and Fertility in Bangladesh: Breastfeeding and Post Partum Amenorrhoea." *Population Studies* 41:447–62.

Huq, Md. N., and J. Cleland. 1990. *Bangladesh Fertility Survey, 1989, Main Report.* Dhaka: National Institute of Population Research and Training.

Johnston, Heidi Bart. 1998. "Measuring Induced Abortion: Integrating Qualitative with Quantitative Research Techniques." Paper presented at the Annual Meeting of the Population Association of America, Chicago.

Johnston, Heidi Bart, and Shefali Akter. 1997. "Induced Abortion: Users and Providers in Matlab, Bangladesh." Paper presented at the Fourth Canadian Conference on International Health, Ottawa, Ontario, Canada.

Koenig, Michael, Ubaidur Rob, Mehrab A. Khan, J. Chakraborty, and Vincent Fauveau. 1994. "Contraceptive Use in Matlab in 1990: Levels, Trends, and Explanations." In *Matlab: Women, Children, and Health,* ed. V. Fauveau, 285–308. Dhaka: International Centre for Diarrhoeal Disease Research, Bangladesh.

Maloney, Clarence, K. M. A. Aziz, and Profulla Sarkar. 1981. *Beliefs and Fertility in Bangladesh.* Dhaka: International Centre for Diarrhoeal Disease Research, Bangladesh.

Mitra, S. N., M. Nawab Ali, Shahidul Islam, Anne R. Cross, and Tulshi Saha. 1994. *Bangladesh Demographic and Health Survey, 1993–94.* Dhaka and Calverton, Md.: National Institute of Population Research and Training (NIPORT), Mitra and Associates, and Macro International Inc.

Mostafa, Golam, M. A. Kashem Shaikh, Jeroen K. van Ginneken, and A. M. Sardar. 1998. *Demographic Surveillance System—Matlab: Registra-*

tion of Demographic Events 1996. Dhaka: International Centre for Diarrhoeal Disease Research, Bangladesh.

NIPORT, Mitra and Associates, and Macro International. 1997. *Bangladesh Demographic and Health Survey, 1996–97: Preliminary Report.* Dhaka and Calverton, Md.: National Institute of Population Research and Training (NIPORT), Mitra and Associates, and Macro International.

Rahman, Mizanur, Mehrab A. Khan, Bruce K. Caldwell, and Thomas T. Kane. 1997. "Factors Associated with Reported Side-effects of Oral Pills and Injectables in Rural Bangladesh." In *Reproductive Health in Rural Bangladesh: Policy and Programmatic Implications,* vol. 1, ed. T. T. Kane, Barkat-e-Khuda, and James F. Phillips, 191–216. Dhaka: International Center for Diarrhoeal Disease Research, Bangladesh.

Ronsmans, Carine, Anne Marie Vanneste, Jyotsnamoy Chakroborty, and Jeroen van Ginneken. 1997. "Decline in Maternal Mortality in Matlab, Bangladesh." *The Lancet* 350 (December 20/27):1810–14.

Simmons, Ruth, Rezina Mita, and Michael Koenig. 1992. "Employment in Family Planning and Women's Status in Bangladesh." *Studies in Family Planning* 23, no. 2:97–109.

World Bank. 1995. *Integrated Nutrition Project: Staff Appraisal Report.* Washington, D.C.: World Bank.

WHO (World Health Organization and Task Force on Psychosocial Research in Family Planning). 1981a. "A Cross-Cultural Study of Menstruation: Implications for Contraceptive Development and Use." *Studies in Family Planning* 12, no. 1:3–16.

———. 1981b. "Women's Bleeding Patterns: Ability to Recall and Predict Menstrual Events." *Studies in Family Planning* 12, no. 1:17–27.

CHAPTER 13

Bloodmakers Made of Blood: Quechua Ethnophysiology of Menstruation

Patricia J. Hammer

Quechua-speaking women of the South American Andes perceive the show of menstrual blood as an indication of childbearing potential. Menstrual blood is understood to be female fertile substance. The proper amount of blood, and its properties for managing humoral flow, are important to health in general and reproductive health in particular. The Bolivian women in this study hold the view that, by nature, women are made up of larger quantities of blood than are men—that is, they are formed from, born with, and produce more blood.

With regard to menstrual regulation, it is women in families who freely share information about proper diet and particular herbs useful to ensure flows of fertile menstrual blood. They acquire, prepare, and provide one another with foods and herbal mixtures intended to induce menstruation. Such remedies are discussed positively, as measures required to safeguard health. When menstrual blood does not flow, women turn to female relatives in the household for recommendations on curative actions.

SETTING

Data presented in this chapter were gathered as part of dissertation research carried out from 1992 through 1994, focusing on Quechua women's knowledge and experiences of illness, emotion, and the body in their everyday lives (Hammer 1997). The research site discussed is the southern Bolivian community of Cororo, which has a population of 600 inhabitants. The rural settlement is accessible from the nearest city, Sucre, by cattle truck via unpaved roads. The journey takes 3 to 4 hours, dependent upon weather conditions and factors such as mechanical failures, accidents, or floods. Cororo sits in a highland Andean valley at an altitude of 2,800 meters, nestled between two rivers. Residents of the settlement are small-scale farmers who base their livelihoods on the production of grains, vegetables, legumes, tubers, and limited fruit crops (primarily peaches). In addition to agriculture, local farmers also raise herd animals and domestic fowl for home consumption, local trade, and market sale. The study sample consists of 100 women between 15 and 80 years of age.

NOTIONS OF BODY FLOW AND HUMORAL SUBSTANCES

Throughout Latin America, notions of hot and cold as properties of sickness and remedies in informal systems of healing are salient (for Central America, see Cosminsky, this volume). Extensive research by Foster (cf. Foster 1994) suggests that the widespread use of hot and cold oppositions in Latin American healing "is largely a simplified folk variant of classical Greek and Persian humoral pathology" (Foster 1987:355) imported by Spanish colonizers. At the time of Spanish contact in Peru, Father Cobo recorded that Andean healers "did not know the pulse nor to examine the urine . . . they had no knowledge of the four humors" (Foster 1988:377). Foster identifies the simplified humoral notions adapted in Latin America as focused solely on oppositions of hot and cold, leaving aside aspects of wet and dry. He proposes that because indigenous populations in the Americas were illiterate, they were unable to comprehend European medical texts, and, therefore, the subtler characteristics of moistness and dryness were not assimilated into local healing systems (Foster 1987:381).

However, in the Andes region of contemporary South America, properties of wet and dry, along with those of hot and cold, are central to understanding and classifying body processes, illness, and remedies. While indigenous peoples in the Americas may not have employed the specific Western principles of the "four humors," there is evidence that comprehensive local ethnophysiologies that included notions of the movement of body substances were in use in the New World (Classen 1993).

Differences in culture, language, social structures, and natural environment, in addition to contrasting models of the body held respectively by Europeans and indigenous Americans, most likely made the translation of physiological concepts very difficult. For the present-day Andes, Bastien argues that, although Greek humoral pathology certainly is an influence in local physiological concepts, the variant he discovered in his own research among Bolivian healing specialists has indigenous origins (Bastien 1989).

My own research findings verify the integration of Western concepts in highland Quechua understandings of reproductive processes. Other chapters in this book suggest that many concepts in contemporary Andean ways of thought are similar to those presented in Greek, European, and American writings. Notions of the "rising of the mother," the circulating uterus, vicarious menstruation, and the consideration of hot and cold properties to manage body flows are related (see Cosminsky, Levin, and van de Walle, this volume). This is not surprising, given the more than 500 years of European domination in the political centers of the Americas.

Due to the lack of pre-Hispanic written records, it is difficult to trace historical processes of the emergence of particular ways of conceptualizing the balance of health and illness in the Americas at the moment of European contact. Founded on my own contemporary investigations, I maintain that Quechua systems of knowledge are dynamic, continually shaped by information and experiences shared within spheres of human interactions. At present it is evident that salient models of Andean ethnophysiology are based upon principles of body flows. Flows of body airs and fluids are regulated and influenced by balances of hot/cold and wet/dry qualities that are locally defined.

Ethnographic accounts of communities in the Andean region, as well as analyses of the myths of many South American cultures, demonstrate the prevalence of hydraulic models for representing cosmological, environmental, and physiological systems (e.g., Gose 1994; Allen 1992; Arnold 1988; Bastien 1985; Whitten 1985, 1988; Earls and Silverblatt 1976). Data from southern Peru show how celestial movements of the Milky Way, called *mayu* ("river"), are understood to cycle into underground waterways in the earth during the day, and reemerge and travel through the skies at night. Gose's work reveals water's key role as a "cosmological link" between the realms of the living and the dead in Andean perceptions of life cycles. As corpses dry out after death, body fluids are absorbed back into the earth in order to supply living descendants with needed water (Gose 1994:131). Water is a vital substance that mediates spheres of the human body and agricultural processes.

While water in itself is a substance essential to all life forms, its movement is necessary for renewal and revitalization of organisms to sustain and stimulate life. Flows of water and analogous substances penetrate discrete domains, integrating them into the universe as perceived and experienced by Quechua peoples. Metaphoric relations among human and natural processes are portrayed in northern Bolivia, where Bastien finds that the Kallawaya draw analogies between local physiology and the environment: "They understand their own bodies in terms of the mountain, and they consider the mountain in terms of their anatomy" (Bastien 1985:598).

In this sense, it appears that the circulation of water in the natural environment provides models for Andean conceptualizations of the workings of the body. Body flows are of primary concern for well-being. They can be hindered through strong emotional reactions, shock, humoral imbalances, and exposure to environmental conditions. Impeded flow of essential substances (blood, bile, milk, phlegm, urine, semen, feces, sweat, fat, air, water) are causes for bodily disorders. Extreme qualities of hot/cold and wet/dry influence the movement of humoral substances, such as menstrual blood.

REGULATION OF MENSTRUAL FLOWS

When women talk about the onset of menarche, they say that an adolescent girl becomes "accustomed to getting sick each month" *(sapa killa onqokuy yachan)*. This same notion of becoming sick *(onqokuy)* also refers to the act of giving birth. On one level, the sense of menstruation as the onset of sickness refers to the actual physical discomfort and the sick role that demands the attention and treatment of caregivers. On another level, the notion of becoming ill may be an indicator of the overall hardships that women suffer throughout their lifetimes, as the bearers and rearers of children, and as the result of the discrimination associated with their ascribed gender status that limits access to resources.

Elsewhere in the Andes, blood is considered strictly a limited substance in the body. For northern Bolivia, "[Kallawayas] believe that by the age of seven a person has acquired his or her amount of blood for life: if during his lifetime he loses some blood, there is no way of recovering it . . ." (Bastien 1985:599). Bastien's study among the Kallawaya healers of northern Bolivia offers no gender distinctions concerning the implications of a nonregenerative blood supply. However, in nearby Puno in southern Peru, it is shown that, indeed, women suffer weakness and fatigue more often than men as the result of blood loss at childbirth and menstruation. Also, among Puno women and men, blood is understood as replaceable, although "the replacement 'blood' will never be as strong as the original" (Larme 1993:98).

In Cororo, blood is talked about in terms of its qualities: weak/strong, hot/cold, and wet/dry. Blood is fortified in the body's system by consuming milk, meat, and animal hearts. People of the Tarabuco region, to which Cororeños pertain, are called *sonqo mikhuj* ("heart-lung eaters").[1] This designation derives from a nineteenth-century battle between indigenous independence fighters and Spanish nationalists, in which rural warriors defeated Spanish troops, ripping out their hearts and eating them in their victory. Platt provides contemporary ethnographic evidence of the eating of human flesh during moiety conflicts in the neighboring Department of Potosí.[2]

The strong relation between consuming internal organs and blood production may be connected with the pre-Spanish fertility deity, Mama Waku. According to the colonial Spanish chronicler Sarmiento, in conquering territory along the road to Charcas (present-day Sucre, capital of the department to which Cororo pertains), Mama Waku and her husband, Manku Cápac, brutally attacked local inhabitants:

> Mama Waku was so ferocious, that in killing a Gualla Indian she tore him to pieces and ripped out his guts and took the heart and lungs in her mouth. (Sarmiento de Gamboa [1572] 1943:129; my translation)[3]

In Cororo, women tell me that some females have more blood than others. Such women are described as *yawarsapa* (having a great amount of blood).[4] *Yawarsapa* women tend to have longer menstrual periods, lasting 6 or more days, and they say that they never eat the hearts of animals because it will dangerously increase their blood supply. These women point out that they inherited this characteristic from their mothers. While sufficient blood is necessary for reproductive well-being, excessive amounts are related to problems such as hemorrhaging during pregnancy and post partum.

Concerns over menstruation focus on the nature of blood flow, particularly the consistency of flow and the quantity expelled. Women who are sexually active in heterosexual unions as well as those who are not become distressed about irregular and delayed menstrual periods. When menstruation fails to begin in a given month, women worry that the blood is stuck inside the abdomen. This is often attributed to contact with cold environmental elements, usually water. Bathing, or placing the hands in water, is said to induce in the body the state of *chiri* (cold, an intrinsic characteristic rather than one of temperature) that can stop menstrual flow. It is believed that such contact causes blood to coagulate into tight balls; then the abdomen becomes hard to the touch, and one suffers *wijsa nanan* ("bellyache"). Women say that this blood becomes firm "like a baby" *(wawa jina)*, and must be warmed through healing methods so that it can be expelled from the body.

While embryos are formed essentially of blood, lumps of cold blood or other growths that appear in the abdomen unrelated to male insemination are signs of danger to a woman's well-being. Women use the borrowed Western terms, *tumor* and *cancer*, to describe severe, often terminal cases of menstrual malfunction identified with the growth of masses in the belly and throughout the body. Pains that women experience during menstruation are attributed to impeded blood flow. Women frequently take herbal emmenagogues to melt clots and hasten blood flow, which relieves menstrual cramps.

Amenorrhea is understood to stem from blood that is misdirected to other parts of the body. Blood that seeps from orifices other than the vagina, such as the nose, mouth, ears, and anus, is linked to this condition. (See also Introduction, this volume, for "vicarious menstruation.") Dark spots that appear on the face are associated with blood that clots as a result of handling water while menstruating. Lactational amenorrhea is understood to be caused by menstrual blood that is redirected and transformed into breast milk; the suckling infant consumes breast milk to form its own blood supply. Women are concerned about accounting for body fluids, whether detained inside a body cavity or transformed into another substance; this is not surprising, given the preoccupation with the location and movement of humoral substances in Cororo explanations of body processes.

Irregularity in menstrual periods and blood flows are addressed and controlled by women within relationships of trust and mutual support in spheres of household and community interactions. Lack of menstruation or unusually light flows are discussed and treated by nonspecialized women who acquire and share knowledge with one another about measures to induce or increase menstruation. Although Cororo women complain that their own mothers never warned them about the imminent onset of menarche when they were adolescents, they point out that once menstruation begins, it is their mothers who offer care and advice in relation to menstrual disturbances.

Cororo women describe the humoral quality of emmenagogues as "hot." Emmenagogues are used to heat and break up the blood inside that has clotted and ceased to flow. Also, compresses of mud and dung may be applied, tied in a cloth fastened around the abdomen. The pains of menstrual cramps are explained as resulting from clotted menstrual blood. To ease the pain, herbal and plaster treatments must be applied to encourage renewed menstrual blood flow.

During the menstrual period, women observe a number of avoid-
ances (cf. Buckley and Gottlieb 1988). Principally, menstruating
women shun contact with elements of a fundamentally "cold" quality.
They refrain from immersing their body in general, and their hands
in particular, in water. Foods locally categorized as having a "cool"
quality are not consumed because they make the abdomen swell and
cause cramps. The "cold" quality of water, wind, and certain foods can
potentially stop the flow of uterine blood by upsetting the "hot" flowing state of menstruation.

Additional prohibitions relate to menstruating women who cultivate
crops. Women who are experiencing their periods are restricted from
going near newly sprouting fields, as well as from stepping over the
vines of squash plants. It is feared that women's "hot" state of active
blood flow will cause the fields to dry up and the plants to wilt and
die. Menstruation is believed to be a fertile time when substances are
in movement. In the case of young crops, it appears that the fecund,
desiring state of menstruating women may dangerously lure wet and
inseminating natural forces away from the propagation of delicate
crops and toward the women's bodies.

MENSTRUAL BLOOD AS FERTILE SUBSTANCE

Cororo women explain that when the man's seed joins with the mother's blood, the baby begins to form, and thrives by sucking up the
mother's uterine blood. This is why the mother does not menstruate
while she is pregnant. The fetus grows, nourished by the mother's
blood, analogous to how the infant will suckle breast milk.

Sometimes miscarriages that occur within the first months of pregnancy are welcome. Women who are already burdened with full households and limited resources may be relieved when, once again, their
"blood descends" *(yawarniy urashan)*. Women discreetly discuss "late
periods" and may purposefully perform extra-strenuous tasks and take
herbal emmenagogues or abortifacients. Thinking about fertility regulation primarily in terms of postconception birth control is prevalent
throughout rural South America (e.g., Newman 1985).

When the embryo (less than 9 weeks of development) or young fetus
is aborted or miscarries, women examine it for gender characteristics.
Inca medical practices at the time of the Spanish conquest included
the examination and dissection of embryos (Moll 1944:15). Today females are recognized by their bloody appearance, while males are "just

watery" *(yakulla)*. These expelled substances are unceremoniously discarded.

Where pregnancy is unwanted, either for a woman's fear of suffering and the possibility of maternal death or for fear of her inability to adequately provide for another child, unproblematic miscarriage and successful abortion are experienced with relief. According to the Cororo model of body flows, abortion dislodges the obstacle of undesired conception, and allows women to continue the responsibilities and reciprocal obligations with which they are already challenged. Induced abortion is perceived by Cororo women as an acceptable way to flush out unwanted substances that confer new obligations. By way of abortion, uninhibited flow is returned to both the body and to favorable social relationships (cf. Sobo 1996:501).

INFERTILITY

One kind of female infertility is linked to vaginal discharges that are white and watery *(yuraj yaku)*. Watery and pale-colored menstrual blood is considered "weak blood" and is a symptom of infertility and other reproductive malfunctions (see Renne, this volume, for similar associations in Nigeria). Another kind of infertility that persists despite regular menstrual periods is recognized as the *wijsa tijrasqa* ("inverted womb"), in which the fetus, called *wawatiyana* ("baby seat"), cannot settle in the womb and falls out.

Other reasons for female infertility are traced to traumatic events or harsh conditions in childhood or adolescence. For example, a Cororo woman, at the age of seven years, was in a serious truck crash in which her left hand was irreparably damaged and thus was amputated. She and her extended family attribute her infertility to that misfortune and to the severe shock of the accident. Infertility, associated with white menstruation, the inverted womb, and traumatic events, is perceived as the disruption and misdirection of normal body flows that are related to the *madri,* the specific female organ responsible for the production and flow of fertile blood.

THE ROLE OF THE *MADRI* IN REPRODUCTIVE ETHNOPHYSIOLOGY

According to local logic in the community of Cororo, it is because women's bellies contain the female organ *madri* that they are distinct from male bellies. The *madri* is not the womb, but rather a small, round organ, usually nestled in with the intestines. It is not attached to any other part of the body, but moves freely about, according to its will.

The word *madri*, as pronounced and used in Cororo, is derived from the Spanish word *madre*, literally "mother," and used as a synonym for *womb* at the turn of the twentieth century and earlier (Cuyás [1903] 1940). Derivations of the Spanish term *madre* referring to the womb or reproductive potential are widespread throughout Quechua-speaking populations. No native term is currently used to refer to this aspect of the female body (Soto Ruíz, personal communication; Morató Peña 1994). Colonial transcriptions of Quechua vocabulary indicate *quisma* as a term for *womb* (Classen 1993). This is suggestive of, and perhaps shares a linguistic relation with, the term *qesa*, meaning "nest" (Soto Ruíz 1976). The concept of "nest" as a temporary place to nurture a growing fetus closely resembles present-day notions of the protective environment of the female womb.

It is important to emphasize that in order to begin to approach the Quechua ethnophysiology of female reproduction, we must set aside our own preconceptions of the existence and function of the uterus. Through my long-term research among Cororo women, I validated their knowledge of the role, purpose, and character of the *madri* organ in processes of menstruation, conception, and embryonic and early fetal development, in addition to female-specific illnesses throughout the life course. The *madri* is clearly differentiated from the simple place in the belly where babies grow, sit, stretch, and lie. Distinct from Western scientific perspectives, Quechua beliefs are unperturbed by ambiguous concepts. The fact that the *madri* organ is sometimes indicated to be what we refer to as the abdominal aorta and at other times is known to be a hard ball-like entity that drifts about the body, causing severe female ailments and even death, is acceptable in local thought (see Douglas 1966 on the power of ambiguity and crossing boundaries).

When I confessed my ignorance about the nature of the *madri* to 70-year-old Teofila, a respected specialist of *madri* ailments, she took it upon herself to instruct me. She had me undress and lie down on her bed. She seated herself beside me and placed her left hand on top of her right, with fingertips touching. She positioned both hands just below my navel and pressed deeply into my abdomen. With her hands held firmly in place, she kept pressure on my abdominal aorta until we both felt a strong, steady pulsation.

"That's it!" Teofila exclaimed when we both felt the beating. "It's like the heart-lung."

"Do men have a *madri*, too?" I asked.

"No! Only women produce babies, right?"

"Yes," I agreed.

"That's why men don't have the *madri*. Men have only veins and arteries," Teofila clarified, indicating men's lack of the *madri* that endows women with reproductive potential.

Identifying characteristics of the abdominal aorta with female reproductive functions is also found among the Yucatecan Maya (Sheila Cosminsky, personal communication). As a midwife's assistant in southern California in the late 1980s, I found that pregnant immigrants from southeastern Mexico were concerned about the pulsation of the abdominal aorta that they associated with something they called the *tipte*. These women always wore a metal safety pin, sometimes with a metallic adornment attached, fastened on clothing just below the navel. They explained that this protected them from lightning, which the *tipte* attracts when they are pregnant. The principal worry of these immigrant women regarding hospital birth was that doctors would perform a cesarean section and unknowingly sever the vital female pulse, the *tipte*.

The prevalence of indigenous female knowledge that is hidden, or kept out of view of dominant society, was made clear to me by Cororo women, who were not surprised at my ignorance of their understandings of body processes. One woman pointed out to me that especially female-related syndromes cannot be treated by city-trained doctors and nurses:

> They don't know about how our organs tend to move about the body, following birth, or with severe sickness. The doctors don't believe that we must bind our waist post partum so that the *madri* organ won't ascend the chest and choke us. But we know that will happen. Here in the village the old women who are special healers of female ailments know how to cure us.

Cororo women learn from and rely on indigenous female *madri* healers to cope with problems in early pregnancy. Those who pursue remedies to bring on late menses or induce abortion talk in terms of curing ailments of the *madri*.

CONCLUSION

The Quechua women in this study apply humoral concepts in their regulation of blood flows, essential for managing fertility and reproductive processes in general. Downward flow of monthly menstruation, as well as the quality of blood expelled and the length of the period, are significant for the well-being of women. Although adequate blood supply is required to maintain reproductive well-being, an excessive supply is linked to health dangers, such as hemorrhaging. Lack of menstruation alarms women that cold and dry humoral qualities are present, which work to retain blood inside the abdomen. Frequently, herbal emmenagogues, perceived as humorally "hot," are administered to melt clots and encourage blood flow, thereby relieving the pain of menstrual cramps. Health and reproductive potential are characterized by flowing movement of substances, whereas illness and suffering are marked by impeded, disrupted, or misdirected body flows. Humoral properties of hot/cold and wet/dry are taken into account to diagnose maladies, explain illness origins and etiology, and prescribe appropriate remedies to alter body flows.

Fundamentally, the Quechua notion of the *madri* organ serves as a metaphor for female experience and as the locus for the production of blood. Menstruation is a sign of fertility and of women's capability to continue the obligations and responsibilities inherent in their positions as productive beings within a constellation of ongoing and reciprocal relationships, passed from generation to generation and realized in present, everyday interactions.

NOTES

This research was carried out under the auspices of the Social Science Research Council, Wenner-Gren Foundation for Anthropological Research (award #5496), Fulbright-Hays (award #PO22A20014), the Department of Anthropology of the University of Illinois at Urbana-Champaign, and the Graduate College of the University of Illinois at Urbana-Champaign.

1. In the battles of independence from Spain, Yldefonso Carrillo, serving as a guide to Spanish nationalist troops, infiltrated them to spy and relate their movements to his people of Tarabuco. On 12 March 1816, the Tarabuqueños ambushed the Spanish in the famous Batallón Verdes in Huanu Huanu, just outside the town of Tarabuco. The site and event have become known as *el Jumbate*. A fiesta is celebrated annually in memory of the victory over the Spanish; in previous years, dramatic reenactments of the battle have been performed for the occasion. Performances culminate in the victorious act of tearing out the enemy captain's heart and biting into it. (Sonqo Mikus, Miranda Rivera, and Porfirio. n.d. Historical account. Biblioteca Nacional, Sucre.)

2. "In some cases when the national authorities are not present—especially during *ch'ajwas* [ritual moiety violence]—the ferocity of the conflict may reach such a pitch that victims may be torn apart with the bare hands—the use of a knife is disdained—and parts of them eaten: I have heard Macha speak with pride of their reputation as *runamikhuj* (maneaters)" (Platt 1986:240).

3. Description of Mama Waku in original Spanish: "Mama Guaco era tan feroz, que matando un indio gualla le hizo pedazos y le sacó el asadura y tomó el corazón y bofes en la boca" (Sarmiento de Gamboa [1572] 1943:129).

4. The noun *yawar* means "blood." The Quechua suffix *-sapa,* when added to a noun, forms an adjective that provides an augmentative meaning (Herrero and Sánchez de Lozada 1983:388).

REFERENCES

Allen, Catherine. 1992. "The Incas Have Gone Inside: Pattern and Persistence in Quechua Iconography." Unpublished manuscript, American University, Washington, D.C.

Arnold, Denise. 1988. "Matrilineal Practice in a Patrilineal Setting: Rituals and Metaphors of Kinship in an Andean Ayllu." Ph.D. diss., University of London.

Bastien, Joseph. 1985. "Qollahuaya-Andean Body Concepts: A Topographical-Hydraulic Model of Physiology." *American Anthropologist* 87:595–611.

———. 1989. "Differences between Kallawaya-Andean and Greek-European Humoral Theory." *Social Science & Medicine* 28, no. 1:45–51.

Buckley, Thomas, and Alma Gottlieb, eds. 1988. *Blood Magic: The Anthropology of Menstruation.* Berkeley: University of California Press.

Classen, Constance. 1993. *Inca Cosmology and the Human Body.* Salt Lake City: University of Utah Press.

Cuyás, Arturo. [1903] 1940. *Appleton's New English-Spanish and Spanish-English Dictionary.* 3d ed. New York: D. Appleton-Century Company.

Douglas, Mary. 1966. *Purity and Danger.* New York: Praeger.

Earls, John, and Irene Silverblatt. 1976. "La Realidad Física y Social en la Cosmología Andina." *Proceedings of the XLI International Congress of Americanists* 4:299–325.

Foster, George M. 1987. "On the Origin of Humoral Medicine in Latin America." *Medical Anthropology Quarterly* 1, no. 4:355–93.

———. 1988. "The Validating Role of Humoral Theory in Traditional Spanish-American Therapeutics." *American Ethnologist* 15, no. 1:120–35.

————. 1994. *Hippocrates' Latin American Legacy. Humoral Medicine in the New World.* New York: Gordon and Breach.

Gose, Peter. 1994. *Deathly Waters and Hungry Mountains: Agrarian Ritual and Class Formation in an Andean Town.* Toronto: University of Toronto Press.

Hammer, Patricia Jean. 1997. "To Be a Woman Is to Suffer. The Interplay of Illness, Emotion and the Body in Quechua Women's Experiences." Ph.D. diss., University of Illinois at Urbana-Champaign.

Herrero, Joaquín, and Federico Sánchez de Lozada. 1983. *Diccionario Quechua. Estructura Semántica del Quechua Cochabambino Contemporáneo.* Sucre: Qori Llama.

Larme, Anne C. 1993. *Work, Reproduction, and Health in Two Andean Communities (Cuyo Cuyo, Puno).* Working Paper no. 5. Chapel Hill: University of North Carolina, Department of Anthropology.

Moll, Aristides. 1944. *Aesculapius in Latin America.* Philadelphia: W. B. Saunders Company.

Morató Peña, Luis. 1994. *Guía Médica Trilingüe. Qheswa-Castellano-English.* Cochabamba: Los Amigos del Libro.

Newman, Lucile F., ed. 1985. *Women's Medicine: A Cross-Cultural Study of Indigenous Fertility Regulation.* New Brunswick, N.J.: Rutgers University Press.

Platt, Tristan. 1986. "Mirrors and Maize: The Concept of *Yanantin* among the Macha of Bolivia." In *Anthropological History of Andean Polities,* ed. J. Murra, N. Wachtel, and J. Revel, 228–59. Cambridge: Cambridge University Press.

Sarmiento de Gamboa, Pedro. [1572] 1943. *Historia de los Incas.* Buenos Aires: Emecé S.A.

Sobo, Elisa J. 1996. "Abortion Traditions in Rural Jamaica." *Social Science & Medicine* 42, no. 4:495–508.

Soto Ruíz, Clodoaldo. 1976. *Diccionario Quechua: Ayacucho-Chanca.* Lima: Ministerio de Educación.

Whitten, Norman. 1985. *Sicuanga Runa. The Other Side of Development in Amazonian Ecuador.* Urbana: University of Illinois Press.

————. 1988. "Historical and Mythic Evocations of Chthonic Power in South America." In *Rethinking History and Myth,* ed. J. Hill. Urbana: University of Illinois Press.

Zuidema, R. Tom. 1990. *Inca Civilization in Cuzco.* Austin: University of Texas Press.

CHAPTER 14

Midwives and Menstrual Regulation: A Guatemalan Case Study

Sheila Cosminsky

Para conocer cuándo la detención de la regla o
de los meses es natural o de enfermedad, se
observará que cuándo detención fuere por razón
de estar preñadas, entonces habrán precedido las
señales ya sabidas de la preñez. . . . Añádense
estas circunstancias sóla con el fin para que con
los medicamentos se evite la ocasión del aborto.

—Juan de Esteyneffer, *Florilegio medicinal de todas
las enfermedades*

This chapter examines ideas concerning women's health and menstruation, menstrual regulation, and emmenagogue use in rural Guatemala. Although some women possess knowledge of emmenagogues,
they also come to the midwife seeking her assistance for treating delayed menstruation, or *detención*. Some come after they have already
tried various remedies. I suggest that midwives negotiate the ambiguity
and ambivalence inherent in the use of emmenagogues by diagnosing
either *detención* or pregnancy, usually in consultation with the client
and often her mother. The midwives decide whether the use of these
remedies is for bringing on one's menstrual period because a client has
the condition *detención,* which could have implications for the woman's fertility, or as an abortifacient to end a pregnancy. In this role,
they also act as an agent of social control, reinforcing the values of
gender, family, and community, as well as passing on ethnomedical
knowledge and principles.

SETTING

Data for this paper was obtained during the course of ethnographic fieldwork in a Maya community, Chuchexic, in the western highlands of Guatemala, and on a sugar and coffee plantation, Finca San Felipe (a pseudonym), in the Pacific lowlands of Guatemala. Fieldwork was carried out in Chuchexic in 1968–69, 1974, and 1978 and in Finca San Felipe during several trips in 1974–79, 1993, and 1996.

Chuchexic is a rural hamlet, or *aldea,* of the town of Santa Lucia Utatlán and has a population of approximately 1,600, whereas the population of Santa Lucia Utatlán is approximately 8,000. Ninety-six percent of Chuchexic's inhabitants are Kiché-speaking Mayan Indians; the rest are Ladinos.[1] The Indians grow maize as the staple crop, supplementing their incomes by growing wheat and other cash crops and engaging in wage labor, primarily seasonal work on coastal plantations. In contrast, the Ladino residents are landowners, entrepreneurs, and wage laborers. In terms of housing, the Indians live in dispersed households in the rural hamlets, whereas most of the Ladinos live in the town center, which they control politically and economically.

Finca San Felipe is a coffee and sugar plantation with a population of approximately 690. The adults and older children there are agricultural wage laborers working on either Finca San Felipe or nearby plantations. In addition, the entire family participates in cultivating corn and beans on small plots of land or on strips of land in the cane fields provided by the plantation owner. The population is of mixed ethnicity, consisting mainly of second- or third-generation Mayan Indian migrants from different towns in the western highlands; the rest are Ladinos, originally from nearby coastal towns. Many of the Indians are "ladinoized," speaking Spanish as their mother tongue and wearing Western dress, yet they identify themselves as *naturales,* the local word for indigenous Maya.

Despite differences in ethnicity, acculturation, training, location (highland or lowland), and religion (Catholic or Protestant), residents of Chuchexic and Finca San Felipe share many basic concepts and practices, including the use of specific herbal remedies. Plants that do not grow locally are available in the town market, where products from different ecological settings are exchanged. One difference between local and purchased plant products is that herbs grown in the area may be used fresh, whereas those brought in from elsewhere and sold at market have been dried. The influence this preparation has on the efficacy of a particular herbal remedy is unknown.

A previous study by Cosminsky (1977) compared data from the Finca and Chuchexic communities with that compiled from various ethnographies on Guatemala and Mexico, including plants used as emmenagogues or abortifacients and for other aspects of reproduction or birth, such as birth pains, prolonged labor, infertility, and prevention of miscarriage. A number of more recent studies and publications have included discussion and analyses of many different plants used for menstrual regulation and various reproductive problems (Browner 1985a, 1985b; Browner and Ortiz de Montellano 1986; Low and Newman 1985; Kay 1996; Orellana 1987; Morton 1981). Several of the same plants were mentioned as emmenagogues in a number of the communities studied.

ETHNOMEDICAL CONTEXT

Rural Guatemalans understand menstrual regulation and reproduction according to the same principles that they apply to health in general, especially the hot/cold or humoral principle. A healthy body is one that is in balance, including qualities of hot and cold, although in actuality, a warm body is considered normal. All bodily states, foods, plants, medicines, and natural elements are classified according to the qualities of hot and cold. Hotness and coldness are considered innate or inherent characteristics possessed by the substance in question, although they may be influenced by physical temperature. Illnesses are caused by an imbalance in the body of excess cold or heat. Treatment usually involves restoring the balance or equilibrium by administering a substance possessing the opposite quality; alternatively, purgatives or other substances may be administered to unclog the part of the body that may be blocked and preventing proper flow of bodily fluids.

This system of treating illness has been assumed by many to be a variant of the Greek humoral theory, which was carried to Spain with the Moors and then to the New World through the Spanish conquest (Foster 1978). Some investigators have presented detailed rebuttals to Foster, arguing that indigenous concepts of hot and cold balance existed before the Spanish conquest (Lopez Austin 1988; Ortiz de Montellano 1990). They do not deny that Spanish humoral concepts were brought to the New World by the Spanish, but maintain that these were added to, syncretized with, or reinforced by existing hot/cold concepts:

I have never contended, and it would be absurd to do so, that contemporary indigenous medicine has a pure pre-Hispanic tradition. In it, as in any ideological system of rural Mexico, can be found complex combinations of different origins. (Lopez Austin 1988:280)

Bastien (1989) also argues that indigenous origins of hot/cold and wet/dry exist along with influence from Greek humoral pathology among contemporary Andean healers. Tedlock (1987), however, criticizes the use of the conceptual syncretism in her analysis of humoral medicine. Instead, she demonstrates that indigenous healers in Momostenango, Guatemala, do not use hot/cold categories in either etiological concepts or treatment, whereas individuals using self-treatment may do so. Recently, Foster (1994) has written a rebuttal to the indigenous-origin arguments. He and his opponents alike suggest that concepts of wet/dry qualities dropped out or became insignificant in comparison to hot/dry ones. Hammer (this volume), however, argues that wet/dry as well as hot/cold qualities are important in regulating flows of body airs and fluids that are basic to Quechua ethnophysiology in Bolivia, and says that these reflect a dynamic system whose historical process is difficult to trace. Neuenswander and Souder (1977) demonstrate that wet/dry and hot/cold are both salient properties of the Guatemalan Joyabaj Kiché universe, but that "wet" and "dry" are only applied in the domain of disease. "Wet" properties seem to be correlated with "good" diseases or those that come from God, whereas "dry" qualities are associated with "bad" diseases caused by people, such as witchcraft, and are difficult to cure. They consider the persistence of the wet/dry distinctions as inexplicable and unique to the Joyabaj Maya. I suggest that such distinctions may be more widespread but have not been researched; at any rate, the ongoing debate about humoral medicine cannot be resolved in this paper. The important point for this chapter is that the hot/cold classification used both humorally and with respect to physical temperature is pervasive in terms of people's concepts and the accompanying meanings about blood, menstruation, fertility, birth, illness, and food—regardless of where the concepts and practices originate.

In Chuchexic and Finca San Felipe, menstruation, pregnancy, and birth are considered hot conditions due to the body's possessing excessive heat. After giving birth, however, a woman is in a cold condition because of the loss of blood, which is usually thought of as a hot substance. Infertility may be attributed to a "cold womb," so treatment would be aimed at administering "warming" remedies. Menstrual regularity would be an indication that the body is in balance, so a delayed period would signal some type of imbalance. If this condition were believed to stem from too much cold, the emmenagogues and other substances used would be hot, to warm the blood and the body. All the herbs used as emmenagogues or abortifacients or for treating infertility are of a hot quality. Thus if a woman were pregnant, a hot condition, and wanted to have an abortion, she would take hot herbs, since these would make her condition one of excess hotness and possibly induce an abortion. All the herbs that have oxytocic properties are also classified as hot. On the other hand, if a woman had been infertile and wanted children, she might be given remedies to heat her uterus, which would first bring on her menstrual period. One of the midwives in Chuchexic uses the sweatbath:

> The sweatbath is my medicine. Because the womb *(matriz)* is cold, it doesn't want to receive the liquid from the man. Place her in the sweatbath. Put the fire below her, two times. The first day, her period comes; on the third day, give her a sweatbath, blow it, and heat the womb. The next month, her period won't come and she will be pregnant.

Instead of taking the sweatbath remedy, the woman can drink a tea made from 3 sprigs of the plant *eneldo* mixed with liquor.

Browner and Ortiz de Montellano (1986) analyze 5 plants (avocado, pineapple, cinnamon, lemon, and rue) considered effective emmenagogues by informants not only because of their qualities of hotness and coldness but more so because of their quality of being irritating. An irritating substance is needed to "clean" the blood when menstrual delay is believed to be caused by accumulated impurities in the bloodstream of the womb. The authors then discuss the chemical evidence supporting the informants' perceptions.

If a woman is menstruating, she should not bathe in cold water. These hot/cold extremes would make her body cold, causing the bleeding to stop and her abdomen to swell. A menstruating woman's heat can ruin the thick drink made from new fresh corn, *atol de elote,* by causing it to become thin if she passes by while it is being made.

A menstruating or pregnant woman can cause the evil eye, an illness primarily affecting small children. Excess heat from someone having "hot" or "strong" blood, including menstruating or pregnant women, is transmitted intentionally or unintentionally through the eyes or gaze while looking at someone else's child. The illness also may be transmitted by such persons by complimenting or envying the child (Cosminsky 1976).

Beliefs, knowledge, and practices concerning menstrual regularity, and the specific plants and substances used to ensure it, originate from a combination of indigenous and European sources. Thus native plants such as *cihuapahtli (Montanoa tomentosa)*, avocado *(Persea americana)*, and pineapple *(Ananas comosum)* are still widely used, as are European transplants such as chamomile, celery, cinnamon *(Cinnamonum zeylanicum)*, and rue *(Ruta chalepensis)*. Several emmenagogues of the Aztecs and Mayans, some indigenous and some European, were mentioned in early sixteenth-, seventeenth-, and eighteenth-century sources, such as Esteyneffer, Farfan, Sahagun, Hernandez, Ximenez, and Fuentes y Guzman (Orellana 1987:136–38). Also using some of these sources, Quezada (1975) lists several plants that are still used as contraceptives, abortifacients, or fertility enhancers.

Cihuapahtli or *zoapatle (Montanoa tomentosa)* is the best known and best documented of the Aztec plants, and its use continues among Mexicans today. Ortiz de Montellano (1990:185–86) reviews the pharmacological analyses of *cihuapatli,* which produces uterine contractions. Two new compounds, zoapatonol and montanol, along with kaurenedienoic acid are believed to be the effective agents acting synergistically in an aqueous solution.

Margarita Kay (1977) has argued that this widespread usage of certain plants, both indigenous and European, throughout the American Southwest, Mexico, and other parts of Central and South America is due at least in part to a book written by a Jesuit lay brother, Juan de Esteyneffer, titled *Florilegio Medicinal.* A compilation of herbal lore from various Indians missionized by the Jesuits together with materia medica from Europe, the book attached these remedies to diseases that were recognized in the eighteenth century (Esteyneffer [1719] 1978). The text provided a standardization of this knowledge and was then used by other priests in their role as physicians to both Spaniards and Indians. It became both a source for herbal uses in many locations and the basis for diffusion of this knowledge. One section of Esteyneffer focuses on women's health with an extensive discussion of the causes and treatment of *detención,* including the appropriate plant remedies, which are strikingly similar to those found in the aforementioned studies as well as in my Guatemalan research.

Among rural Guatemalans, delayed menstruation may be attributed to a condition called *falta de sangre,* or "lack of blood." This may be a term indicating anemia. Since blood is considered a "hot" quality, lack of blood would be a "cold" condition treatable with "heating" substances. Lack of blood also causes *debilidad,* or weakness, in which case fortifying substances would need to be taken. Hence another dimension of the balance of the body system is the weak/strong principle. Lack of blood, therefore, not only is "cold" but also causes weakness, whereas sufficient blood is needed for a healthy or balanced body.

One woman from Finca San Felipe was concerned about her 16-year-old daughter, who had not gotten her period for 4 months. The girl, who began menstruating when she was 15 years of age, was asked by her mother if she had a boyfriend, and she said no. The mother said her daughter was afraid of men, and thought the amenorrhea might be from *falta de sangre*. Another woman who had missed her period went to the clinic because she didn't have any appetite. They examined her and said she was pregnant but also had "lack of blood," or *falta de sangre*. In such cases, iron pills are usually prescribed by the clinic. Anemia is a problem among women on the plantation, especially during pregnancy.

Women also spend long periods of postpartum amenorrhea in a pregnancy-lactation cycle, going from pregnancy to lactation to another pregnancy. At least 70 percent of females between 20 and 30 years of age were either pregnant, lactating, or both. A woman might get pregnant after her first ovulation while nursing and not actually experience a menstrual period. Although bottle-feeding has increased in both locations, initial breast-feeding is almost universal. Babies are usually nursed at least for a year and often up to 2 years, with increasing supplementation of solid foods. Delgado et al. (1982) found that maternal nutritional status, which affected the amount of breast milk available, was negatively associated with the length of postpartum amenorrhea. The combination of longer periods of breast-feeding, which suppresses ovulation, and poor nutritional status results in longer periods of postpartum amenorrhea. Although I do not have specific data on length of postpartum amenorrhea for the Finca San Felipe women, the above conditions exist. One survey in 1976 found that only 8 percent of pregnant women and none of the lactating women were meeting the recommended dietary level for calories, and none of the women had protein intakes reaching the levels recommended by the Food and Agriculture Organization of the United Nations (Gilbert 1976).

THE MIDWIFE

In both locations, more than 85 percent of births take place in the mother's home, attended by a midwife (or so-called Traditional Birth Attendant; *iyom* in Kiché, *comadrona* in Spanish). Although these figures refer to births in the 1970s, the rates are still extremely high today. Warren et al. (1987) report that more than 80 percent of "interior" Indians and more than one-half of "interior" Ladinos use midwives; according to Schieber et al. (1994), midwives manage more than 90% of deliveries in their study of a rural community in Quezaltenango, western Guatemala.

Many of the local midwives are ritual as well as obstetrical specialists. Training is usually through apprenticeship and experience, although many midwives have also taken formal midwifery training courses. These courses are offered by the government or various nongovernmental organizations so that the midwife may receive her license to practice, a legal requirement in Guatemala.

Some midwives are recruited through supernatural calling, as revealed by birth signs, dreams, illness, and the discovery of strange objects. These signs are interpreted by a diviner or shaman as signifying a woman's destiny as a midwife, and the objects are considered messages sent by spirits or by God. If she does not follow her calling, she would suffer supernatural sanctions in the form of illness or death, either to herself or to members of her family (Paul 1975; Cosminsky 1982). Others become midwives by helping a woman deliver successfully in an emergency or by delivering their own baby successfully. As word spreads of this achievement, more people request their help. Even midwives who do not believe in divine calling believe they receive assistance in their work from God, the spirits of dead midwives, Saint Ann (patroness of childbirth), or Mary. In addition, some experience premonitions of an imminent birth in the form of bodily twitches or trembling in the fingers or legs.

Along with providing prenatal and postpartum care and managing deliveries, midwives are also consulted for various reproductive problems, including amenorrhea, sterility, hemorrhaging, and uterine prolapse. Women consult midwives when their adolescent daughters have not reached menarche or have missed their period for a few months, or when they themselves have missed their period. In some cases, the mothers are concerned about their own or their daughter's future fertility, whereas in others they are worried about a possible pregnancy. Married and unmarried women who have missed their periods come to the midwife concerned about their condition. Midwives interviewed mentioned herbs that were used to bring on one's menstrual period, but insisted that they would not use substances that caused an abortion. However, several herbs can be used for both purposes. They repeatedly emphasized that abortion is a sin, since the number of children one has is up to God. Interestingly, no one, midwives or mothers, mentioned that abortion is illegal in Guatemala; instead, they always used a religious or moral discourse. While it is acceptable to administer something to "bring on one's period" if one has *detención* or delayed menstruation, it is a sin otherwise.

DETENCIÓN

A woman who has not gotten her period, but is not pregnant, may have *detención,* according to the plantation residents. In this situation certain villages in the highlands use the term *retención*—probably related to the ancient Greek concept of menstrual retention, based on the belief that the amenorrhea is from retained blood (van de Walle, this volume)—although the general term *atrazo* ("delay") is more common (Hurtado, personal communication). *Atrazo* is similarly used in Colombia to refer to menstrual delay and suggests possible cultural acceptance of a terminated unwanted pregnancy (Browner 1985a). In Chuchexic, people tended to use the phrase *la regla no baja* ("her menstruation doesn't fall") or *no tiene su costumbre* (a euphemism using the term *custom* or *ritual* for menstrual period).

The midwife on the plantation, Doña Maria, explained that *detención* is for unmarried girls; a woman who has a husband is less likely to get *detención* because she is probably pregnant. Therefore, by not treating a woman she suspects is pregnant, the midwife avoids the stigma attached to performing abortions. Doña Maria consequently examines the girl or woman first to see if she is pregnant. She is particularly suspicious if her client is unmarried. Some women are actually pregnant but are ashamed because they are not married and are hoping to get medicines that will cause an abortion:

> They ask, "Please do me a favor and give me the remedy for *detención.*"
> Then I say, "Let me see, come here. I am going to see if it is *detención.*"
> If it is above here [abdomen] and it is hard, hard, then one knows it is *detención.* If she is pregnant, it is lower and one can see it in the chest, in the breast. It becomes bigger and the nipples darken. Then it is not *detención.*

Doña Maria uses several signs to detect pregnancy, including the size and color of the nipples and the hardness and height of the abdomen. If the fetus is male, the woman gets dark spots or a "mask" across her nose and cheeks, because a boy's blood is stronger. Even if the girl is thin and doesn't "show," Doña Maria says she can tell by the girl's eyes:

they look strange, pale, and empty *(huero)*. The woman also salivates a good deal after missing the first menstrual period. If she looks at eggs to cook, she feels nauseous and gets much saliva.

If she decides that her client is pregnant, Doña Maria will not give the woman anything to induce abortion because she considers it a sin "and the health center forbids it." On the other hand, if her diagnosis is the illness *detención,* she will treat the client. First, Doña Maria gives the woman a firm massage in the stomach and along with a tea of boiled *Salvia santa (Lippia dulcis)*[2] leaves with oregano, white honey, rum, and *esencia maravaillosa.*[3] After drinking the tea for 9 days,[4] the woman should get her menses.

Delayed menarche also is believed to cause illness. Doña Maria says that some girls on the plantation have yet to get their first period at the age of 14, 15, or even 18 years of age. Then the illness may suddenly rise upwards in the body. Symptoms of delayed menarche include an enlarged, swollen stomach, wheezing, and difficulty breathing when walking. As with *detención,* Doña Maria massages the affected girl and treats her with *Salvia santa* and oregano. She boils 3 twigs and adds white honey to this mixture. The girl takes this remedy 3 times. However, this treatment has to be followed when the moon is full; it doesn't work at any other time.

Salvia is also used by one of the midwives in Chuchexic in treating delayed menarche. Other remedies used as emmenagogues by the Chuchexic midwives include a tea made from boiling 3 sprigs of *artemisia (Artemisia mexicana)* and a tea made from mustard leaves *(Brassica negra),* pink honey *(miel rosado)* from the pharmacy, and the root of *escorcionera (Erygium carlinae).* This latter plant was also used in Verapaz to regulate menstruation (mentioned in Orellana 1987:137), and Aguilar Giron (1966:350) says it is considered a strong emmenagogue and may also cause abortion. Artemisia can also be used if a woman is getting her period every 15 or 20 days, to regulate it to once a month.

Another herb that is used as an emmenagogue is *sanguinaria* or *botoncillo (Gomphrena dispersa)*; dosage is 9 flowers taken in a tea for 9 days. Low and Newman (1985:154) mention that *sanguinaria* or *sangranita* is used in Costa Rica, where it is thought to have powerful effects and "bring down the period." *Sanguinaria* is a symbolic plant whose name denotes blood, indicating its emmenagogic use, and it is unclear whether the name is derived from the plant's physical effects or from its appearance.

The midwives interviewed mentioned several cases of women who had come to them because they had not gotten their menses. Below is one such case:

One woman showed Doña Maria a dress she bought for her daughter. Doña Maria said it would be better if it were pleated because her daughter was very pale and maybe she was pregnant. The mother said she was pale because she doesn't cover herself in the night. Doña Maria asked her, "Aren't the girl's eyes very strange?" The mother said it was because she got fever in the night from bathing. Doña Maria said, "Look, don't get angry at what I am going to say, but Martha is pregnant." The mother said, "No! How could that be, she's still studying." Doña Maria said to me jokingly, "Maybe this is what she studied." "No," the mother said, "the child doesn't know anything yet because she hasn't had her period yet. She is 15 years old." "Take care because she is pregnant," Doña Maria said. The mother insisted that her daughter couldn't be pregnant. Then in 1 month and 15 days, she gave birth to a little girl. The mother asked her who the father was. She mentioned 3 different boys, 2 of whom denied doing anything. The third was a boy who was staying with them in the same house who did "this bad thing."

This incident indicates the values placed on premarital chastity and pregnancy that the mother is trying to enforce, and the family's attempts to keep up appearances and their reputation. The mother's presumed lack of complicity in and ignorance of the daughter's condition also reflect the lack of communication between daughters and mothers about sex, which is culturally unacceptable to discuss, until it is too late. In some cases, the ignorance may be real. According to Reina (1966), among the Maya in Chinautla, Guatemala, menstruation is generally not known to be related to fertility or pregnancy, reflecting the young woman's ignorance on sexual matters. Paul (1975:451) reports similar ignorance and shame in the Maya community of San Pedro la Laguna, resulting in the woman being unprepared for her first menstruation, her wedding night, and the birth of her first baby. The negative attitudes toward premarital sex are reflected in the discourse used; for example, it was that boy who did "the bad thing" *(malita)*. The midwife's refusal to provide a remedy in this situation may also be related to the girl's advanced stage of pregnancy by the time she was brought in by her mother.

According to Doña Maria, most girls on the plantation get their period at 14 years of age, but some don't have it until 16. A survey done in 1970 in which reproductive histories were taken of women of reproductive age on a sample of 77 women, found that the median age at menarche was 14 years. This figure was based on the women's recollection, often after many years, which is methodologically problematical.

Table 14.1   Age of Menarche, Finca San Felipe, 1970

Age (in years)	Number	Percentage
12	5	6.6
13	8	10.5
14	37	48.7
15	18	23.7
16	7	9.2
17	1	1.3
Total, 12–17	76	100.0

In addition, if women perceive that 14 is the normal age, then they may say that or round off the number even though they may not remember the actual date or age of their own menarche. One woman, who said she did not menstruate until she was 21, attributed this delay to her being orphaned at a very young age, neglected, and malnourished.

Table 14.1 shows the distribution of menarche on the Finca. There was no association of age at menarche with age of the mother or ethnicity (Ladino or Maya). According to Saquic Calel (1973), some Mayan women say that menstruation begins between 12 and 14 years of age, but older women say that 40 or 50 years ago, it began at 15 to 16 years of age, perhaps indicating a secular trend.

For cases of delayed menstruation (indicating possible fertility problems) when the woman wants a child but has been unable to conceive, Doña Maria mentioned a remedy using a piece of dried umbilical cord. (When a baby's umbilical cord dries and falls off, it is saved and guarded, for it is thought to influence the child's future.) A piece of the dried cord is cooked with *pimiento de castilla,* clove, cinnamon, cumin, oregano, *balsamito de aire,* and two 8-ounce bottles of rum; then white honey is added. This mixture is put in a bottle and a cup of it drunk each morning until it is consumed. According to Doña Maria, the period soon begins, and pregnancy will occur in the next month. She says she doesn't use this remedy anymore, however, because she considers the dried umbilical cord dirty. This statement may reflect the influence of medicalization on her ideas about cleanliness.

Doña Maria is about 80 years of age now and no longer practices midwifery, though she still continues her work as a diviner and healer. One of her daughters, Doña Ciriaca, is a practicing midwife. She apprenticed with her mother and has taken a biomedical midwifery training course, for which she received a license from the Ministry of Health.

Doña Ciriaca said she hasn't seen much *detención.* Sometimes women come to her and say it is 2 or 3 months since they have seen their periods and they have *detención*. However, she insists on examining them first to see if they are pregnant. She went on to mention examples very similar to those given by her mother 20 years earlier.

- Case 1: A girl came to Doña Ciriaca because she had not gotten her period. She insisted that she did not have a boyfriend and was not pregnant. She was afraid her brothers would beat her up if she was. Doña Ciriaca spoke to the girl's mother to tell her she was pregnant. Finally, the girl said there was a man who was fixing the road who had spoken to her from the other side of the river, but that was all. Doña Ciriaca laughed when relating this story as she said the man must have been very powerful. She said that the baby was born dead, maybe because the girl had taken so many medicines from different people in trying to abort it.

- Case 2: A woman came in and said she had not gotten her period for 3 months. She said she was not pregnant, but had *detención*. She had 6 children and didn't want more. Doña Ciriaca looked at her and told her she was pregnant. The woman insisted she was not, maintaining that she had *detención*. She asked Doña Ciriaca to do her a favor and make her a remedy. Doña Ciriaca agreed to do so and made up a bottle of medicine of *balsamito de aire* with white honey to strengthen the child instead of aborting it. The woman eventually gave birth to a boy. Doña Ciriaca said, "Look what you wanted to kill. Doesn't your heart hurt that you wanted to kill your son. I am not a murderer of children." She added that she would make up a remedy to give strength to a child because it is a sin to terminate the pregnancy. According to Doña Ciriaca, the woman thanked her because she cured her.

- Case 3: I asked Doña Ciriaca about a child who had been extremely malnourished in 1978. He was admitted to the hospital's nutrition center and had recovered, but remained deaf. He went to a school for the deaf and in 1996 was working with the deaf in Guatemala City. Doña Ciriaca said that he was born with health problems because his mother took a lot of medicines to induce abortion, including aspirin, which harmed the child. Thus 20 years later, gossip about this woman's attempted abortion and the supposedly negative results of trying different remedies was still part of the "community lore" being perpetuated by the midwife as well as others, and that would serve as a warning to other women.

Although most of the cases mentioned by the midwives were of pregnant women seeking remedies for an abortion under the guise of having delayed menstruation, there were cases in which amenorrhea was related to fertility problems. For example, a married woman still childless after 12 years came to see Doña Ciriaca. She was having a bitter life and was very thin because her abusive husband beat for not bearing any children. Doña Ciriaca said she cured her by giving her a massage, then a remedy of *balsamito de aire* boiled with oregano and sweetened with honey to drink before each meal. The next time the woman came in, she said her period was coming. She was told that if she did not menstruate again in the next 2 months, she could be pregnant or just delayed. She became pregnant and gave birth to twins.

Doña Ciriaca, in her role as midwife, was acting as an arbiter of moral values and an agent of social control. Like her mother before her, she was reinforcing the norms of the society including the role of motherhood and the value placed on children, through preventing abortions, gossiping about and passing on news from case histories, and treating menstrual problems and possible infertility with her knowledge of emmenagogues and remedies for regulating menstruation. But as Willats (1995) points out, the midwife also has "social permission" to induce menstruation in unmarried women by diagnosing *detención*. This authorization provides the opportunity to reduce the number of pregnancies of unwed mothers, which carry a social stigma. In sum, the midwife can interpret and manipulate the physiological concept of delayed menstruation because of its ambiguity: abortion is a sin, but inducing menstruation is socially and culturally acceptable.

THE FAMILY PLANNING PROGRAM

Despite informants' statements that the number of children born to them is "up to God" and "abortion is a sin," their behavior in requesting emmenagogues and abortifacients indicates that at least some women would like to regulate their fertility despite cultural constraints. Fatalistic notions of reproduction in rural Guatemala are not as rigid when it comes to people's reproductive decisions. The region has low rates of contraceptive usage, reflecting problems of accessibility in addition to sociocultural factors (Ward et al. 1992; Warren et al. 1987). Various studies on family planning have emphasized the latter, especially attitudinal "barriers" to accepting modern contraceptive methods. However, a program that existed on the plantation from 1971 to 1974 demonstrated that despite rumors, fears, and negative attitudes about pills, IUDs, and injections, many women (at least 45) used contraceptives when available.

During that time, a private physician held a monthly health clinic and family planning program on the plantation. Initially, he distributed contraceptive pills at a low cost of 15 cents per month. In the middle of 1972, he began giving injections of Depo-Provera, which lasted for 3 months, for 1 dollar. Despite the higher costs, people preferred the injections to the pills because of the convenience. Even though the doctor said he had explained the possibility of amenorrhea if the injections were taken, some users expressed concern because they did not get their period. This concern might reflect ambiguous reactions to amenorrhea in that the women did not know whether it was caused by the injection or by pregnancy. On the other hand, the few women who had IUDs experienced heavy bleeding, and this loss of blood was of more concern than not menstruating at all. This reaction might be related to the belief that the body has a limited amount of nonrenewable blood, so that such a loss leaves the body weak and cold and thus susceptible to various illnesses.

The midwife was initially supportive of the family planning program. However, one of her daughters had used an IUD. She then became very ill, was diagnosed as having a tumor, and underwent a hysterectomy. The midwife, as well as everyone else who knew about it, attributed the tumor to the IUD and began expressing more negative opinions about the contraceptive. Instead, she advises women not to have intercourse during their period or for 5 days before or 5 days afterward if they do not want children. Browner and Ortiz de Montellano (1986) similarly report that in Mexico and Colombia, women consider the most likely time for conception to be just before, during, and after menstruation, when semen can enter the womb because it is "open." What the midwife considers the "fertile" period, however, is the "safe" period, according to biomedicine.

In addition to fears about tumors and cancer, the pills and injections were considered "hot" and "strong," thus causing inflammation and making one sick. Even so, these were not mentioned as reasons for rejecting or not participating in the program. Several women did discontinue because of side effects they experienced and others stopped when the doctor no longer held the clinic, yet they still expressed interest in some form of family planning.

Today, the Association for Family Well-being *(Asociacion Pro Bienestar de la Familia),* or APROFAM, an affiliate of the International Planned Parenthood Federation, is the primary source of contraceptives and family planning information at Finca San Felipe. The organization works through community distributors as well as at clinics. According to Doña Ciriaca, many of the plantation women are now practicing family planning; workers from APROFAM come to the Finca, and some women go to APROFAM in Retalhuleu. When women come to her, however, she continues to recommend natural methods, especially the use of the avocado pit, which she says doesn't have the harmful side effects of some of the other contraceptive methods:

> What I recommend is to mash the avocado pit, boil it, and drink the water for 3 days during her period. On the third day, drink a cup of water. I told one woman to keep her avocado pits when it is the season for avocados. She had 2 bagfuls. She mashed and boiled them every 3 days of her period, and she did not get pregnant. But she finished them and didn't have any more and then she got pregnant. (Interview, July 1996)

I do not know the current situation concerning the availability or utilization of family planning in Santa Lucia Utatlán. In some countries, indigenous midwives have been incorporated in family planning programs, in terms of either disseminating information or distributing contraceptives. Some pilot programs for midwifery training in Guatemala in the late 1970s included family planning, but these were interrupted by the violence of the early 1980s. Recent programs have included family planning but in a limited manner. Willats (1995) describes the tension, conflict, and misunderstandings between midwives and community family planning workers in 1994 in the indigenous community of San Antonio Aguas Calientes. These issues have implications not only for the effectiveness of family planning programs but for health programs in general.

CONCLUSION

Many ethnographies and botanical studies mention plants and substances used for menstrual regulation. However, little ethnobotanical information is provided, such as details of preparation, dosage, reported effectiveness, and so on. Similarly, little analysis is given of the way the use of these plants relates to the ethnomedical system; demographic variables such as infant mortality, fertility behavior, or migration; and the broader social and cultural context. Research in these areas is needed, and I hope this book will stimulate such future investigations.

Browner (1985a) argues that the knowledge of plants and various methods of menstrual regulation is shared and horizontally distrib-

uted. All women in her study, as well as many of the men, knew various
remedies to induce menstruation; such knowledge, in other words, was
not limited to herbalists or midwives. My research has focused on the
midwife's knowledge and thus the vertical distribution of knowledge.
Even when people have knowledge of some of these plant remedies,
they seek out the midwife, possibly because they have already tried
remedies that failed or because they regard information from her as
more authoritative. It is this knowledge for which people come to her
and with which she maintains her authority, autonomy, and ability
to negotiate the ambiguity of *detención*. However, this knowledge is
also constantly attacked and denigrated by the biomedical authorities
and in midwifery training courses. The midwife is repeatedly told by
physicians and nurses not to use such plants, nor the sweatbath, nor
the massage, all of which are critical aspects of her practice and used
to treat menstrual irregularity, fertility problems, and pregnancy.
Meanwhile, midwives are increasingly using pharmaceuticals and
oxytocic injections, sometimes with disastrous results (Schieber et al.
1994). The loss of knowledge of medicinal plants and their applications
means a curtailment of the midwife's role and a loss of her autonomy,
making her more dependent on biomedicine. Research focusing on
these plants is needed, not only because it may provide us with new
medical knowledge, but also because of the increasing possibility that
both the knowledge and the source of that knowledge may be dying
out.

NOTES

Support for the research in Guatemala was provided by Rutgers University Research Council Grants and the International Nutrition Program, Department of Nutrition and Food Science, Massachusetts Institute of Technology. I wish to express my appreciation to the owner and people of the plantation; the people of Santa Lucia Utatlán, for their cooperation and hospitality; my coinvestigator, Mary Scrimshaw; and Dr. Nevin Scrimshaw, for his support and encouragement.

1. The term *Ladino* refers to descendants of Spanish or mixed Spanish-Indian ancestry and to people following Spanish or Western culture, in contrast to those oriented toward Indian culture. It is used generally to refer to non-Indians.

2. Botanical identifications were made by Dr. Lorin Nevling of the Field Museum of Chicago from plant specimens collected by the author.

3. *Esencia maravaillosa* is a liquid sold in the pharmacies. According to

the information enclosed with a bottle, each 100 cubic centimeters contains alcohol, 67 cubic centimeters; aloes, 852 milligrams; pear, 852 milligrams; rhubarb, 852 milligrams; sassafras, 852 milligrams; manzanilla, 852 milligrams; jaborandi, 426 milligrams; alcotán, 426 milligrams; and water. It is supposedly an antipyretic, diphoretic, expectorant, antispasmodic, and eupeptic.

4. The numbers three and nine appear in many remedies that refer to the number of leaves in the preparation or the number of times or days the remedy is to be taken. These are considered sacred numbers. Three symbolizes the 3 hearthstones in the Mayan household. Nine may refer to the 9 months of pregnancy. It also may signify the 9 layers of the underworld and the corresponding 9 Lords of the Dead, who were believed by the ancient Maya to influence the effectiveness of the treatment. The numbers three and nine are also sacred numbers in the Catholic tradition as well, symbolizing the Trinity, the novena, and the 9-day wake.

REFERENCES

Aguilar Giron, Jose. 1966. *Relacion de unos aspectos de la flora util de Guatemala.* 2d ed. Guatemala: Tipografia Nacional.

Bastien, Joseph. 1989. "Differences between Kallawaya-Andean and Greek-European Humoral Theory." *Social Science & Medicine* 28, no. 1: 45–51.

Browner, Carole. 1985a. "Traditional Techniques for Diagnosis, Treatment, and Control of Pregnancy in Cali, Colombia." In *Women's Medicine,* ed. Lucille Newman, 99–123. New Brunswick, N.J.: Rutgers University Press.

———. 1985b. "Plants Used for Reproductive Health in Oaxaca, Mexico." *Economic Botany* 39, no. 4:482–504.

Browner, Carole, and Bernard Ortiz de Montellano. 1986. "Herbal Emmenagogues Used by Women in Colombia and Mexico." In *Plants in Indigenous Medicine and Diet: Biobehavioral Approaches,* ed. Nina Etkin, 32–47. New York: Gordon and Breach Science.

Cosminsky, Sheila. 1976. "The Evil Eye in a Guatemalan Indian Village." In *The Evil Eye,* ed. Clarence Maloney, 163–174. New York: Columbia University Press.

———. 1977. "El papel de la comadrona en mesoamerica." *America Indigena* 37:305–35.

———. 1982. "Knowledge and Body Concepts of Guatemalan Midwives." In *Anthropology of Human Birth,* ed. Margarita Kay, 233–52. Philadelphia: F. A. Davis.

Delgado, Hernan, Reynoldo Martorell, and Robert Klein. 1982. "Nutri-tion, Lactation, and Birth Interval Components in Rural Guatemala." *The American Journal of Clinical Nutrition* 35:1468–76.

Esteyneffer, Juan de. [1719] 1978. *Florilegio medicinal de todas las en-fermedades*. Edited by Carmen Anzures de Bolanos. Mexico City: Aca-demia Nacional de Medicina.

Farnsworth, Norman. 1975. "Potential Value of Plants as Sources of New Antifertility Agents." *Journal of Pharmaceutical Sciences* 64, no. 4:535–98; 64, no. 5:717–54.

Foster, George. 1978. "Hippocrates' Latin American Legacy: 'Hot' and 'Cold' in Contemporary Folk Medicine." In *Colloquia in Anthropology* 2:3–19, ed. R. K. Wetherington. Dallas: Southern Methodist Univer-sity, Fort Burgwin Research Center.

———. 1994. *Hippocrates' Latin American Legacy: Humoral Medicine in the New World*. New York: Gordon and Breach.

Gilbert, D. 1976. "A Dietary Survey of Guatemalan Women on the Finca San Luis." Unpublished manuscript, Department of Nutrition, Massa-chusetts Institute of Technology.

Kay, Margarita. 1976. "The Fusion of Utoaztecan and European Ethnogy-necology in the Florilegio Medicinal." In *Actas del XLI Congreso Interna-cional de Americanistas*, vol. 3. Mexico City: Instituto Nacional de An-tropologia e Historia.

———. 1977. "The *Florilegio Medicinal:* Source of Southwest Ethnomedi-cine." *Ethnohistory* 24:251–59.

———. 1996. *Healing with Plants in the American and Mexican West*. Tuc-son: University of Arizona Press.

Lopez Austin, Alfredo. 1988. *The Human Body and Ideology: Concepts of the Ancient Nahuas*, trans. T. Ortiz de Montellano and B. R. Ortiz de Mon-tellano. 2 vols. Salt Lake City: University of Utah Press.

Low, Setha, and Bruce Newman. 1985. "Indigenous Fertility Regulating Methods in Costa Rica." In *Women's Medicine*, ed. Lucile Newman, 147–60. New Brunswick, N.J.: Rutgers University Press.

Morton, Julia. 1981. *Atlas of Medicinal Plants of Central America:Bahamas to Yucatan*. Springfield, Ill.: Charles C. Thomas.

Neuenswander, Helen, and Shirley Souder. 1977. "The Hot-Cold-Wet-Dry Syndrome among the Quiché of Joyabaj: Two Alternative Cognitive Models." In *Cognitive Studies of Southern Mesoamerica*, ed. Helen Neuenswander and Dean Arnold, 96–125. SIL Museum of Anthropol-ogy Publication no. 3. Dallas: Summer Institute of Linguistics.

Orellana, Sandra. 1987. *Indian Medicine in Highland Guatemala*. Albuquer-que: University of New Mexico Press.

Ortiz de Montellano, Bernard. 1990. *Aztec Medicine, Health, and Nutrition*. New Brunswick, N.J.: Rutgers University Press.

Paul, Lois. 1974. "The Mastery of Work and the Mystery of Sex in a Gua-temalan Village." In *Women, Culture and Society*, ed. Michelle Rosaldo and Louise Lamphere, 281–99. Stanford, Calif.: Stanford University Press.

———. 1975. "Recruitment to a Ritual Role: The Midwife in a Maya Community." *Ethos* 3, no. 3:449–67.

Quezada, Noemi. 1975. "Metodos anticonceptivos, and abortivos tradicionales." *Anales de Antropologia* 12:223–242.

Reina, Ruben. 1966. *The Law of the Saints.* Indianapolis: Bobbs-Merrill Co.

Saquic Calel, Felipe Rosalio. 1973. "La Mujer Indigena Guatemalteca," *Guatemala Indigena* 8, no. 1:82–110.

Schieber, Barbara, et al. 1994. "Risk Factor Analysis of Peri-Neonatal Mortality in Rural Guatemala." *Bulletin of PAHO* 23, no. 3:229–38.

Tedlock, Barbara. 1987. "An Interpretive Solution to the Problem of Humoral Medicine in Latin America." *Social Science & Medicine* 24: 1069–83.

Ward, Victoria M., Jane T. Bertrand, and Francisco Puac. 1992. "Exploring Sociocultural Barriers to Family Planning Among Mayans in Guatemala." *International Family Planning Perspectives* 18, no. 2:59–65.

Warren, Charles, et al. 1987. "Use of Maternal-Child Health Services and Contraception in Guatemalan and Panama." *Journal of Biosocial Sciences* 19:229–43.

Willats, Amy. 1995. "Midwives and Community Workers in Conflict: Exploring the Cultural Appropriateness of Family Planning Programs." Master's thesis, Vanderbilt University, Nashville.

CONTRIBUTORS

JANET FARRELL BRODIE is an associate professor in the Department of History, Claremont Graduate University, Claremont, Calif.

SHEILA COSMINSKY is associate professor of anthropology, Department of Sociology, Anthropology, and Criminal Justice, Rutgers University, Camden, N.J.

AISSE DIARRA is a researcher for the Population Council, Bamako, Mali.

PATRICIA J. HAMMER is director of the Center for the Promotion of Social Well Being, Lima, Peru.

TERENCE H. HULL is a fellow at Australian National University, Canberra.

VALERIE J. HULL is a director in the Australian Agency for International Development (AusAID) in Canberra.

HEIDI BART JOHNSTON is a research associate, Health Systems Research, at Ipas, Chapel Hill, N.C.

SUSAN E. KLEPP is professor of history at Temple University, Philadelphia.

ELISE LEVIN is a doctoral candidate in the Department of Anthropology, Northwestern University, Evanston, Ill.

SANGEETHA MADHAVAN is Mellon Post-Doctoral Fellow, Department of Anthropology, Brown University, Providence, R.I.

LINDA S. POTTER is a health behavior consultant at Family Health Research, Princeton Junction, N.J.

ELISHA P. RENNE is assistant professor in the Department of Anthropology and the Center for Afroamerican and African Studies at the University of Michigan, Ann Arbor.

GIGI SANTOW is professor of demography and chair of the Demography Unit at Stockholm University.

STEFANIA SIEDLECKY is a retired medical practitioner and a member of the Demography Research Group, Macquarie University, Sydney, Australia.

ETIENNE VAN DE WALLE is professor of demography and a member of the Population Studies Center at the University of Pennsylvania, Philadelphia.

INA WARRINER is a social scientist in the Reproductive Health Research Department of the World Health Organization in Geneva, Switzerland.

to, xxxix, 40, 41, 65–66, 67, 87, 114; physiological emphasis of Western texts on, xx; pollution and impurity associated with, xviii–xix, xxv, 220; as precondition to fertility, xxii, xxv, xxvi; and productive labor, xv–xvi; as purifying, xix, xxv, 16, 18, 175, 220; Quechua ethnophysiology of, 241–53; recording of, 44–45, 57n. 6; seasonal variation in, 129, 136n. 8; sexual intercourse during, xix, 175; venesection compared with, xxxiiin. 3; vicarious menstruation, xiv, 243, 246; why menstruate at all, 146–48, 150–51. *See also* amenorrhea; menstrual regulation

Mentha pulegium. See pennyroyal
mercury, 68, 98
Meuvret, Jean, 114
Midwifery and the Diseases of Women (Shew), 41
Midwife's Practical Directory, The (Hersey), 44
midwives: abortions performed by Indonesian, 216n. 3; in Guatemala, 254, 258, 260–67, 268, 269, 270; Hippocrates' influence in books on, xxi; Hippocratic treatises reflecting influence of, 8; Western-trained in Guinea, 181–82
mifepristone (RU-486), xxxiiin. 1, 109
Mill, John Stuart, 74
Millspaugh, Charles, 52–53, 58n. 16
mint, 17, 27
miscarriage, xli, 13–14, 47, 53, 83–84
Monari, Paola, 121
Montanari, Angela, 121
Montanoa tomentosa (cihuapahtli; zoapatle), 259
montanol, 259
Montgomery, Edward, 66–67, 71, 79
Moran, H. M., 75
Mother's Own Book and Practical Guide to Health . . . Designed for Females only, The (Hall), 42
Muchtar, A., 208
mugwort, xv, 50
Munster, K., 124
Muscion, 11
myrrh, 28

Naphey, George H., 45, 57n. 8
Nardi, Enzo, 13
Narodetzki, A., 71, 80

Native Americans, 27
Nature of Woman (Hippocrates), 6, 7, 8, 10
Ndembu, xxvii
Neuenswander, Helen, 257
New Age medicine, 73
New York Academy of Medicine, 83
New York and London Drug Co., 75
Ngaglik (Indonesia), 205, 210, 216nn. 3, 4, 217n. 8
Nigeria: menstrual regulation in southwestern, 187–201. *See also* Ekiti Yoruba
Nillius, Sven Johan, 127
Nkula ritual, xxvii
norethindrone, xvii, 143
norethynodrel, xvii
Novak, Edmund R., 57n. 3
nutrition, and secondary amenorrhea, 114–15, 124–25, 228
nutritional supplements, 88
nyama, 162, 163, 164, 170n. 3
Nyonya Meneer, P. T., 208

Observations (Bourgeois), xxi, xxiii
Ogino, Kyusaku, 67, 87
oral contraceptives, 141–54; ambivalence about using, 150; attitudes about menstruation changed by, 87; in Bangladesh, xxx, 220, 225–26, 227, 229, 232, 234–35, 236; bicycle (honeymoon) regimen, 147; as cycle deregularizer, 144–46; going off the Pill to have a "real bleed," xxxivn. 6; Indonesian use of, 213; as initially approved for menstrual regulation, 93; Latin American use of, xxix; and menstrual irregularity, 67, 114, 143–44; number of women using, 149; pill-induced amenorrhea, 130; as postcoital contraceptive, 141, 148–49; and regular menstrual periods, xxiv, 67, 141, 193; release of blood incorporated with, xxiv; "resting from," 145–46; side effects of, 143; Sunday start with, 144; as ultimate menstrual regulator, 141; withdrawal (breakthrough) bleeding with, xl, 130, 142, 143, 144, 145–46, 150
oregano, 263, 267
Organon, 199n. 5
Ortiz de Montellano, Bernard R., xxviii, 258, 259, 268
ovarian cysts, 117

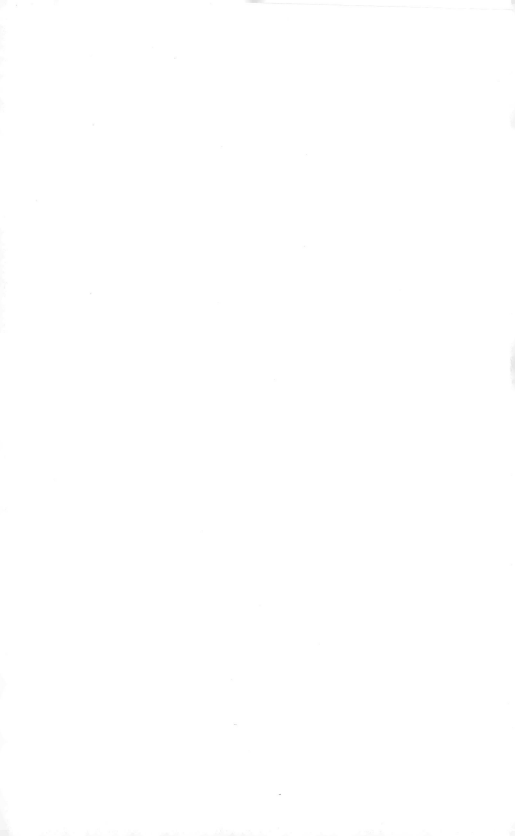